COVID-19 Lung Disease: Lessons Learned

Editors

GUANG-SHING CHENG
CHARLES DELA CRUZ

CLINICS IN CHEST MEDICINE

www.chestmed.theclinics.com

June 2023 • Volume 44 • Number 2

ELSEVIER

1600 John F. Kennedy Boulevard • Suite 1800 • Philadelphia, Pennsylvania, 19103-2899

http://www.theclinics.com

CLINICS IN CHEST MEDICINE Volume 44, Number 2
June 2023 ISSN 0272-5231, ISBN-13: 9780323961776

Editor: Joanna Gascoine
Developmental Editor: Karen Justine S. Dino

Clinics in Chest Medicine (ISSN 0272-5231) is published quarterly by Elsevier Inc., 360 Park Avenue South, New York, NY 10010-1710. Months of issue are March, June, September, and December. Periodicals postage paid at New York, NY and additional mailing offices. Subscription prices are $420.00 per year (domestic individuals), $895.00 per year (domestic institutions), $100.00 per year (domestic students/residents), $449.00 per year (Canadian individuals), $1112.00 per year (Canadian institutions), $514.00 per year (international individuals), $1112.00 per year (international institutions), $100.00 per year (Canadian Students), and $230.00 per year (International Students). International air speed delivery is included in all Clinics subscription prices. All prices are subject to change without notice. **POSTMASTER:** Send address changes to Clinics in Chest Medicine, Elsevier Health Sciences Division, Subscription Customer Service, 3251 Riverport Lane, Maryland Heights, MO 63043. **Customer Service: Telephone: 1-800-654-2452** (U.S. and Canada); **1-314-447-8871** (outside U.S. and Canada). **Fax: 1-314-447-8029. E-mail: journalscustomerservice-usa@elsevier.com (for print support); journalsonlinesupport-usa@elsevier.com (for online support).**

Reprints. For copies of 100 or more of articles in this publication, please contact the Commercial Reprints Department, Elsevier Inc., 360 Park Avenue South, New York, NY 10010-1710. Tel.: 212-633-3874; Fax: 212-633-3820; E-mail: reprints@elsevier.com.

Clinics in Chest Medicine is covered in *MEDLINE/PubMed (Index Medicus), Current Contents/Clinical Medicine, EMBASE/ Excerpta Medica, Science Citation Index,* and *ISI/BIOMED.*

Contributors

EDITORS

GUANG-SHING CHENG, MD
Associate Professor, Clinical Research
Division, Fred Hutchinson Cancer Research
Center, University of Washington, Seattle,
Washington, USA

CHARLES S. DELA CRUZ, MD, PhD
Associate Professor, Department of Internal
Medicine, Section of Pulmonary, Critical Care
and Sleep Medicine, Yale School of Medicine,
New Haven, Connecticut, USA

AUTHORS

DARRYL ABRAMS, MD
Division of Pulmonary, Allergy, and Critical
Care Medicine, Department of Medicine,
Columbia University Vagelos College of
Physicians and Surgeons, New York, New
York, USA

CARA AGERSTRAND, MD
Division of Pulmonary, Allergy, and Critical
Care Medicine, Department of Medicine,
Columbia University Vagelos College of
Physicians and Surgeons, New York, New
York, USA

PETA M.A. ALEXANDER, MBBS
Department of Cardiology, Boston Children's
Hospital, Department of Pediatrics, Harvard
Medical School, Boston, Massachusetts, USA

MARWAN M. AZAR, MD
Section of Infectious Diseases, Department of
Laboratory Medicine, Yale School of Medicine,
New Haven, Connecticut, USA

JENELLE BADULAK, MD
Department of Emergency Medicine, Division
of Pulmonary, Critical Care and Sleep
Medicine, University of Washington, Seattle,
Washington, USA

MARK BARASH, DO
Assistant Professor, Division of Pulmonary,
Critical Care and Sleep Medicine, Medical
College of Wisconsin, HUB for Collaborative
Medicine, Milwaukee, Wisconsin, USA

ANKIT BHARAT, MD
Chief, Department of Thoracic Surgery,
Northwestern University Feinberg School of
Medicine, Chicago, Illinois, USA

CLEMENTE BRITTO-LEON, MD
Pulmonary, Critical Care and Sleep Medicine,
Yale School of Medicine, New Haven,
Connecticut, USA

DANIEL BRODIE, MD
Department of Intensive Care, Alfred Health,
Melbourne, Australia

MARIO CALDARARO, MD, MS
Veteran's Affairs Connecticut Healthcare
System, West Haven, Connecticut, USA

JESSICA FAE CALVER, BSc (Hons)
University of Nottingham, Medical School,
Nottingham, United Kingdom

MAURIZIO H. CECCONI, MD
Department of Anesthesia and Intensive Care,
IRCCS Instituto Clinico Humanitas, Milan, Italy

JUAN C. CELEDÓN, MD, DrPH
Division of Pediatric Pulmonary Medicine,
UPMC Children's Hospital, University of
Pittsburgh, Pittsburgh, Pennsylvania, USA

EMILY CERIER, MD
Surgery Resident, Department of Thoracic
Surgery, Northwestern University Feinberg
School of Medicine, Chicago, Illinois,
USA

JAPJOT CHAHAL, MD
Department of Pulmonary and Critical Care
Medicine, SUNY Upstate Medical University,
Syracuse, New York, USA

MATTHEW W. DAVIS, PharmD
Department of Pharmacy Services, Yale
New Haven Hospital, New Haven, Connecticut,
USA

CHARLES S. DELA CRUZ, MD, PhD
Associate Professor, Department of Internal
Medicine, Section of Pulmonary, Critical Care
and Sleep Medicine, Yale School of Medicine,
New Haven, Connecticut, USA

ALEJANDRO A. DIAZ, MD, MPH
Division of Pulmonary and Critical Care
Medicine, Brigham and Women's Hospital,
Harvard Medical School, Boston,
Massachusetts, USA

RODRIGO DIAZ, MD
Clinica Las Condes, Clinica Red Salud
Santiago CCHC, Santiago, Chile

CHRISTOPHER D. BERTINI, Jr, MD
Department of Internal Medicine, UTHealth
Houston McGovern Medical School, Houston,
Texas, USA

LAURA DRAGOI, MD, MHSc
Interdepartmental Division of Critical Care,
University of Toronto, Toronto General
Hospital–MaRS Centre, Toronto, Ontario,
Canada

AMY DZIERBA, PharmD
Department of Pharmacy, NewYork-
Presbyterian Hospital, New York, New York,
USA

LAURA FABBRI, MD
National Heart and Lung Institute, Imperial
College London, London, United Kingdom

EDDY FAN, MD, PhD
Interdepartmental Division of Critical Care
Medicine, University of Toronto, Toronto
General Hospital–MaRS Centre, Institute of
Health Policy, Management and Evaluation,
University of Toronto, Toronto, Ontario,
Canada

HEIKE GEDULD, MBCHb
Division of Emergency Medicine, Faculty of
Medicine and Health Sciences, Stellenbosch
University Tygerberg Campus, Cape Town,
South Africa

GAYATRI GUPTA, DO
Department of Internal Medicine, Section of
Pulmonary and Critical Care Medicine, Yale
School of Medicine, New Haven, Connecticut,
USA

CHARLES C. HARDIN, MD, PhD
Associate Professor, Division of Pulmonary
and Critical Care Medicine, Massachusetts
General Hospital, Boston, Massachusetts,
USA

DIEGO R. HIJANO, MD, MSc
St. Jude Children's Research Hospital,
Memphis, Tennessee, USA

CAROL HODGSON, PhD
Department of Epidemiology and Preventive
Medicine, Australian and New Zealand
Intensive Care Research Centre, Monash
University, Melbourne, Australia

JOE HSU, MD, MPH
Assistant Professor, Division of Pulmonary,
Allergy, and Critical Care Medicine, Stanford
University, Stanford, California, USA

R. GISLI JENKINS, MD, PhD, FRCP, FERS
National Heart and Lung Institute,
Imperial College London, London, United
Kingdom

DAVID A. KAMINSKY, MD
Pulmonary and Critical Care, University of
Vermont Larner College of Medicine,
Burlington, Vermont, USA

VIREN KAUL, MD
Department of Pulmonary and Critical Care
Medicine, Crouse Health/Upstate Medical
University, Syracuse, New York, USA

LETICIA KAWANO-DOURADO, MD, PhD
Hcor Research Institute, Hospital do Coracao,
Sao Paulo, Pulmonary Division, InCor,
University of Sao Paulo, Sao Paulo,
Brazil

FAREED KHAWAJA, MD
Department of Infectious Diseases, Infection Control, and Employee Health, Assistant Professor, The University of Texas MD Anderson Cancer Center, Houston, Texas, USA

DANAI KHEMASUWAN, MD, MBA, FCCP, ATSF
Pulmonary and Critical Care, Virginia Commonwealth University Health System, Richmond, Virginia, USA

CHITARU KURIHARA, MD
Instructor, Department of Thoracic Surgery, Northwestern University Feinberg School of Medicine, Chicago, Illinois, USA

ASHLEY LOSIER, MD
Department of Internal Medicine, Section of Pulmonary and Critical Care Medicine, Yale School of Medicine, New Haven, Connecticut, USA

KALVIN LUNG, MD
Assistant Professor, Department of Thoracic Surgery, Northwestern University Feinberg School of Medicine, Chicago, Illinois, USA

MARICAR MALINIS, MD
Section of Infectious Diseases, Yale School of Medicine, New Haven, Connecticut, USA

MELISSA M. MARKOSKI, PhD
UFCSPA - Federal University of Health Sciences of Porto Alegre, Porto Alegre, Brazil

DAYNA MCMANUS, PharmD
Department of Pharmacy Services, Yale New Haven Hospital, New Haven, Connecticut, USA

JAMES MAY, BSc (Hons), MBBS, MRCP
Guy's and St Thomas' NHS Trust, Westminster Bridge, United Kingdom

JEZID MIRANDA, MD, PhD
Intensive Care and Obstetric Research Group (GRICIO), Department of Obstetrics and Gynecology, Universidad de Cartagena, Department of Obstetrics and Gynecology, Maternal-Fetal Medicine Division, Centro Hospitalario Serena del Mar, Cartagena, Colombia

DANA MULLIN, MS, CCP, LP
Department of Clinical Perfusion and Anesthesia Support Services, NewYork-Presbyterian Hospital, New York, New York, USA

SHAIKH M. NOOR HUSNAIN, MD
Interventional Pulmonary Section, Department of Medicine, Westchester Medical Center, New York Medical College, Valhalla, New York, USA

ALEX ORTIZ, MD, MS
Pulmonary, Critical Care and Sleep Medicine, Yale School of Medicine, New Haven, Connecticut, USA

MADHAVI PAREKH, MD
Division of Pulmonary, Allergy, and Critical Care Medicine, Department of Medicine, Columbia University Vagelos College of Physicians and Surgeons, New York, New York, USA

MINA PIRZADEH, MD
Assistant Professor, Department of Internal Medicine, University of Michigan, Staff Physician, Veterans Affairs Ann Arbor Healthcare System, Ann Arbor, Michigan, USA

HALLIE C. PRESCOTT, MD, MSc
Associate Professor, Department of Internal Medicine, Staff Physician, Veterans Affairs Ann Arbor Healthcare System, VA Center for Clinical Management Research, University of Michigan, Ann Arbor, Michigan, USA

SUSANNA PRICE, MBBS
Adult Intensive Care Unit, Royal Brompton and Harefield Hospitals, Guy's and St Thomas' NHS Foundation Trust, London, United Kingdom

CHRISTOPHER RADCLIFFE, MD
Section of Infectious Diseases, Yale School of Medicine, New Haven, Connecticut, USA

VIJAYA RAMALINGAM, MD, FCCP
Division of Pulmonary, Critical Care and Sleep Medicine, Medical College of Wisconsin, HUB for Collaborative Medicine, Milwaukee, Wisconsin, USA, Adjunct Associate Professor, Department of Pulmonary and Critical Care Medicine, Northeast Georgia Health System, Gainesville, Georgia, USA

JOSE ROJAS-SUAREZ, MD, MSc
Intensive Care and Obstetric Research Group
(GRICIO), Department of Obstetrics and
Gynecology, Universidad de Cartagena,
Colombia

ISAAC N. SCHRARSTZHAUPT
Capixaba Institute of Health Education,
Research and Innovation (ICEPi), Rede de
Analise, Rua Duque de Caxias, Brazil

HUSHAM SHARIFI, MD, MS
Clinical Assistant Professor, Division of
Pulmonary, Allergy, and Critical Care Medicine,
Stanford University, Stanford, California,
USA

YINZHONG SHEN, MD
Department of Infection and Immunity,
Shanghai Public Health Clinical Center, Fudan
University, Shanghai, China

AJAY SHESHADRI, MD, MS
Department of Pulmonary Medicine, Associate
Professor, The University of Texas MD
Anderson Cancer Center, Houston, Texas,
USA

ANDRE M. SIQUEIRA, MD, PhD
Instituto Nacional de Infectologia Evandro
Chagas , Fundação Oswaldo Cruz, Rio de
Janeiro, Brazil

MATTHEW T. SIUBA, DO, MS
Department of Critical Care Medicine,
Respiratory Institute, Cleveland Clinic,
Cleveland Clinic Main Campus, Cleveland
Clinic Lerner College of Medicine of Case
Western Reserve University, Cleveland, Ohio,
USA

KAI E. SWENSON, MD
Division of Thoracic Surgery and Interventional
Pulmonology, Beth Israel Deaconess Medical
Center, Division of Pulmonary and Critical Care
Medicine, Massachusetts General Hospital,
Boston, Massachusetts, USA

NEETA THAKUR, MD, MPH
Department of Medicine, University of
California San Francisco, San Francisco,
California, USA

JEFFREY E. TOPAL, MD
Department of Pharmacy Services, Yale
School of Medicine, New Haven, Connecticut,
USA

ALPANA WAGHMARE, MD
University of Washington/Fred Hutchinson
Cancer Center, Department of Infectious
Diseases, Seattle Children's Hospital, Seattle,
Washington, USA

Contents

Because of the potential for high aerosol transmission during pulmonary function testing and pulmonary procedures, performing these tests and procedures must be considered carefully during the coronavirus disease-2019 (COVID-19) pandemic. Much has been learned about the transmission of severe acute respiratory syndrome coronavirus 2 (SARS-CoV-2) by aerosols and the potential for such transmission through pulmonary function tests and pulmonary procedures, and subsequently preventative practices have been enhanced and developed to reduce the risk of transmission of virus to patients and personnel. This article reviews what is known about the potential for transmission of SARS-CoV-2 during pulmonary function testing and pulmonary procedures and the recommended mitigation steps to prevent the spread of COVID-19.

Coronavirus disease-2019 (COVID-19) pneumonia has diverse clinical manifestations, which have shifted throughout the pandemic. Formal classifications include presymptomatic infection and mild, moderate, severe, and critical illness. Social risk factors are numerous, with Black, Hispanic, and Native American populations in the United States having suffered disproportionately. Biological risk factors such as age, sex, underlying comorbid burden, and certain laboratory metrics can assist the clinician in triage and management. Guidelines for classifying radiographic findings have been proposed and may assist in prognosis. In this article, we review the risk factors, clinical course, complications, and imaging findings of COVID-19 pneumonia.

As the pandemic has progressed, our understanding of hypoxemia in coronavirus disease 2019 (COVID-19) lung disease has become more nuanced, although much remains to be understood. In this article, we review ventilation-perfusion mismatching in COVID-19 and the evidence to support various biologic theories offered in explanation. In addition, the relationship between hypoxemia and other features of severe COVID-19 lung disease such as respiratory symptoms, radiographic abnormalities, and pulmonary mechanics is explored. Recognizing and understanding hypoxemia in COVID-19 lung disease remains essential for risk stratification, prognostication, and choice of appropriate treatments in severe COVID-19.

(COVID-19) acute respiratory distress syndrome (ARDS) changed over the course of the pandemic, being adjusted as more evidence became available. This article will review how the ventilatory management of COVID-19 ARDS evolved and will conclude with current evidence-based recommendations.

The coronavirus disease 2019 (COVID-19) pandemic has seen an increase in global cases of severe acute respiratory distress syndrome (ARDS), with a concomitant increased demand for extracorporeal membrane oxygenation (ECMO). Outcomes of patients with severe ARDS due to COVID-19 infection receiving ECMO support are evolving. The need for surge capacity, practical and ethical limitations on implementing ECMO, and the prolonged duration of ECMO support in patients with COVID-19-related ARDS has revealed limitations in organization and resource utilization. Coordination of efforts at multiple levels, from research to implementation, resulted in numerous innovations in the delivery of ECMO.

Coronavirus-19 (COVID-19) can result in irrecoverable acute respiratory distress syndrome (ARDS) or life-limiting fibrosis for which lung transplantation is currently the only viable treatment. COVID-19 lung transplantation has transformed the field of lung transplantation, as before the pandemic, few transplants had been performed in the setting of infectious disease or ARDS. Given the complexities associated with COVID-19 lung transplantation, it requires strict patient selection with an experienced multidisciplinary team in a high-resource hospital setting. Current short-term outcomes of COVID-19 lung transplantation are promising. However, follow-up studies are needed to determine long-term outcomes and whether these patients may be predisposed to unique complications.

Severe acute respiratory syndrome coronavirus-2 (SARS-CoV-2) infection is common in children, and clinical manifestations can vary depending on age, underlying disease, and vaccination status. Most children will have asymptomatic or mild infection, but certain baseline characteristics can increase the risk of moderate to severe disease. The following article will provide an overview of the clinical manifestations of coronavirus disease 2019 in children, including the post-infectious phenomenon called multisystem inflammatory syndrome in children. Currently available treatment and prophylaxis strategies will be outlined, with the caveat that new therapeutics and clinical efficacy data are constantly on the horizon.

Coronavirus disease-2019 (COVID-19) infection during pregnancy is associated with severe complications and adverse effects for the mother, the fetus, and the neonate. The frequency of these outcomes varies according to the region, the gestational age, and the presence of comorbidities. Many COVID-19 interventions, including oxygen therapy, high-flow nasal cannula, and invasive mechanical ventilation, are challenging and require understanding physiologic adaptations of pregnancy. Vaccination is safe during pregnancy and lactation and constitutes the most important intervention to reduce severe disease and complications.

Severe acute respiratory syndrome coronavirus 2 (SARS-CoV-2) is a novel coronavirus that causes an acute respiratory tract infection known as coronavirus disease 2019 (COVID-19). SARS-CoV-2 enters cells by binding the ACE2 receptor and coreceptors notably TMPRSS2 or Cathepsin L. Severe COVID-19 infection can lead to acute lung injury. Below we describe the impact of common chronic lung diseases (CLDs) on the development of COVID-19. The impact of treatment of CLD on COVID-19 and any the importance of COVID-19 vaccination in patients with CLD are considered.

Immunocompromised hosts, which encompass a diverse population of persons with malignancies, human immunodeficiency virus disease, solid organ, and hematologic transplants, autoimmune diseases, and primary immunodeficiencies, bear a significant burden of the morbidity and mortality due to coronavirus disease-2019 (COVID-19). Immunocompromised patients who develop COVID-19 have a more severe illness, higher hospitalization rates, and higher mortality rates than immunocompetent patients. There are no well-defined treatment strategies that are specific to immunocompromised patients and vaccines, monoclonal antibodies, and convalescent plasma are variably effective. This review focuses on the specific impact of COVID-19 in immunocompromised patients and the gaps in knowledge that require further study.

Although coronavirus disease 2019 (COVID-19) remains an ongoing threat, concerns regarding other respiratory infections remain. Throughout the COVID-19 pandemic various epidemiologic trends have been observed in other respiratory viruses including a reduction in influenza and respiratory syncytial virus infections following onset of the COVID-19 pandemic. Observations suggest that infections with other respiratory viruses were reduced with social distancing, mask wearing, eye protection, and hand hygiene practices. Coinfections with COVID-19 exist not only with other respiratory viruses but also with bacterial pneumonias and other nosocomial and opportunistic infections. Coinfections have been associated with increased severity of illness and other adverse outcomes.

In the United States, the coronavirus disease-2019 (COVID-19) pandemic has disproportionately affected Black, Latinx, and Indigenous populations, immigrants, and economically disadvantaged individuals. Such historically marginalized groups are more often employed in low-wage jobs without health insurance and have higher rates of infection, hospitalization, and death from COVID-19 than non-Latinx White individuals. Mistrust in the health care system, language barriers, and limited health literacy have hindered vaccination rates in minorities, further exacerbating health disparities rooted in structural, institutional, and socioeconomic inequities. In this article, we discuss the lessons learned over the last 2 years and how to mitigate health disparities moving forward.

Viren Kaul, Japjot Chahal, Isaac N. Schrarstzhaupt, Heike Geduld, Yinzhong Shen, Maurizio H. Cecconi, Andre M. Siqueira, Melissa M. Markoski, and Leticia Kawano-Dourado

Coronavirus disease-2019 has impacted the world globally. Countries and health care organizations across the globe responded to this unprecedented public health crisis in a varied manner in terms of public health and social measures, vaccination development and rollout, the conduct of research, developments of therapeutics, sharing of information, and in how they continue to deal with the widespread aftermath. This article reviews the various elements of the global response to the pandemic, focusing on the lessons learned and strategies to consider during future pandemics.

CLINICS IN CHEST MEDICINE

SERIES OF RELATED INTEREST

Infectious Disease Clinics
Available at: https://www.id.theclinics.com/
Critical Care Clinics
Available at: https://www.criticalcare.theclinics.com/

THE CLINICS ARE AVAILABLE ONLINE!
Access your subscription at:
www.theclinics.com

Preface
COVID-19 Lung Disease: Lessons Learned

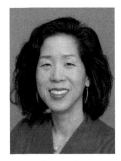   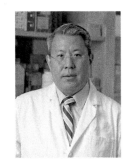

Guang-Shing Cheng, MD   Charles Dela Cruz, MD, PhD
Editors

Like so many aspects of medicine, pulmonary and critical care has been inexorably changed, for better or worse, by COVID-19. The learning curve has been steep and often challenging. Now, 3 years after the World Health Organization declared COVID-19 a global pandemic, we can afford to reflect on recent history and ask: what have we learned from this unprecedented experience? What will we need to do to confront the next respiratory viral epidemic/pandemic? What do we need to continue to learn?

In this issue of *Clinics in Chest Medicine*, we review the collective knowledge of COVID-19 lung disease, particularly as experienced in the first 2 years of the pandemic. We assembled a diverse group of authors from multiple disciplines, all of whom were on the frontline caring for patients with COVID-19 in the intensive care unit and in the clinic, in operating rooms, and in the community. Many of our authors were also leading the charge in composing clinical guidelines, conducting clinical trials, and innovating and advocating for the care of patients with COVID-19. Everyone synthesized a great deal of new data in a short period of time, and we thank our panel of authors for sharing their insights while managing ever busier schedules.

As detailed in our opening article, we learned how to mitigate the risk of SARS-CoV-2 transmission posed by the chest physician's basic tools of the trade: pulmonary function tests, bronchoscopies, and other aerosol-generating procedures. The collective experience of COVID-19 has forced us to evaluate all aspects of our understanding of infectious pneumonia, including atypical clinical presentations, the role of infection versus inflammation in the pathophysiology of COVID-19 lung disease, the protean manifestations that set COVID-19 apart from other respiratory viral illnesses, and how different aspects of the disease should be managed. We continue to learn about the long-term effects of SARS-CoV-2 infection on health. So much of medical practice was tested, stretched, and now accepted because of COVID-19. This includes the use of corticosteroids, novel immunomodulatory and antiviral agents, noninvasive oxygen support strategies, extracorporeal membrane oxygenation, and even lung transplantation.

We have learned about the unexpected manifestations of COVID-19 in special populations, including children, pregnant women, those with chronic lung disease, and the immunocompromised host. Importantly, we have learned (and relearned) how our behaviors and social structures make us vulnerable to respiratory viral illnesses, and how we can mitigate the spread of the virus with simple precautions. These measures have also altered the usual epidemiology of other respiratory viruses and infections. We have learned

Clin Chest Med 44 (2023) xiii–xiv
https://doi.org/10.1016/j.ccm.2023.03.001
0272-5231/23/© 2023 Published by Elsevier Inc.

hard lessons about the social determinants of health, laid painfully bare as health care systems struggled to handle surges of critically ill patients in the early phases of the pandemic. The outsized burden of COVID-19 on socially disadvantaged populations highlights racial and socioeconomic disparities that exist here in the United States as well as in countries around the world.

By nature, COVID-19 is a fluid and evolving topic. What we offer in this issue of *in Chest Medicine* is not the last word, but a point of departure for understanding the lessons learned from the pandemic so as to better prepare us for the future.

In addition to our authors, we would like to thank Jo Gascoine and Karen Dino of Elsevier as well as all of the production staff for shepherding this issue to fruition. Last but not least, we are grateful for the family, friends, and colleagues who have supported us through this project.

Guang-Shing Cheng, MD
Fred Hutchinson Cancer Center
University of Washington
1100 Fairview Avenue N
Mailstop D5-366
Seattle, WA 98109, USA

Charles Dela Cruz, MD, PhD
Yale University School of Medicine
300 Cedar Street
TAC S441-D
New Haven, CT 06513, USA

E-mail addresses:
gcheng2@fredhutch.org (G.-S. Cheng)
charles.delacruz@yale.edu (C. Dela Cruz)

What Have We Learned About Transmission of Coronavirus Disease-2019

Implications for Pulmonary Function Testing and Pulmonary Procedures

David A. Kaminsky, MD[a],*, Shaikh M. Noor Husnain, MD[b],
Danai Khemasuwan, MD, MBA, FCCP, ATSF[c]

KEYWORDS

- COVID-19 • SARS-CoV-2 • Aerosol transmission • Pulmonary function testing • Bronchoscopy
- Tracheostomy • Pleural procedures

KEY POINTS

- Pulmonary function testing and procedures represent important challenges during the coronavirus disease-2019 (COVID-19) pandemic because they have the potential for high aerosol generation and transmission of severe acute respiratory syndrome coronavirus 2.
- Important considerations in operating the pulmonary function laboratory and conducting pulmonary procedures are local prevalence and risk of COVID-19, clinical importance of the test, relative risk of the test for aerosol generation, and availability of resources to enhance mitigation of viral transmission to patients and staff.
- Lessons learned during the COVID-19 pandemic will be helpful in managing pulmonary function testing and pulmonary procedures during any similar circumstances in the future.

INTRODUCTION

One of the unique features of pulmonary function testing is the effort dependence of testing and the reliance of spirometry on a forced exhalation. By necessity this creates the potential for high aerosol generation, which is of primary concern for transmission of infectious agents. This concern quickly resulted in the abandonment of pulmonary function testing (PFT) at the beginning of the coronavirus disease-2019 (COVID-19) pandemic. Subsequently, many authorities issued summary statements, recommendations, and guidelines on how to best proceed with pulmonary function testing and other pulmonary procedures during the pandemic, especially in cases that were felt to be necessary for proper and appropriate patient care.[1–9] This article reviews the key principles involved in the development of such statements and guidelines as well as review the guidelines themselves. A detailed international document has just been issued that likewise reviews these topics.[10]

Basics of Aerosol Science

Aerosols are collections of particles that settle out very slowly by gravity because of their small size (Fig. 1). Aerosols are characterized by their mass

[a] Pulmonary and Critical Care, University of Vermont Larner College of Medicine, Given D213, 89 Beaumont Avenue, Burlington, VT 05405, USA; [b] Department of Pulmonary and Critical Care, Section of Interventional Pulmonary, Westchester Medical Center, 100 Woods Road, Valhalla, NY 10595, USA; [c] Pulmonary and Critical Care, Virginia Commonwealth University Health System, 1200 East Broad Street, Richmond, VA 23298, USA
* Corresponding author.
E-mail address: david.kaminsky@uvm.edu

Clin Chest Med 44 (2023) 215–226
https://doi.org/10.1016/j.ccm.2022.11.005
0272-5231/23/© 2022 Elsevier Inc. All rights reserved.

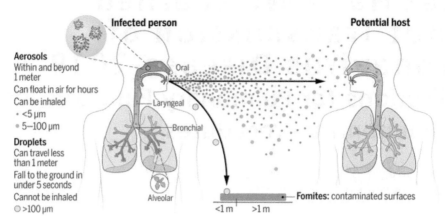

Fig. 1. Overview of aerosol generation and transport. Aerosols and droplets are emitted during exhalation, including breathing, speaking, and coughing/sneezing. Larger droplets will settle out quickly to surfaces, whereas smaller aerosols may travel significant distances. (*From* Wang CC, Prather KA, Sznitman J, et al. Airborne transmission of respiratory viruses. Science. 2021;373(6558):eabd9149.)

median aerodynamic diameter (MMAD), which can by described by the diameter at which 50% of the particles are larger, and 50% are smaller. Particles of MMAD = 0.5 to 5 μ are considered the respirable fraction because they are most likely to be inhaled and settle into the lung. Larger particles are considered droplets and are typically > 5 to 10 μ in size. Aerosol particles are thought to be generated during inhalation from the reopening of small, collapsed airways during quiet breathing, but additional mechanisms including shear stress and vibration of airway walls contribute to particle generation during coughing or sneezing.[11] These aerosols are then emitted during exhalation together with droplets in the range of 0.1 to 1000 μ in size.[12] Humans emit aerosols through not only forced exhalation but also quiet breathing and speaking. The factors that determine how droplets and aerosols behave in the air are their size, inertia, gravity, and evaporation.[12] If they undergo gravitational settling before evaporation, they can contaminate surfaces on contact. If they undergo evaporation faster than they settle, they remain buoyant and can be transported across distances in the air. Small particles on the order of 0.5 μ in size settle out slowly, whereas larger particles of 20 μ size settle out much more quickly.[13]

Evidence that Severe Acute Respiratory Syndrome Coronavirus 2 is Transmitted by Aerosols

Most studies of viral transmission by aerosols have involved influenza. Influenza A, as well as rhinovirus, respiratory syncytial virus (RSV), influenza B, parainfluenza 1, 2, and 3, and human metapneumovirus, have been detected mainly in smaller particles < 5 μ in size. Like these other viruses, severe acute respiratory syndrome coronavirus 2 (SARS-Co-V-2), which is 80 to 160 nm in size,[14] is thought to transmit primarily by aerosols.[13,15]

Production of Aerosols by Spirometry

Previous work has shown that microbiological contamination of spirometers by aerosol is quite uncommon, with minimal risk of transmission after 5 min of time between tests.[16] However, this work was performed using a volume spirometer and did not specifically investigate aerosol transmission of virus, only transmission of non-pathogenic bacteria. To our knowledge, there has never been a reported outbreak of viral infection associated with a PFT laboratory. The first study to show aerosol transmission during spirometry was published based on data from five volunteers at Mayo Clinic.[17] Spirometry resulted in an increase in respirable 0.3 μ particles when measured near the exhalation port of the spirometer, but none were detected at 1.5 or 3 feet away. In a subsequent study of 28 patients conducted in 3 PFT laboratories, there was a small increase in ambient small particles (<0.5 μ) with return to pretest baseline within 25 to 30 min.[18] Larger particles were also detected. As expected, particles took longer to return to baseline in smaller rooms or those with less ventilation. With the use of bacterial filters, particles were not detected during testing, only after when patients removed the mouthpiece and started talking or breathing without a face mask.[19] Another study found small particle emission increases during simple breathing maneuvers that might be used during lung function testing, as well as during cough.[20]

Production of Aerosols by Other Pulmonary Function Procedures

One study has shown that aerosol generation increases not only during spirometry, but also with measurement of lung volumes and diffusing capacity (D_LCO) while the patient sat in a body plethysmograph. There were no differences in particle emissions between tests, although the sample size was small ($n = 25$).[15] Aerosol transmission is increased during peak flow testing, as expected, but the concentration is small.[21] Also as expected, methacholine challenge testing, which involves repeated spirometry, results in high emission of ultrafine particles (0.02–1 μ), but particle generation was significantly reduced by using a breath-actuated dosimeter with viral filter.[21] Importantly, this study showed significant variability between patients, with most particles detected only a short distance from the mouth despite likely inadequate room ventilation. Of note, the estimated number of viral gene copies emitted was about one order of magnitude higher than would be expected from quiet breathing and the same order of magnitude as expected from normal speaking.

Aerosol generation is also documented after exercise. A study of 8 healthy volunteers showed significant aerosol generation with exercise, although there was considerable heterogeneity between participants.[22] Similarly, exercise involved in cardiac rehabilitation resulted in aerosol generation that peaked at 35 to 40 min after the start of each class, even though patients wore procedural masks.[23] However, lower levels of exercise did not generate excess particles while participants in a different study wore procedural masks.[24] Wearing a surgical mask has been shown to have negative consequences on exercise performance during maximal cardiopulmonary exercise testing (CPET) in young healthy people, including increased dyspnea, lower peak oxygen consumption, and lower anaerobic threshold.[25] Aerosol generation during exercise is significantly reduced by use of an high efficiency particulate air (HEPA) filter with fume hood.[26]

To date, no studies have documented the extent to which aerosols are generated during other pulmonary function tests such as inert gas washout, measurement of fractional excretion of nitric oxide (FeNO), or oscillometry, although oscillometry, in particular, has been suggested as a relatively safe, low aerosol-generating procedure to use during lung function testing.[27]

Mitigation of Transmission of Severe Acute Respiratory Syndrome Coronavirus 2 by Aerosols

The primary way to reduce COVID transmission is through masking and social distancing.[28] Masks are of critical importance to protect people from viral transmission through droplets and aerosols.[28] The WHO recommendation for social distancing of 6 feet is based on studies of respiratory droplets performed in the 1930s.[28] We now know 100 μ droplets will settle to the ground as far away as 8 feet and a 1 μ aerosol may take up to 12 hours to settle in still air. Coughs and sneezes can result in particles traveling at 8 m/s that can propel particles more than 20 feet.[11] Transmission of virus is much less likely outdoors due to air movement, dilution and the effects of UV radiation and concomitant air pollution.[28]

Recommendations for Operation of the Pulmonary Function Testing Laboratory

Initial guidelines for operation of the PFT laboratory during the pandemic were issued by major medical societies such as American Thoracic Society (ATS), European Respiratory Society (ERS), Occupational Safety and Health Administration (OSHA), and others.[1–5,7,9,14] A comprehensive literature review of available statements at the time was published by Crimi and colleagues.[29] An international guideline statement has now been published and is based on the consensus opinion of 23 experts.[10] The first section focuses on transmission, environmental and equipment considerations, with specific recommendations for the type of inline filter and personal protective equipment (PPE) to be used during different PFTs. For common procedures such as spirometry, lung volumes and D_LCO, these recommendations include use of an inline filter, N95 or equivalent mask, apron/gown and goggles/shield. For high aerosol potential procedures, such as bronchial challenge testing or bronchodilator testing with a nebulizer and CPET, an N99 mask is recommended, and such procedures should ideally be conducted with a filter on the expiratory port and in a negative pressure room, if available. An important point that is emphasized in the document is the proper consideration of room ventilation, as discussed below.

The second section focuses on referral, triage, and PCR testing. The need for the PFT must be weighed against the potential risks of exposing test personnel and other patients to the virus. Low-priority need might include routine screening or monitoring of stable patients, whereas high-priority need might include monitoring of patients with heart or lung transplant, those on potentially pulmonary toxic drugs, or those with severe symptoms for whom diagnostic testing is important to help with diagnosis of dyspnea. High aerosol generation procedures should be avoided, such as bronchial challenge testing and CPET. If a bronchodilator is administered, it is thought better to use a metered dose inhaler than a nebulizer to minimize exogenous aerosol emission from the device, although evidence for this is lacking.[19,30] Using biofilters on the exhalation port of a nebulizer will effectively reduce escape of aerosols from the device.[19] Doing testing in a body plethysmograph could theoretically reduce environmental aerosol exposure. A protocol must be in place for assessing symptoms and need for COVID testing before pulmonary function testing. The timing of testing should consider local prevalence of COVID-19 and the most recent evidence for infectivity, with current recommendations suggesting performing PFTs no earlier than 10 days after onset of illness in mild-moderate COVID if there are 2 negative PCR tests after disease available, no earlier than 20 days in severe patients who have one negative PCR, and no earlier than 30 days with no PCR needed. The latter guideline seems the most sensible since the CDC recommends against repeat PCR testing up to 90 days after acute illness due to persistent positivity that may last that long even though a patient is no longer infectious.[31]

The third section focuses on operational issues, including staffing and waiting area. Patients should wear a mask in the waiting area after passing the pre-screening procedure. Patients should be distanced at least 6 feet apart, although this may be flexible depending on room configuration and ventilation. There should be physical barriers such as plexiglass shields and equipment covers to prevent cross-contamination and protect both patients and staff.

The fourth section focuses on testing room precautions including air conditioning and ventilation. It is recommended there be at least 6 air changes per hour but 12 to 15 is better,[14,32] and testing in a negative pressure room is preferable. Recently, the value of portable HEPA filters in reducing aerosol contamination has been shown.[33] Reducing viral transmission by UV light also holds promise.[34]

The fifth section focuses on lung function testing procedures, with detailed instructions for spirometry, bronchodilator testing, lung volume measurement, $D_L CO$, FeNO, oscillometry, capnography, muscle pressures, 6-min walk test, CPET, and bronchial challenge tests. Of particular importance is the proper use of in-line filters, which should be of sufficient efficacy in screening out viral-sized

particles smaller than SARS Co-V-2 (<0.8 μ) while maintaining low enough airway resistance to allow high peak expiratory flows of up to 700 L/min. Manufacturers should provide testing data to show that their filters have at least 99.9% efficiency.

The sixth section focuses on the management of special populations, such as pediatrics, elderly, lung cancer and surgery patients, immunocompromised patients. Precautions should be taken to prevent infection and cross-contamination in each context, and caregivers of these patients should be adequately protected as well.

The final section focuses on testing outside the hospital, for example, in community and primary care offices. In non-hospital settings, it is important to consider the availability and proper use of in-line filters vs. disposable sensors, PPE, room ventilation, and screening and waiting room policies. In this context, telemedicine or remote, video-coached spirometry is becoming more prevalent. New techniques, such as the use of wearable electromagnetic sensors, have also been described to allow for non-contact, point-of-care monitoring of pulmonary function during the COVID-19 pandemic.[35]

Outcomes in Pulmonary Function Testing Laboratories So Far

There is no evidence to date that the PFT laboratory has been the source of an outbreak of COVID-19, which is remarkable considering the high-aerosol-generating potential of the procedures involved. Only one study has specifically analyzed the incidence of COVID-19 after lung function testing.[36] In a retrospective analysis of 278 patients tested between April and September 2020, the cumulative incidence of COVID-19 within 15 days of testing was 0.36%, with none of the technicians developing symptomatic disease. This finding is very encouraging and speaks to the efficacy of following protocols and guidelines to mitigate spread of COVID-19.

Regarding PFT laboratory performance and adherence to guidelines, a survey of 132 laboratories conducted between August and October of 2020 found that nearly all laboratories required adequate PPE for their technologist, including the use of N95 masks for at least some procedures.[37] Likewise, nearly all laboratories used in-line filters, used proper recommended room and equipment cleaning and 83% provided time for air exchange. Although screening for COVID-19 symptoms and temperature checks were nearly universal, PCR testing was variable depending on local COVID prevalence. By the close of the survey, 71% of laboratories were fully operational, demonstrating how PFT laboratories were able to cope with the pandemic in its early phases.

A qualitative review of international practices among pediatric PFT laboratories has also been published.[38] A unique feature of this review included the concern of both patients and parents in terms of symptom screening, waiting room conditions, and use of face masks, which is especially challenging for younger children. In addition, special mention was made of the sequence of testing, with the most aerosol-generating procedures such as forced exhalation and exercise testing done last to be able to leave the room as soon as such testing is completed.

Another review of PFT laboratory practices during the pandemic revealed a sharp decline in total number of PFTs performed starting in March 2020, reaching a maximum decline in April 2020, and then variably rebounding since then.[39] Bronchoscopies showed the smallest decline, and there were more ambulatory exercise tests and CPETs than compared with before the pandemic.

Pulmonary Procedures Other Than Pulmonary Function Testing

The following section will review pulmonary procedures in the context of COVID-19, including bronchoscopy, tracheostomy, and pleural procedures. The pulmonologist may be in a unique position of risk due to the nature of the procedures performed involving the airway and hence the high aerosol-generating potential of these procedures. In addition, pulmonologists may be involved not only in the care of acutely ill patients with COVID-19, but also of those recovering from the illness who may require post-tracheostomy care or diagnostic bronchoalveolar lavage (BAL) or lung biopsy in the setting of persistent pulmonary fibrosis.[40]

Bronchoscopy

Bronchoscopy is classified as a high aerosol-generating procedure, which could lead to accidental transmission of droplet and airborne particles to health care professionals.[41] In the COVID-19 era, indications for bronchoscopy have not changed apart from following a more cautious approach and careful selection of the procedure if absolutely needed.

Safety of Bronchoscopy in Patients with Coronavirus Disease-2019

In a review published by Saha and colleagues,[42] 12 cohorts (9 retrospective and 3 prospective) reported on the safety of bronchoscopy and transmission of virus among bronchoscopists. A total of 2245 bronchoscopies were performed among 1345 patients. Eleven of 12 studies (92%) specified the use of PPE. All the health care workers used full PPE, including gown, face shield, eye protector, shoe cover, double gloves, filtering face pieces (FFP2/FFP3), N95 mask, and, sometimes, a powered air-purifying respirator. Only 57% reported the use of negative pressure rooms for all their procedures.[42] Only one study reported 1 bronchoscopist who developed COVID-19 during the 3 weeks of study.[43]

Recommendations for Bronchoscopy from Major Respiratory Societies

American College of Chest Physicians/American Association for Bronchology and Interventional Bronchoscopy (CHEST/AABIP) guidelines suggest avoiding invasive methods like bronchoscopy with BAL to establish diagnosis unless necessary.[8] A nasopharyngeal specimen should be obtained first in patients suspected of having COVID-19 infection. In patients with severe respiratory failure who require intubation, specimens from an endotracheal aspirate or bronchoscopy with BAL can be performed.[8] In terms of therapeutic bronchoscopy, this guideline-recommended four indications for emergent bronchoscopy regardless of COVID-19 status which included (1) moderate to severe tracheobronchial stenosis; (2) symptomatic central airway obstruction; (3) massive hemoptysis and (4) stent migration. Meanwhile, in patients with confirmed COVID-19 infection and undergoing elective bronchoscopy, the guideline recommended waiting at least 30 days from the resolution of symptoms with two, negative consecutive nasopharyngeal swab PCR specimens collected > 24 hours apart.[8] However, local practice varies by the waiting time for negative tests and the number of tests before elective procedures.

The Society for Advanced Bronchoscopy (SAB) provided similar recommendations to CHEST/AABIP,[6] with combined recommendations for urgency of bronchoscopy shown in **Table 1**. The SAB described the advantages of single-use (disposable) flexible bronchoscopes, which, in addition to avoiding reprocessing equipment, requires less equipment to set up, and only needs a single user to operate, decreasing the number of contact personnel. However, the access to disposable bronchoscopes may vary based on local resources.[44] Other procedural recommendations include intubation with general anesthesia rather than conscious sedation, using an endotracheal tube rather than laryngeal mask airway for a tighter airway seal, and consideration of use of paralytics to abolish coughing.[8,45,46] For rigid bronchoscopy, a recommendation is made for a

Table 1
Relative urgency and timing of indications for bronchoscopy

Emergent (Same day)	Urgent (1–2 d)	Non-urgent (>2 d)
Acute foreign body aspiration	Infiltrates in neutropenic or immunocompromised host with fever	Airway inspection for cough or minor hemoptysis
Massive hemoptysis (without obvious source for embolization)	Lung mass or mediastinal/hilar adenopathy suspicious for cancer	Mild central airway stenosis
Severe symptomatic central airway obstruction or stenosis	Non-massive hemoptysis	Clearance of mucus
Migrated stent	Whole lung lavage	Suspected sarcoidosis
	Acute lobar atelectasis	Detection of chronic infection (eg, mycobacterial, fungal)
		Chronic interstitial lung disease
		Bronchoscopic lung volume reduction or bronchial thermoplasty
		Evaluation for tracheobronchomalacia
		Tracheostomy changes
		Surveillance transplant bronchoscopy

Data from Wahidi MM, Shojaee S, Lamb CR, et al. The Use of Bronchoscopy During the Coronavirus Disease 2019 Pandemic: CHEST/AABIP Guideline and Expert Panel Report. Chest. 2020;158(3):1268-1281 and Pritchett MA, Oberg CL, Belanger A, et al. Society for Advanced Bronchoscopy Consensus Statement and Guidelines for bronchoscopy and airway management amid the COVID-19 pandemic. J Thorac Dis. 2020;12(5):1781-1798.

closed-circuit ventilation system rather than jet ventilation.[47] Other international expert panels from Europe and Asia also provided recommendations for bronchoscopy which were very similar to other respiratory societies as mentioned above.[48]

Lastly, decontamination of the procedural area is important. Recent literature shows that the SARS-CoV-2 virus can remain aerosolized for up to 3 hours and can be found on surfaces for up to 3 days, depending on the surface type.[49] The room turnover time will depend on changing of room air volume. The negative-pressure bronchoscopy rooms require a minimum of 12 total air exchanges per hour to provide dilution and exhaust of contaminated air.[31] At this rate, after 23 min 99% of particles will be cleared.[6]

In conclusion, flexible bronchoscopy must be cautiously performed amid the COVID-19 crisis. Judicious case selection and meticulous contact and airborne precautions are important to minimize infection transmission. Mandatory universal PPE, pre-bronchoscopy PCR tests, dedicated protective barriers and disposable bronchoscopes might be the safest and simplest way to perform bronchoscopy in the setting of COVID-19.

Tracheostomy

Tracheostomy is another high aerosol-generating procedure with risk of infectious transmission for health care workers.[50]

Optimal Time to Perform Tracheostomy in Coronavirus Disease-2019 Patients

Since the start of the pandemic, the duration of mechanical ventilation for COVID-19-related acute respiratory distress syndrome (ARDS) has been longer compared with non-COVID-19-related ARDS, with many COVID-19 patients remaining intubated for at least one to 2 weeks or longer.[51–53] This observation has been true for patients with asymptomatic COVID-19 infection as well, who have been admitted to intensive care unit (ICU) for trauma-related causes.[54] Despite this observation of prolonged ventilation, there is insufficient evidence on optimal timing to perform tracheostomy on COVID patients. The CHEST/AABIP guidelines did not recommend a specific timing of tracheostomy due to insufficient evidence to suggest performing a tracheostomy either early (<10 days) or late (>14 days).[55]

The early tracheostomy strategy accelerates weaning from the ventilator and may have a critical role in freeing up ventilators, ICU beds, and staff during surges.[56] However, there was a concern of COVID-19 transmission for operators and health care workers. The early report of case series for tracheostomy from New York University showed a median of 10.6 days from intubation to tracheostomy. There were no team members testing positive for SARS-CoV-2.[57] A multicenter, retrospective study included 118 COVID-19 patients who underwent tracheostomy.[58] Early tracheostomy (≤14 days) was associated with decreased ventilator days, decreased ventilator-associated pneumonia, and shorter ICU duration and shorter hospital length of stay (LOS) among patients who were discharged. The median time from intubation to tracheostomy was 22 days with 78% of patients undergoing percutaneous dilatational technique vs. 22% surgical technique. Although there was a concern of COVID-19 infection risk for health care workers, a high rate of infection has not been reported. The systematic review and meta-analysis of 69 studies indicated that enhanced PPE is associated with low rates of SARS-CoV-2 transmission during tracheostomy.[59]

Meanwhile, delaying tracheostomy may reduce the risk to health care workers because the viral load of severe acute respiratory syndrome coronavirus 2 (SARS-CoV-2) may be lower, but that reduction in risk must be weighed against prolonged intubation.[56] SARS-CoV-2 infectivity peaks 3 to 4 days after infection, and infectivity is diminished by waiting 10 days before performing tracheostomy.[56] In addition, SARS-CoV-2 viral loads are highest in upper respiratory tract mucosa, particularly the nasopharynx.[60] Thus, aerosolization may be less in patients with mechanical ventilation. A cross-sectional review of institutional protocols and practices from 26 countries showed timing for tracheostomy varied from 3 to >21 days depending on risk of implied infectivity to personnel performing and handling tracheostomy.[61] In this study, over 90% of protocols recommended 14 days of intubation before tracheostomy. Most protocols advocate delaying tracheostomy until COVID-19 testing was negative. A report from a single tertiary care institution reviewed 258 invasive mechanical ventilation patients out of whom 46 (18%) required tracheostomy (**Table 2**). Although tracheostomy placement in patients with COVID did not decrease overall LOS, duration of mechanical ventilation, or ICU LOS, patients with a tracheostomy experienced a significantly lower number of deaths vs. those without tracheostomy.[62] A systematic review and meta-analysis of 18 studies exploring 3234 COVID-19 patients showed that only 5.2% of tracheostomies were performed within 7 days (early), and 21.2% were performed between days 8 and 13, whereas most (71.5%) of the tracheostomies were performed 14 days or later post-intubation. The meta-analysis did not reveal the benefit of early tracheostomy in terms of duration of mechanical ventilation or time to decannulation, nor was late tracheostomy associated with increased mortality.[63,64]

Based on above studies, there is evidence supporting both strategies. Thus, a specific timing of tracheostomy cannot be recommended. When COVID-19 overwhelms capacity in ICUs, early timing of tracheostomy may accelerate ventilator weaning and free up critical care resources. General decisions surrounding optimal timing in the critically ill patient can be complex outside of the pandemic, but given the clinical evidence so far, one may conclude that early tracheostomy may be a better option for these patients given the overall benefits to patients and the health care system. However, more data and research are required.

Tracheostomy Techniques in the Coronavirus Disease Era

As for other high aerosol-generating procedures, patient selection for tracheostomy is important. Contraindications including hemodynamic instability, hypoxemia (Pao_2/Fio_2 <200), high intracranial pressure (>20 mm Hg), multi-organ failure, coagulopathy, platelet dysfunction or anticoagulation, surgical site infection, history of major cervical surgery that alters cervical flexion-extension, and abnormal cervical anatomy apply to COVID patients just as any patient.[65] Patients who are in the prone position or likely to be placed prone for respiratory failure should not be considered for tracheostomy due to the increased risk of complications that is, tube displacement, occlusion, or impaired ability to identify complications.[56]

Multiple factors influence the technique for this procedure. The first consideration is the location of the patients. These patients are critically ill and usually admitted to the ICU, hence percutaneous technique is preferred as it minimizes transfer. Ideally aerosolizing procedures should be performed in a negative pressure room but those are not always available. Performing tracheostomy at the bedside offers advantages of time availability as compared with needing to schedule in the operating room. Some disadvantages include less trained ancillary staff, and less equipment to control complications. To minimize aerosolization, Angel and colleagues have developed a modified percutaneous technique where the flexible bronchoscope was passed alongside the endotracheal

Table 2
Suggested requirements for safe testing in the pulmonary function testing laboratory and selective pulmonary procedures

Test/Procedure	In-Line Antimicrobial Filter	Mask (N95 or Equivalent)	Gown	Eye Protection	Other
Spirometry	+	+	+	+	
Lung volumes body box gas dilution	+	+	+	+	
DLCO	+	+	+	+	
Bronchodilator	–	+	+	+	Filter on expiratory port
MDI nebulizer	+	+	+	+	
Bronchial challenge testing	+	+	+	+	Negative pressure room if available
6 min walk	–	+	+	–	
CPET	–	+	+	+	Negative pressure room if available
Oscillometry	+	+	+	+	
FeNO	+	+	+	+	
MIP/MEP	+	+	+	+	
Bronchoscopy	NA	+	+	+	Negative pressure room if available
Tracheostomy	NA	+	+	+	Negative pressure room if available
Pleural procedures	+ (in suction tubing)	+	+	+	

+, required; - , not required.
Modified from McGowan A, Laveneziana P, Bayat S, et al. International consensus on lung function testing during the COVID-19 pandemic and beyond. ERJ Open Res. 2022;8(1):00602-2021. Published 2022 Mar 7.

tube (through vocal cords) and not inside the tube as in conventional percutaneous tracheostomy.[57] This modified technique permitted the operator to perform uninterrupted mechanical ventilation after re-positioning the inflated endotracheal tube cuff to the distal trachea. It offered significant mitigation of the risk of virus aerosolization during the procedure. Another modification described is percutaneous tracheostomy using an acrylic box as an aerosol shield (**Fig. 2**).[66] This technique had the least aerosolization and contamination but has a long procedure time compared with standard technique with or without a ventilator pause. Another prospective single-system multicenter observational cohort study was conducted examining safety for both patients and health care workers.[67] In this series, 29 percutaneous tracheostomies were performed; 19 cases used a conventional technique with intermittent ventilator pause and 10 cases used a modified technique. There was no report of health care worker transmissions resulting from performing the procedure.

These proposed modifications of standard percutaneous tracheostomy provide minimal aerosolization which may mitigate viral transmission to operator and health care workers. The selection of the technique should depend on the expertise of operator, availability of team and resources, and overall safety of patient and providers. It is imperative that appropriate PPE is always used by every member of the procedural team.[68]

Pleural Procedures

All pleural procedures, including thoracentesis, chest tube insertion and pleural biopsy by thoracostomy or pleuroscopy, might be considered aerosol-generating as patients may cough, and theoretically virus-containing aerosols may be emitted from a chest drain with an air leak.[40] SARS-CoV-2 viral RNA has also been detected in pleural fluid,[40] making direct transmission by contact also a potential risk due to fluid splashing and contamination. A statement from the American Association for the Surgery of Trauma (AAST) Acute Care Surgery and Critical Care Committees recommends putting in-line antimicrobial filters on

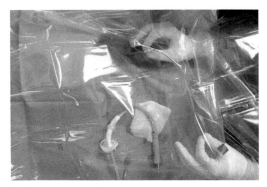

Fig. 2. A clear plastic coverage is used to provide an additional barrier to contamination during percutaneous dilatational tracheostomy. Shown are the positions of the bronchoscopist at the side of a surgical field. (*Adapted from* Majid A, Ayala A, Uribe JP, et al. Protective Strategies in a Simulated Model When Performing Percutaneous Tracheostomies in the COVID-19 Era. Ann Am Thorac Soc. 2020;17(11):1486-1488.)

the suction line of a chest tube drainage system while on suction or on water seal.[69] Although no other special techniques are described to perform these procedures, the usual precautions in terms of stratifying by current risk of active infection and prioritization of the procedure should apply, with personnel wearing appropriate PPE in all circumstances where a patient has COVID-19 or their COVID-19 status is unknown A summary of suggested requirements for safe testing in the pulmonary function laboratory and selective pulmonary procedures is provided in **Table 2**.

Transitioning Back to Normal Operations

To date, there are no formal guidelines about how to make the transition back to normal operations of the PFT laboratory or pulmonary procedures, other than some societies recommending "return to pre-COVID standards" in the post-pandemic phase.[5,70] However, the Canadian Thoracic Society has explicitly stated that "return to pre-pandemic infection control practices in the PFT testing will not provide acceptable risk mitigation", and lessons learned and additional precautions taken during COVID-19 should result in updated PFT laboratory testing protocols to protect against SARS CoV-2 as well as other emerging pathogens.[71] It makes sense that any transition back to normal operations will need to include ongoing consideration of local prevalence of COVID-19, immune or vaccination status of the community, and importance of testing or procedure for patient relative to risk to PFT and proceduralist staff. Screening procedures will, and already have, become less involved, with many

institutions no longer requiring PCR testing and only relying on symptom screening. A selective rather than universal approach to PCR testing before elective surgery has been shown to be safe.[72] The role of antigen testing is unclear although has been proposed.[73] Individual institutional policy will dictate local PPE and infection control procedures, such as wearing N95 or procedural masks, eye protection, contact precautions, cleaning and disinfection, and procedure room ventilation.

SUMMARY

The COVID-19 pandemic has caused us to carefully reconsider all that we do in the PFT laboratory, from the importance of ordering the test, to the screening of patients, waiting room conditions, testing environment, personnel protection, and decontamination procedures. Although like many aspects of health care the PFT laboratory initially had to stop operations for all but the most urgent conditions, laboratories around the world have adapted to COVID-19, and are most are back in full operation. It is a tribute to the testing personnel and the careful attention and care to infection prevention that the PFT laboratory has not been a source of community spread during the COVID-19 pandemic despite the high aerosol-generating potential of its many procedures. Similarly, regarding pulmonary procedures, it is mandatory that contact precautions and proper training on donning and doffing of PPE be provided to all health care workers. Another key element is advanced planning and keeping each procedure unit well-organized. Although the reduction in the number of elective procedures represents one of the central strategies to improve safety, it is crucial that patients not suffer unnecessary delays in diagnostic or therapeutic procedures. The lessons learned so far regarding the impact of the COVID-19 pandemic on PFTs and pulmonary procedures will certainly apply to any potential future outbreaks.

CLINICS CARE POINTS

- Whether and how to perform pulmonary function testing during the COVID-19 pandemic depends on many factors related to importance of test, risk of aerosol spread, prevalence of local disease, and adequacy of safe testing environment.

- Environmental safety features related to pulmonary function testing include adequate room ventilation, proper PPE for testing personnel, in-line mouth filters, cleaning and disinfecting of equipment, and use of meter dose inhalers rather than nebulizers for administration of aerosolized bronchodilators.

- Whether and how to perform pulmonary procedures also relies on balancing risk vs. benefit with careful attention to protection of health care workers.

- Special protection of health care workers during pulmonary procedures includes adequate PPE and room ventilation, minimizing exposure to staff, intubation rather than concious sedation, use of closed-circuit ventilation rather than jet ventilation during rigid bronchoscopy, and performance of percutaneous tracheostomy with physical shielding from aerosol exposure.

DISCLOSURE

Dr D.A. Kaminsky is a speaker for MGC Diagnostics, Inc. and a contributor to UptoDate, Inc. Dr S.M. Husnain has no conflicts of interest and any funding sources Dr D. Khemasuwan has no conflicts of interest and any funding sources.

FUNDING SOURCES

Dr D.A. Kaminsky is funded, in part, by the Vermont Lung Center.

REFERENCES

1. Harber P, MC T, Levine M. Occupational spirometry and fit testing in the COVID-19 era: 2021 interim recommendations from the american college of occupational and environmental medicine. Available from: https://acoem.org/Guidance-and-Position-Statements/Guidance-and-Position-Statements/Occupational-Spirometry-and-Fit-Testing-in-the-COVID-19-Era-2021-Interim-Recommendations-from-the-American-Collegeof-Occupational-and-Environmental-Medicine.
2. American thoracic society. May 18, 2022. Available from: https://www.thoracic.org/professionals/clinical-resources/disease-related-resources/pulmonary-function-laboratories.php.
3. Association for respiratory technology and physiology and british thoracic society. May 18, 2022. Available from: org.uk/write/MediaUploads/Standards/COVID19/Respiratory_Function_Testing_During_Endemic_COVID_V1.5.pdf.
4. Canadian society of respiratory therapists. May 18, 2022. Available from: https://www.csrt.com/csrt-novel-coronavirus-resources/.
5. European respiratory society. May 18, 2022. Available from: https://ers.app.box.com/s/zs1uu88wy51monr0ewd990itoz4tsn2h.
6. Pritchett MA, Oberg CL, Belanger A, et al. Society for advanced bronchoscopy consensus statement and guidelines for bronchoscopy and airway management amid the COVID-19 pandemic. J Thorac Dis 2020;12:1781–98.
7. Thoracic society of Australia and New Zealand. May 18, 2022. Available from: https://www.thoracic.org.au/information-public/tsanz-update.
8. Wahidi MM, Shojaee S, Lamb CR, et al. The use of bronchoscopy during the coronavirus disease 2019 pandemic: CHEST/AABIP guideline and expert panel report. Chest 2020;158:1268–81.
9. Wilson KC, Kaminsky DA, Michaud G, et al. Restoring pulmonary and sleep services as the covid-19 pandemic lessens. from an association of pulmonary, critical care, and sleep division directors and american thoracic society-coordinated task force. Ann Am Thorac Soc 2020;17:1343–51.
10. McGowan A, Laveneziana P, Bayat S, et al. International consensus on lung function testing during the COVID-19 pandemic and beyond. ERJ Open Res 2022;8. 00602-2021.
11. Dhand R, Li J. Coughs and sneezes: their role in transmission of respiratory viral infections, including SARS-CoV-2. Am J Respir Crit Care Med 2020;202:651–9.
12. Wang CC, Prather KA, Sznitman J, et al. Airborne transmission of respiratory viruses. Science 2021;373(6558):eabd9149.
13. Scheuch G. Breathing is enough: for the spread of influenza virus and SARS-CoV-2 by breathing only. J Aerosol Med Pulm Drug Deliv 2020;33:230–4.
14. Federation of european heating ventilation and air conditioning associations. 2022. Available from: https://www.rehva.eu/activities/covid-19-guidance/rehva-covid-19-guidance.
15. Tomisa G, Horváth A, Farkas Á, et al. Real-life measurement of size-fractionated aerosol concentration in a plethysmography box during the COVID-19 pandemic and estimation of the associated viral load. J Hosp Infect 2021;118:7–14.
16. Hiebert T, Miles J, Okeson GC. Contaminated aerosol recovery from pulmonary function testing equipment. Am J Respir Crit Care Med 1999;159:610–2.
17. Helgeson SA, Lim KG, Lee AS, et al. Aerosol generation during spirometry. Ann Am Thorac Soc 2020;17:1637–9.
18. Li J, Jing G, Fink JB, et al. Airborne particulate concentrations during and after pulmonary function testing. Chest 2021;159:1570–4.
19. Fink JB, Ehrmann S, Li J, et al. Reducing aerosol-related risk of transmission in the era of COVID-19: an interim guidance endorsed by the international

society of aerosols in medicine. J Aerosol Med Pulm Drug Deliv 2020;33:300–4.

20. Greening NJ, Larsson P, Ljungström E, et al. Small droplet emission in exhaled breath during different breathing manoeuvres: implications for clinical lung function testing during COVID-19. Allergy 2021;76:915–7.

21. Subat YW, Guntupalli SK, Sajgalik P, et al. Aerosol generation during peak flow testing: clinical implications for COVID-19. Respir Care 2021;66:1291–8.

22. Sajgalik P, Garzona-Navas A, Csécs I, et al. Characterization of aerosol generation during various intensities of exercise. Chest 2021;160:1377–87.

23. Helgeson SA, Taylor BJ, Lim KG, et al. Characterizing particulate generation during cardiopulmonary rehabilitation classes with patients wearing procedural masks. Chest 2021;160:633–41.

24. Helgeson SA, Lee AS, Patel NM, et al. Cardiopulmonary exercise and the risk of aerosol generation while wearing a surgical mask. Chest 2021;159:1567–9.

25. Zhang G, Li M, Zheng M, et al. Effect of surgical masks on cardiopulmonary function in healthy young subjects: a crossover study. Front Physiol 2021;12:710573.

26. Garzona-Navas A, Sajgalik P, Csécs I, et al. Mitigation of aerosols generated during exercise testing with a portable high-efficiency particulate air filter with fume hood. Chest 2021;160:1388–96.

27. Gupta N, Sachdev A, Gupta D. Oscillometry-A reasonable option to monitor lung functions in the era of COVID-19 pandemic. Pediatr Pulmonol 2021;56:14–5.

28. Prather KA, Wang CC, Schooley RT. Reducing transmission of SARS-CoV-2. Science 2020;368:1422–4.

29. Crimi C, Impellizzeri P, Campisi R, et al. Practical considerations for spirometry during the COVID-19 outbreak: literature review and insights. Pulmonology 2021;27:438–47.

30. Goldstein KM, Ghadimi K, Mystakelis H, et al. Risk of transmitting coronavirus disease 2019 during nebulizer treatment: a systematic review. J Aerosol Med Pulm Drug Deliv 2021;34:155–70.

31. Centers for Disease Control and Prevention. 2022. Available from: https://www.cdc.gov/media/releases/2021/s1227-isolation-quarantine-guidance.html.

32. Centers for Disease Control and Prevention. May 18, 2022. Available from: https://acoem.org/Guidance-and-Position-Statements/Guidance-and-Position-Statements/Occupational-Spirometry-and-Fit-Testing-in-the-COVID-19-Era-2021-Interim-Recommendations-from-the-A.

33. Lindsley WG, Derk RC, Coyle JP, et al. Efficacy of portable air cleaners and masking for reducing indoor exposure to simulated exhaled SARS-CoV-2 Aerosols - United States, 2021. MMWR Morb Mortal Wkly Rep 2021;70:972–6.

34. Chiappa F, Frascella B, Vigezzi GP, et al. The efficacy of ultraviolet light-emitting technology against coronaviruses: a systematic review. J Hosp Infect 2021;114:63–78.

35. Shahrestani S, Chou TC, Shang KM, et al. A wearable eddy current based pulmonary function sensor for continuous non-contact point-of-care monitoring during the COVID-19 pandemic. Sci Rep 2021;11:20144.

36. Wainstein EJ, Peroni HJ, Ferreyro BL, et al. Incidence of COVID-19 after pulmonary function tests: a retrospective cohort study. Rev Fac Cien Med Univ Nac Cordoba 2021;78:367–70.

37. Saunders MJ, Haynes JM, McCormack MC, et al. How local SARS-CoV-2 Prevalence shapes pulmonary function testing laboratory protocols and practices during the COVID-19 pandemic. Chest 2021;160:1241–4.

38. Beydon N, Gochicoa L, Jones MJ, et al. Pediatric lung function testing during a pandemic: an international perspective. Paediatr Respir Rev 2020;36:106–8.

39. Call JT, Lee AS, Haendel MA, et al. The effect of the COVID-19 pandemic on pulmonary diagnostic procedures. Ann Am Thorac Soc 2022;19:695–7.

40. Piro R, Casalini E, Livrieri F, et al. Interventional pulmonology during COVID-19 pandemic: current evidence and future perspectives. J Thorac Dis 2021;13:2495–509.

41. Zietsman M, Phan LT, Jones RM. Potential for occupational exposures to pathogens during bronchoscopy procedures. J Occup Environ Hyg 2019;16:707–16.

42. Saha BK, Saha S, Chong WH, et al. Indications, clinical utility, and safety of bronchoscopy in COVID-19. Respir Care 2022;67:241–51.

43. Torrego A, Pajares V, Fernández-Arias C, et al. Bronchoscopy in patients with COVID-19 with invasive mechanical ventilation: a single-center experience. Am J Respir Crit Care Med 2020;202:284–7.

44. Barron SP, Kennedy MP. Single-use (Disposable) flexible bronchoscopes: the future of bronchoscopy? Adv Ther 2020;37:4538–48.

45. Lentz RJ, Colt H. Summarizing societal guidelines regarding bronchoscopy during the COVID-19 pandemic. Respirology 2020;25:574–7.

46. Ost DE. Bronchoscopy in the age of COVID-19. J Bronchology Interv Pulmonol 2020;27:160–2.

47. Ozturk A, Sener MU, Yılmaz A. Bronchoscopic procedures during COVID-19 pandemic: experiences in Turkey. J Surg Oncol 2020;122:1020–6.

48. Luo F, Darwiche K, Singh S, et al. Performing bronchoscopy in times of the COVID-19 pandemic: practice statement from an international expert panel. Respiration 2020;99:417–22.

49. van Doremalen N, Bushmaker T, Morris DH, et al. Aerosol and surface stability of SARS-CoV-2 as compared with SARS-CoV-1. N Engl J Med 2020;382:1564–7.

50. Tay JK, Khoo ML, Loh WS. Surgical considerations for tracheostomy during the COVID-19 pandemic: lessons learned from the severe acute respiratory

syndrome outbreak. JAMA Otolaryngol Head Neck Surg 2020;146:517–8.

51. Bain W, Yang H, Shah FA, et al. COVID-19 versus Non-COVID-19 acute respiratory distress syndrome: comparison of demographics, physiologic parameters, inflammatory biomarkers, and clinical outcomes. Ann Am Thorac Soc 2021;18:1202–10.

52. Grasselli G, Zangrillo A, Zanella A, et al. Baseline characteristics and outcomes of 1591 patients infected with SARS-CoV-2 admitted to ICUs of the lombardy region, Italy. Jama 2020;323:1574–81.

53. Saad M, Laghi FA Jr, Brofman J, et al. Long-term acute care hospital outcomes of mechanically ventilated patients with coronavirus disease 2019. Crit Care Med 2022;50:256–63.

54. Klutts GN, Squires A, Bowman SM, et al. Increased lengths of stay, ICU, and ventilator days in trauma patients with asymptomatic COVID-19 infection. Am Surg 2022;88(7):1522–5.

55. Lamb CR, Desai NR, Angel L, et al. Use of tracheostomy during the COVID-19 pandemic: american college of chest physicians/american association for bronchology and interventional pulmonology/association of interventional pulmonology program directors expert panel report. Chest 2020;158:1499–514.

56. McGrath BA, Brenner MJ, Warrillow SJ, et al. Tracheostomy in the COVID-19 era: global and multidisciplinary guidance. Lancet Respir Med 2020;8:717–25.

57. Angel L, Kon ZN, Chang SH, et al. Novel percutaneous tracheostomy for critically ill patients with COVID-19. Ann Thorac Surg 2020;110:1006–11.

58. Mahmood K, Cheng GZ, Van Nostrand K, et al. Tracheostomy for COVID-19 respiratory failure: multidisciplinary, multicenter data on timing, technique, and outcomes. Ann Surg 2021;274:234–9.

59. Staibano P, Levin M, McHugh T, et al. Association of tracheostomy with outcomes in patients with COVID-19 and SARS-CoV-2 transmission among health care professionals: a systematic review and meta-analysis. JAMA Otolaryngol Head Neck Surg 2021;147:646–55.

60. Zou L, Ruan F, Huang M, et al. SARS-CoV-2 viral load in upper respiratory specimens of infected patients. N Engl J Med 2020;382:1177–9.

61. Bier-Laning C, Cramer JD, Roy S, et al. Tracheostomy during the COVID-19 pandemic: comparison of international perioperative care protocols and practices in 26 countries. Otolaryngol Head Neck Surg 2021;164:1136–47.

62. Molin N, Myers K, Soliman AMS, et al. COVID-19 tracheostomy outcomes. Otolaryngol Head Neck Surg; 2022. 1945998221075610.

63. Benito DA, Bestourous DE, Tong JY, et al. Tracheotomy in COVID-19 patients: a systematic review and meta-analysis of weaning, decannulation, and survival. Otolaryngol Head Neck Surg 2021;165:398–405.

64. Mattioli F, Fermi M, Ghirelli M, et al. Tracheostomy in the COVID-19 pandemic. Eur Arch Otorhinolaryngol 2020;277:2133–5.

65. Smith D, Montagne J, Raices M, et al. Tracheostomy in the intensive care unit: guidelines during COVID-19 worldwide pandemic. Am J Otolaryngol 2020;41:102578.

66. Majid A, Ayala A, Uribe JP, et al. Protective strategies in a simulated model when performing percutaneous tracheostomies in the COVID-19 Era. Ann Am Thorac Soc 2020;17:1486–8.

67. Chao TN, Harbison SP, Braslow BM, et al. Outcomes after tracheostomy in COVID-19 patients. Ann Surg 2020;272:e181–6.

68. Chee VW, Khoo ML, Lee SF, et al. Infection control measures for operative procedures in severe acute respiratory syndrome-related patients. Anesthesiology 2004;100:1394–8.

69. Pieracci FM, Burlew CC, Spain D, et al. Tube thoracostomy during the COVID-19 pandemic: guidance and recommendations from the AAST acute care surgery and critical care Committees. Trauma Surg Acute Care Open 2020;5(1):e000498. PMID: 32411822; PMCID: PMC7213907.

70. Rodríguez Moncalvo JJ, Brea Folco JC, Arce SC, et al. Recommendations for pulmonary function laboratories in the COVID-19 era. Medicina (B Aires) 2021;81:229–40.

71. Stanojevic S, Beaucage F, Comondore V, et al. Resumption of pulmonary function testing during the post-peak phase of the COVID-19 pandemic. a position statement from the canadian thoracic society and the canadian society of respiratory therapists. Can J Respir Crit Care Sleep 2020;4.

72. Moreno-Pérez O, Merino E, Chico-Sánchez P, et al. Effectiveness of a SARS-CoV-2 infection prevention model in elective surgery patients - a prospective study: does universal screening make sense? J Hosp Infect 2021;115:27–31.

73. Fouzas S, Gidaris D, Karantaglis N, et al. Pediatric pulmonary function testing in COVID-19 pandemic and beyond. a position statement from the hellenic pediatric respiratory society. Front Pediatr 2021;9:673322.

Coronavirus Disease-2019 Pneumonia
Clinical Manifestations

Husham Sharifi, MD, MS*, Joe Hsu, MD, MPH

KEYWORDS

- COVID-19 • SARS-CoV-2 • Pneumonia • Clinical manifestations • CT chest

KEY POINTS

- Social risk factors for coronavirus disease-2019 (COVID-19) pneumonia such as race, ethnicity, income inequality, and living environment correlate with infection and severity of infection.
- Biological risk factors are numerous and highly correlate with cardiovascular disease and its risk factors.
- COVID-19 pneumonia has a broad presentation, ranging from mild illness to critical illness.
- Post-acute sequelae of severe acute respiratory syndrome coronavirus 2 has protean manifestations that can persist for months to over a year and is receiving increasing attention into its physiology and potential treatments.
- Imaging findings of pneumonia can be categorized as typical, indeterminate, and atypical and may differ according to vaccine status and viral variant.

INTRODUCTION

The global disease burden from coronavirus disease-2019 (COVID-19) infection has been unprecedented in recent history, with 619 million recorded cases and 6.55 million recorded deaths worldwide as of October 5, 2022[1] and with studies showing that these figures are likely underestimates.[2–4] Our understanding of its clinical manifestations has evolved due to increasing insight into risk factors, ability to triage, evolution of viral variants,[5,6] and imaging findings during and after acute infection.[7] Changes in the manifestations of COVID-19 pneumonia have also occurred, which has relevance for clinical care in ambulatory and hospital settings. Our approach to recognizing and managing COVID-19 will require ongoing study to adjust appropriately to the shifting disease burden that the global pandemic has created.

RISK FACTORS
Social Risk Factors for Infection and Severe Disease

Since the onset of the pandemic, racial and ethnic minorities—in particular the non-Hispanic black, Hispanic, and Native American communities—have experienced increased rates of infection, hospitalization, and mortality from severe acute respiratory syndrome coronavirus 2 (SARS-CoV-2). Given that SARS-CoV-2 is spread through respiratory droplets, socioeconomic conditions have contributed to the disproportionate burden of COVID-19 in these underserved communities. Contributing factors that have been posited include a self-perpetuating system of income inequality, a disproportionate burden of underlying comorbidities, population-dense neighborhoods, family dense households, greater likelihood to work in public-facing occupations, less ability to

Division of Pulmonary, Allergy, and Critical Care Medicine, Stanford University, 300 Pasteur Drive, Stanford, CA 94305, USA
* Corresponding author.
E-mail address: husham@stanford.edu

Clin Chest Med 44 (2023) 227–237
https://doi.org/10.1016/j.ccm.2022.11.006
0272-5231/23/© 2022 Elsevier Inc. All rights reserved.

stop working or to accept a furlough from work, and fewer health care resources in the neighborhoods of these communities.[8–13]

Income inequality has been strongly associated with increased case rate and mortality. One study examined COVID-19 cases and mortality and their association with the Gini index, a measure of income inequality, from January to April 2020 in a cohort of 577,414 cases and 23,424 deaths across 50 states. Multivariate regression with adjustment for multiple confounders (eg, older age, sex, race, health care resources, shelter-in-place order) revealed that a one-unit increase in the Gini index (ie, greater inequality of income) was associated with approximately a 27% increase in mortality.[14] This study did not adjust for comorbidities.

Race has been shown to correlate with increased risk of infection and hospitalization in multiple studies, even after adjustment for income level and other confounders. One study examined a cohort of 20,228 patients with SARS-CoV-2 in Houston in 2020, with covariate adjustment for age, sex, race, ethnicity, household income, residence population density, Charlson Comorbidity Index, hypertension, diabetes, and obesity. Higher likelihood of infection was found in non-Hispanic black individuals compared with non-Hispanic white (odds ratio [OR] 2.23, 95% confidence interval [CI] 1.90 to 2.60) and in Hispanic compared with non-Hispanic (OR 1.95, 95% CI 1.72 to 2.20).[8] A retrospective cohort study of 5698 patients from the University of Michigan from March to April 2020 and with an outcome update in July 2020 assessed the risk of hospitalization with statistical adjustment for multiple confounders, including a customized comorbidity score from seven known risk factors for disease severity: respiratory conditions, circulatory conditions, any cancer, type 2 diabetes, kidney disease, liver disease, and autoimmune disease.[15] Non-Hispanic black patients were more likely to be hospitalized for SARS-CoV-2 infection than non-Hispanic white patients (OR, 1.72, 95% CI 1.15 to 2.58, $P = .009$).

Vaccination Status

Reduced access to health care resources includes reduced access to vaccination, an issue that has persisted even after the widespread availability of vaccines for SARS-CoV-2. Large placebo-controlled trials have found a lower risk of asymptomatic, symptomatic, and severe COVID-19 with vaccinations,[16–18] and subsequent observational studies from national vaccine deployments have supported these findings.[19–21] In one study in the United Kingdom (UK) on vaccination of health care workers (23,324 participants from 104 sites),

rates of effectiveness—as defined by not becoming infected—for the BNT162b2 vaccine were found to be 70% (95% CI 55% to 85%) at 21 days after the first dose and 85% (95% CI 74% to 96%) at 7 days after the second dose.[20] The study included asymptomatic and symptomatic infection and was conducted during a time of high prevalence of the Alpha variant. In a subsequent large study in England investigating effectiveness of various vaccine boosters against the Delta versus Omicron variant (204,154 individuals with Delta, 886,774 individuals with Omicron, 1,572,621 individuals with negative tests), vaccination effectiveness was uniformly higher for Delta than for Omicron.[20] **Table 1** shows the effectiveness of vaccine booster combinations.[22] One can see that booster vaccination with BNT162b2 or mRNA-1273 after either ChAdOx1 nCoV-19 or BNT162b2 primary vaccine courses improved effectiveness in a short time period (ie, 2 to 4 weeks) against Omicron. That effectiveness waned rapidly, however, dropping to as low as 39.6% to 45.7% at 10 or more weeks.

Worse clinical outcomes are much more likely to occur in persons with no vaccination versus booster vaccine and in persons with primary vaccination versus booster vaccine. In a study in Northern California including 118,078 persons that adjusted for confounders such as age, sex, comorbid burden, prior infection, and receipt of prior treatment of SARS-CoV-2, risk of hospitalization was higher in persons who were unvaccinated (adjusted hazard ratio [aHR] 8.34, 95% CI 7.25 to 9.60) and who had the primary vaccine course (aHR 1.72, 95% CI 1.49 to 1.97) compared with those who received the primary vaccine course plus a booster.[23]

Biological Risk Factors for Severe Disease

Early in the pandemic, patients with advanced age and certain underlying comorbidities were noted to be at higher risk of admission and severe disease. In an analysis of 208 acute care hospitals in England, Wales, and Scotland from February to April 2020, the median age of admission was 73 years (interquartile range [IQR] 58 to 82), and men constituted 60% of admissions ($n = 12,068$, from 18,525 total).[24] Comorbid burden was common, with only 23% of patients having no major comorbidity. Cardiovascular disease and its risk factors were common in patients: cardiac disease 31%; diabetes 21%; and chronic kidney disease 16%. Non-asthmatic chronic pulmonary disease was noted in 18% of patients. These findings were similar to data on adult hospitalization in 14 states in the United States in March 2020,

Table 1
Effectiveness of coronavirus disease-2019 vaccine series with subsequent combination boosters

Primary Course Vaccine[a]	Booster Vaccine	Effectiveness at 2 to 4 wk (%, 95% CI)	Effectiveness at 5 to 9 wk (%, 95% CI)	Effectiveness at 10 or More Weeks (%, 95% CI)
ChAdOx1 nCoV-19	BNT162b2	62.4 (61.8 to 63.0)	Not measured	39.6 (38.0 to 41.1)
BNT162b2	BNT162b2	67.2 (66.5 to 67.8)	Not measured	45.7 (44.7 to 46.7)
ChAdOx1 nCoV-19	mRNA-1273	70.1 (69.5 to 70.7)	60.9 (59.7 to 62.1)	Not measured
BNT162b2	mRNA-1273	73.9 (73.1 to 74.6)	64.4 (62.6 to 66.1)	Not measured

[a] Single vaccination for ChAdOx1 nCoV-19 and two vaccinations for BNT162b2.
Adapted from Andrews N, Stowe J, Kirsebom F, et al. Covid-19 Vaccine Effectiveness against the Omicron (B.1.1.529) Variant. N Engl J Med. 2022;386(16):1532-1546.

where 89.3% of patients had at least one underlying condition: 50% hypertension; 48% obesity; 35% chronic lung disease; 28% diabetes; 28% cardiovascular disease; and 13% renal disease.[25]

Ongoing caution is important for individuals with certain risk factors even after vaccination. In a prospective, nested, case-control study from the UK using self-reported data via phone from 6,030 adults with the first vaccine dose and 2370 adults with the second vaccine dose, infection 14 days or more after the first dose was found to be associated with frailty in individuals greater than or equal to 60 years of age (OR 1.93, 95% CI 1.50 to 2.48, $P < .0001$).[26] As before the era of widespread vaccination, residence in economically-deprived areas was associated with a greater risk of infection (OR 1.11, 95% CI 1.01 to 1.23, $P = .03$), and not being obese as defined by body mass index < 30 was associated with less risk of infection (OR 0.84, 95% CI 0.75 to 0.94, $P = .0030$). Of note, the association of increased infection risk persisted even after adjustment for compliance with preventative measures such as mask wearing. The above findings suggest than greater resources for re-vaccination, booster vaccination, and screening may be warranted in care facilities for individuals with high frailty (eg, long-term care homes) and in lower income neighborhoods.

Laboratory Abnormalities Associated with Severe Disease

There are numerous laboratory abnormalities that have been found to associate with severe disease. Leukocytosis has been associated with disease progression and severity,[27–29] and studies have found that lymphopenia is associated with disease severity and with worse outcomes.[29–33] Thrombocytopenia has been routinely observed in patients with COVID-19, with lower platelets manifesting in severe and critical illness[34] and being associated with higher mortality.[35] Additionally, worse outcomes

have been observed in patients with elevations in numerous, routinely available inflammatory markers: D-dimer, C-reactive protein, lactate dehydrogenase, and ferritin.[36,37] Specific cytokines have also been implicated with decreased patient survival—in particular interleukin 6, 8 and Tumor-Necrosis-Factor-alpha (TNF-alpha).[38] The presence of viral RNA in the blood has been associated with increased end-organ damage, including the lung, and mortality.[39,40] Higher plasma nucleocapsid antigen level has also been found to be strongly associated with the need for noninvasive positive pressure ventilation or supplemental oxygen by high-flow nasal cannula.[41]

CLINICAL COURSE
Spectrum of Disease

The spectrum of presentation for SARS-CoV-2 infection is broad. The National Institutes of Health (NIH) definitions for infection severity are detailed in **Table 2**.[42]

Presymptomatic infection and mild to moderate illness are seen in the outpatient setting. A standard approach for outpatients is to note the date of symptom onset and the date of dyspnea onset, if any. This addresses the difficulty of measuring the incubation period, which has median estimates of approximately 3 days for the Omicron variant[6,43] to 4 to 5 days for older variants.[44] Patients who progress from mild disease to dyspnea have been observed to do so in the range of 5 to 8 days after the onset of mild illness.[45,46] In a prospective cohort study in Baltimore of 118 outpatients infected with SARS-CoV-2 and followed from April to June 2020, most of the patients (63.7%) had no symptoms or mild symptoms in the first week of illness.[47] Of those who had symptoms, fatigue or weakness were the most common (65.7%). This was followed by cough (58.8%), headache (45.6%), chills (38.2%), and anosmia (27.9%). These individuals reported returning to

Table 2
National Institutes of Health classification of infection with severe acute respiratory syndrome coronavirus 2[42]

Infection Severity	Criteria
Presymptomatic infection	Positive nucleic acid amplification test or antigen test but no symptoms.
Mild illness	Fever, cough, or sore throat but no dyspnea or abnormal imaging.
Moderate illness	Evidence of lower respiratory disease by auscultation of lungs or imaging and oxygen saturation $\geq$ 94% on room air at sea level.
Severe illness	Oxygen saturation $\leq$ 94% on room air at sea level, a ratio of arterial partial pressure of oxygen to fraction of inspired oxygen $\leq$ 300 mm Hg, respiratory frequency > 30 per minute, or lung opacities on imaging that have increased by 50% or more in 24 to 48 h.
Critical illness	Respiratory failure, shock due to sepsis, with or without non-pulmonary end-organ dysfunction.

their baseline health at a median of 20 days (IQR 13 to 38) after the onset of symptoms. After 28 to 99 days from symptom onset, 83.3% of patients reported returning to their baseline health. A total of 7.6% required hospitalization. In contrast, a large Cochrane review of 42 prospective studies with 52,608 participants found that most symptoms have low diagnostic accuracy on presentation, although anosmia and ageusia can provide unique triggers for screening and cough can warrant additional testing.[48] In this review the summary likelihood ratio (LR) of anosmia as a presenting symptom to be associated with SARS-CoV-2 infection was 4.55 (95% CI 3.46 to 5.9); for ageusia 3.14 (95% CI 1.79 to 5.51); for cough 1.14 (95% CI 1.04 to 1.25); for fever 1.52 (95% CI 1.10 to 2.10); and for sore throat 0.814 (95% CI 0.714 to 0.929). The authors point out that this latter LR suggests sore throat increases the odds of an alternative infectious process, implying that isolated upper respiratory symptoms such as sore throat or rhinorrhea do not support polymerase chain reaction testing for SARS-CoV-2.

Patients with severe illness require admission, and common presenting symptoms in these individuals are fatigue, cough, fever, and hypoxemia. In a retrospective study from Germany of 57 patients admitted to the medicine ward from February to April 2020, the median age was 72 years (IQR 60 to 81), with 23% women.[49] Fifty-six patients had at least 1 comorbid condition, and all patients required supplemental oxygen (median 2 L/min, IQR 2 to 4) to maintain oxygen saturation levels $\geq$ 94%. Fever was the most common presenting symptom (68%), followed by cough (60%), dyspnea (44%), and

fatigue (37%). A majority (77%) had bilateral opacities on initial imaging. Median fever lasted 7 days (IQR 2 to 11), hospitalization 12 days (IQR 7 to 20), and oxygen supplementation 8 days (IQR 5 to 13). In this study and in numerous reports since the beginning of the pandemic, hypoxemia without dyspnea has been described. Some authors posit that the observation may be due to known physiologic principles such as isocapnic hypoxia having a nonlinear ventilatory response in which minute ventilation increases markedly only after arterial oxygen drops below a specific threshold (eg, Pao_2 60 mm Hg).[50–52] It is notable that a study conducted years before this pandemic by Moosavi and colleagues[53] also found that dyspnea exhibits the same response mechanism, with a sharp increase in reported "air hunger" ratings seen primarily in isocapnic patients with Pao_2 less than 60 mm Hg.

Critical illness also manifests with profound hypoxemia but has, in contrast to severe illness, the distinguishing feature of acute respiratory failure.[24,54] Presenting symptoms of these patients are similar to those who do not progress to critical disease (eg, fever, cough).[24,55,56] In patients who develop Acute Respiratory Distress Syndrome (ARDS) after infection with SARS-CoV02, the median time from confirmation of infection to the onset of dyspnea has been reported as 6.5 days.[57,58] The median time from the onset of dyspnea to ARDS has been reported as 2.5 days. Complications such as pneumothorax and barotrauma in patients with ARDS secondary to COVID-19 pneumonia may be higher compared with other patients with ARDS.[59,60] Mechanical ventilation for ARDS in COVID-19 may be an independent risk factor for death compared with ARDS patients who experience barotrauma from noninvasive positive pressure ventilation.[61,62] In a small study comparing ARDS secondary to COVID-19 (n = 27) to non-COVID-19 ARDS (other viral n = 14, bacterial n = 21, culture-negative pneumonia n = 30), time to ventilator liberation was longer for patients with COVID-19 after adjustment for age, sex, and nursing home residence (aHR 0.48, 95% CI 0.24 to 0.98, $P < .05$).[63] No significant difference was found in 2-month mortality between the groups (aHR 0.71, 95% CI 0.33 to 1.56; $P = .39$). Similarly, no difference in mortality at 28 days was found in a second study comparing 130 patients with COVID-19 ARDS to 382 patients with non-COVID-19 ARDS (adjusted risk ratio 1.01, 95% CI 0.72 to 1.42).[64]

Post-Acute Sequelae of Severe Acute Respiratory Syndrome Coronavirus 2 (SARS-CoV-2)

Recovery from acute COVID-19 ranges along a spectrum, with no clear consensus on what constitutes Post-Acute Sequelae of SARS-CoV-2 (PASC). A clinical case definition by the World Health Organization makes the distinction that acute COVID-19 lasts up to 4 weeks after the onset of illness; whereas PASC can develop during or after COVID-19 and must continue at least 3 months after the onset of illness.[65] Common symptoms include fatigue, cognitive impairment, and dyspnea. In a study from Germany of 96 patients with symptom onset between February 2020 and April 2020 and who had follow-up visits at 5, 9, and 12 months, the most frequent symptoms at 5 months were reduced exertional ability (53.1%), fatigue (41.7%), insomnia (32.3%), cognitive impairment (31.3%) and dyspnea (27.1%).[66] From 5 to 12 months, reported fatigue increased from 41.7% to 53.1% ($P = .043$); dyspnea increased from 27.1% to 37.5% ($P = .041$). All other symptoms did not change significantly. This and a second prospective study of 968 patients in France found that 80% to 85% of patients still reported symptoms 1 year after symptom onset.[67] Research into the characteristics of PASC and potential treatments is ongoing.

Associated Infections

Bacterial infections in patients with COVID-19 pneumonia are uncommon and can be distinguished between co-infection and superinfection. The former is diagnosed at the time of COVID-19 pneumonia diagnosis and is presumably acquired in the community. The latter is diagnosed during the period of management for COVID-19 pneumonia. One study in Spain in 2020 reported a co-infection rate of 3.1%, primarily with *Streptococcus pneumoniae* and *Staphylococcus aureus*, and a superinfection rate of 4.7%, primarily with *Pseudomonas aeruginosa* and *Escherichia coli*.[68] A meta-analysis including 2390 patients found higher rates of bacterial co-infections (8%, 95% CI 5% to 11%) and bacterial superinfections (20%, 95% CI 13% to 28%).[69] Significant rates of viral and fungal secondary infections were also noted: viral co-infections, 10% (95% CI 6% to 14%); viral superinfections, 4% (95% CI 0% to 10%); fungal co-infections, 4% (95% CI 2% to 7%); and fungal superinfections, 8% (95% CI 4% to 13%). The most common bacterial pathogens for co-infection were *Klebsiella pneumoniae* (9.9% of all co-infections), *S pneumoniae* (8.2%), and *S aureus* (7.7%). The most common bacterial pathogens for superinfection were *Acinetobacter spp.* (22.0%), *Pseudomonas* (10.8%), and *E coli* (6.9%).[69] Aspergillus was found in 6.7% of co-infections and 13.5% of superinfections.

RADIOGRAPHIC FINDINGS

Chest X-ray can be normal in early or mild disease, and when radiographic findings develop, they typically reveal bilateral opacities that are predominant in the lower lobes.[70] Pulmonary opacities can become more extensive and confluent thereafter, followed by the consolidation seen in acute lung injury.[71] Most patients will experience resolution, but some can progress to a more structured parenchymal injury manifesting as reticular opacities and associated fibrosis.[72] **Fig. 1** illustrates typical chest x-ray findings during initial stages of infection with COVID-19 pneumonia and the evolution to fibrotic changes over time.

Early in the pandemic, temporal stages of CT findings in COVID-19 pneumonia were proposed and included ultra-early, early, rapid progression, consolidation, and dissipation.[73] The ultra-early stage can occur within 2 weeks of exposure and can present with no or scant ground glass opacities (GGOs) on imaging. Symptomatic presentation occurs during the early phase, which may include single or multiple GGOs with interlobular septal thickening. Rapid progression is expected 3 to 7 days after symptomatic presentation and manifests with consolidations and air bronchograms. The consolidation phase occurs 7 to 14 days after symptomatic presentation, when the size and density of consolidations decrease. Dissipation may occur thereafter. It can include reticulations with opacities, thickening of the bronchial wall, and interlobular septal thickening.

Typical chest CT abnormalities are consistent with viral pneumonia, with one large review finding

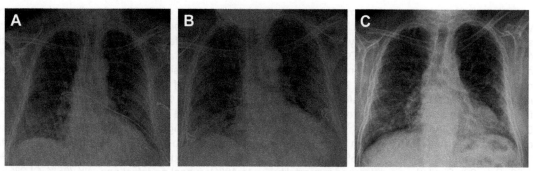

Fig. 1. Serial chest radiographs of a 62-year-old gentleman with a history of essential hypertension with COVID-19 pneumonia and requiring hospital admission and oxygen support by non-rebreather mask. He received remdesivir, dexamethasone, ceftriaxone, and azithromycin in hospital and was discharged on home oxygen. (*A*) Day of first positive SARS-CoV-2 polymerase chain reaction test, taken 9 days after onset of symptoms. Bilateral opacities on the left greater than the right. Air bronchograms and bronchial wall thickening is noted in the right lower lobe. (*B*) Two days after positive test. Slight worsening of bilateral opacities is seen; (*C*) Eleven months after infection. Bilateral opacities and prominent interstitial markings are consistent with fibrotic lung disease, likely a sequelae of lung injury from acute infection.

GGOs to be the most prominent feature (83%), followed by GGOs with mixed consolidation (58%), pleural thickening (52%), and interlobular septal thickening (48%).[7] Criteria have been proposed by the Radiological Society of North America (RSNA) to categorize CT chest findings as *typical*, *indeterminate*, and *atypical*.[74] *Typical* is defined as either multifocal rounded GGOs or peripheral bilateral GGOs with or without consolidation or the superimposed interlobular septal lines that constitute "crazy paving." (**Fig. 2**) A later stage of typical pneumonia is defined as having reverse halo sign or other signs of organizing pneumonia. *Indeterminate* is defined as absence of these typical features with the addition of GGOs that are nonrounded, non-peripheral and either diffuse, perihilar, unilateral, or simply lacking a specific distribution. *Atypical* is defined as lacking the features of typical and indeterminate and having lobar or

segmental consolidation, centrilobular nodules, or lung cavitation. These acute insults can evolve into a chronic phase of inflammation, resulting in subpleural reticulation and bronchiectasis (**Fig. 3**).

Vaccinations attenuate the radiographic presentations of COVID-19, consistent with the impact of vaccinations on disease severity. In a multicenter Korean study, infected patients were divided into groups of unvaccinated, partially vaccinated, and fully vaccinated and had their clinical metrics and radiographic features analyzed for comparative differences.[75] Vaccine status (fully vaccinated vs unvaccinated) was associated with less risk of needing supplemental oxygen (OR 0.24, 95% CI 0.09 to 0.64, $P = .005$) or intensive care unit (ICU) admission (OR 0.08, 95% CI 0.09 to 0.78, $P = .02$). Of the 761 patients, 412 received chest CT and 75% of these were diagnosed with pneumonia. The percentage of patients with negative

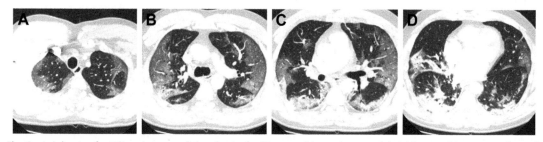

Fig. 2. Axial cuts of a CT angiogram of the chest of a 50-year old gentleman with a history of hyperparathyroidism with typical COVID-19 pneumonia per Radiological Society of North America criteria, taken 1 day after first positive polymerase chain reaction for SARS-CoV-2. The patient required ICU admission and oxygen support by high flow nasal cannula. He was discharged on home oxygen. (*A*) Bilateral, peripheral GGOs in the left upper lobe; (*B*) bilateral GGOs with mild consolidations and mild traction bronchiectasis at the level of the carina; (*C*) Increasing consolidative opacities intermixed with GGOs and more severe bronchiectasis; and (*D*) Bibasilar, posterior, peripheral consolidative opacities with peripheral GGOs.

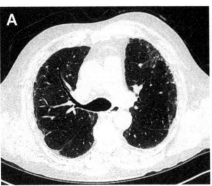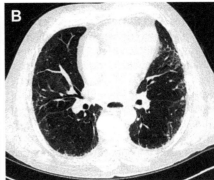

Fig. 3. CT chest scan 5 months after COVID-19 pneumonia in the same patient presented in **Fig. 1**. (*A*) Subpleural peripheral reticulations seen in the bilateral upper lobes. Traction bronchiectasis in left upper lobe takeoff; (*B*) Peripheral GGOs with reticulation in bilateral lower lobes. These findings seem to represent fibrotic lung disease.

CT chest significantly increased with vaccine status—22% of unvaccinated compared with 59% of fully vaccinated. Most of the patients in each vaccine group had typical CT chest findings as defined by RSNA criteria, but these percentages decreased from unvaccinated (72%) to partially vaccinated (60%) to fully vaccinated (56%). This trend was largely due to a greater percentage of fully vaccinated persons having atypical CT chest findings (11%) compared with partially vaccinated (2%) and unvaccinated (3%).

A subsequent study in Korea examined CT chest findings for COVID-19 pneumonia in patients during the Delta wave (*n* = 88) compared with the Omicron wave (*n* = 88).[76] After adjustment for the confounders of age, comorbid burden, vaccination status, and infection duration, patients with Omicron were found to have a less typical CT appearance for COVID-19 pneumonia per RSNA criteria (OR 0.34, 95% CI 0.16 to 0.74, *P* = .006) and more peribronchovascular involvement than patients with Delta (OR 9.2, 95% CI 2.9 to 29, *P* < .001). By using a neural network algorithm, the authors found that pulmonary vascular volume in vessels 5 mm or less in diameter (ie, vessels in the periphery of the lung) was greater for patients with Omicron than patients with Delta (3.8, 95% CI 0.92 to 6.8, *P* = .01). Together, these findings reinforced prior studies that Omicron replicates more predominantly in the bronchi than in the lung parenchyma and that the differing physiologic mechanisms of the variant resulted in distinct radiographic findings.[77] The higher volume of peripheral pulmonary vascular volume in patients with Omicron was consistent with it causing less severe pneumonia than Delta, given that lower peripheral vascular volume (ie, blood vessel volume less than 5 mm in diameter) has been found to associate with worse outcomes for COVID-19 pneumonia.[78] The study was significant in its

implication that emerging variants of concern may produce radiographic findings that are increasingly atypical and therefore at risk of delayed detection.

LESSONS LEARNED

COVID-19 has posed an unprecedented challenge to our diagnostic and prognostic approaches of viral respiratory illness. Since the beginning of the pandemic in late 2019, we have acquired knowledge in the protean manifestations of the disease and in the social and biological risk factors for infection and severe disease. This includes elucidation of critical social and biological determinants of health and codification of disease severity and imaging findings. A commitment to continuing and advancing such research will be crucial for ameliorating the impact of newer viral variants on individual and population health and for preparing for future pandemics.

As viral variants evolve and vaccines continue to be developed, we will be presented with new challenges in identifying and managing upper and lower respiratory tract infection with COVID-19. Phenomena such as post-acute sequelae of COVID-19 have already become prominent, and longer-term morbidity from physiologic damage caused by acute disease will continue to accumulate. The international coordination shown by SARS-CoV-2 vaccine development offers a model for cooperation and scientific knowledge dissemination in these crucial domains. In a similar collaborative vein, the US Centers for Disease Control and Prevention (CDC) has established a Center for Forecasting and Outbreak Analytics in April 2022 to integrate analysts from previously siloed fields of computer science, mathematics, physics, and epidemiology and to allow for a more preemptive approach to future pandemics.[79] To ensure greater equity in vaccine distribution, the CDC has partnered with the Health Resources & Services Administration (HRSA) to deliver vaccines directly to HRSA-funded health centers. These centers serve 30 million individuals in the United States, 93% of them are below 200% of the federal poverty level, and 63% of them identify as racial or ethnic minorities.[80] As societies have reopened and the virus has become endemic, we should continue to pay heed to the suffering and harm that could have been mitigated by this pandemic and apply these difficult lessons to such committed advancement of improved pathways for clinical care.

CLINICS CARE POINTS

- Social risk factors for coronavirus disease-2019 (COVID-19) pneumonia such as race, ethnicity, income inequality, and living environment correlate with infection and severity of infection.

- Biological risk factors are numerous and highly correlate with cardiovascular disease and its risk factors.

- COVID-19 pneumonia has a broad presentation, ranging from mild illness to critical illness.

- Post-acute sequelae of severe acute respiratory syndrome coronavirus 2 has protean manifestations that can persist for months to over a year and is receiving increasing attention into its physiology and potential treatments.

- Imaging findings of pneumonia can be categorized as typical, indeterminate, and atypical and may differ according to vaccine status and viral variant.

ACKNOWLEDGMENTS

The authors would like to thank our patients in the post-acute COVID-19 clinic in Stanford University.

DISCLOSURE

There are no relevant financial relationships to disclose.

REFERENCES

1. University of Oxford. Our World in data. Available at: https://ourworldindata.org/explorers/coronavirus-data-explorer. Accessed October 5, 2022.

2. Wu SL, Mertens AN, Crider YS, et al. Substantial underestimation of SARS-CoV-2 infection in the United States. Nat Commun 2020;11(1):4507. https://doi.org/10.1038/s41467-020-18272-4.

3. Tanne JH. Covid-19: US cases are greatly underestimated, seroprevalence studies suggest. BMJ 2020;370:m2988. https://doi.org/10.1136/bmj.m2988. Published online July 24.

4. Mwananyanda L, Gill CJ, MacLeod W, et al. Covid-19 deaths in Africa: prospective systematic postmortem surveillance study. BMJ 2021;17:n334. https://doi.org/10.1136/bmj.n334. Published online February.

5. Menni C, Valdes AM, Polidori L, et al. Symptom prevalence, duration, and risk of hospital admission in individuals infected with SARS-CoV-2 during periods of omicron and delta variant dominance: a prospective observational study from the ZOE COVID Study. The Lancet 2022;399(10335):1618–24. https://doi.org/10.1016/S0140-6736(22)00327-0.

6. Jansen L, Tegomoh B, Lange K, et al. Investigation of a SARS-CoV-2 B.1.1.529 (omicron) variant cluster — Nebraska, november–december 2021. MMWR Morb Mortal Wkly Rep 2021;70(5152):1782–4. https://doi.org/10.15585/mmwr.mm705152e3.

7. Bao C, Liu X, Zhang H, et al. Coronavirus disease 2019 (COVID-19) CT findings: a systematic review and meta-analysis. J Am Coll Radiol 2020;17(6):701–9. https://doi.org/10.1016/j.jacr.2020.03.006.

8. Vahidy FS, Nicolas JC, Meeks JR, et al. Racial and ethnic disparities in SARS-CoV-2 pandemic: analysis of a COVID-19 observational registry for a diverse US metropolitan population. BMJ Open 2020;10(8):e039849. https://doi.org/10.1136/bmjopen-2020-039849.

9. Gross CP, Essien UR, Pasha S, et al. Racial and ethnic disparities in population-level covid-19 mortality. J Gen Intern Med 2020;35(10):3097–9. https://doi.org/10.1007/s11606-020-06081-w.

10. Webb Hooper M, Nápoles AM, Pérez-Stable EJ. COVID-19 and racial/ethnic disparities. JAMA 2020;323(24):2466. https://doi.org/10.1001/jama.2020.8598.

11. Wiley Zanthia, Ross-Driscoll Katie, et al. Racial and ethnic differences and clinical outcomes of COVID-19 patients presenting to the emergency department. Clin Infect Dis 2022;74(3):387–94.

12. Musshafen LA, El-Sadek L, Lirette ST, et al. In-hospital mortality disparities among American Indian and Alaska native, black, and white patients with COVID-19. JAMA Netw Open 2022;5(3):e224822. https://doi.org/10.1001/jamanetworkopen.2022.4822.

13. Kanter GP, Segal AG, Groeneveld PW. Income Disparities in Access to Critical Care Services: study examines disparities in community intensive care unit beds by US communities' median household

income. Health Aff (Millwood) 2020;39(8):1362–7. https://doi.org/10.1377/hlthaff.2020.00581.

14. Oronce CIA, Scannell CA, Kawachi I, et al. Association between state-level income inequality and COVID-19 cases and mortality in the USA. J Gen Intern Med 2020;35(9):2791–3. https://doi.org/10.1007/s11606-020-05971-3.

15. Gu T, Mack JA, Salvatore M, et al. Characteristics associated with racial/ethnic disparities in COVID-19 outcomes in an academic health care system. JAMA Netw Open 2020;3(10):e2025197. https://doi.org/10.1001/jamanetworkopen.2020.25197.

16. Polack FP, Thomas SJ, Kitchin N, et al. Safety and efficacy of the BNT162b2 mRNA covid-19 vaccine. N Engl J Med 2020;383(27):2603–15. https://doi.org/10.1056/NEJMoa2034577.

17. Frenck RW, Klein NP, Kitchin N, et al. Safety, immunogenicity, and efficacy of the BNT162b2 covid-19 vaccine in adolescents. N Engl J Med 2021;385(3):239–50. https://doi.org/10.1056/NEJMoa2107456.

18. Thomas SJ, Moreira ED, Kitchin N, et al. Safety and efficacy of the BNT162b2 mRNA covid-19 vaccine through 6 months. N Engl J Med 2021;385(19):1761–73. https://doi.org/10.1056/NEJMoa2110345.

19. Haas EJ, Angulo FJ, McLaughlin JM, et al. Impact and effectiveness of mRNA BNT162b2 vaccine against SARS-CoV-2 infections and COVID-19 cases, hospitalisations, and deaths following a nationwide vaccination campaign in Israel: an observational study using national surveillance data. The Lancet 2021;397(10287):1819–29. https://doi.org/10.1016/S0140-6736(21)00947-8.

20. Hall VJ, Foulkes S, Saei A, et al. COVID-19 vaccine coverage in health-care workers in England and effectiveness of BNT162b2 mRNA vaccine against infection (SIREN): a prospective, multicentre, cohort study. The Lancet 2021;397(10286):1725–35. https://doi.org/10.1016/S0140-6736(21)00790-X.

21. Chodick G, Tene L, Patalon T, et al. Assessment of effectiveness of 1 dose of BNT162b2 vaccine for SARS-CoV-2 infection 13 to 24 Days after immunization. JAMA Netw Open 2021;4(6):e2115985. https://doi.org/10.1001/jamanetworkopen.2021.15985.

22. Andrews N, Stowe J, Kirsebom F, et al. Covid-19 vaccine effectiveness against the omicron (B.1.1.529) variant. N Engl J Med 2022;386(16):1532–46. https://doi.org/10.1056/NEJMoa2119451.

23. Skarbinski J, Wood MS, Chervo TC, et al. Risk of severe clinical outcomes among persons with SARS-CoV-2 infection with differing levels of vaccination during widespread Omicron (B.1.1.529) and Delta (B.1.617.2) variant circulation in Northern California: a retrospective cohort study. Lancet Reg Health - Am 2022;12:100297. https://doi.org/10.1016/j.lana.2022.100297.

24. Docherty AB, Harrison EM, Green CA, et al. Features of 20 133 UK patients in hospital with covid-19 using the ISARIC WHO Clinical Characterisation Protocol: prospective observational cohort study. BMJ 2020;369:m1985. https://doi.org/10.1136/bmj.m1985. Published online May 22.

25. Garg S, Kim L, Whitaker M, et al. Hospitalization rates and characteristics of patients hospitalized with laboratory-confirmed coronavirus disease 2019 — COVID-NET, 14 states, March 1–30, 2020. MMWR Morb Mortal Wkly Rep 2020;69(15):458–64. https://doi.org/10.15585/mmwr.mm6915e3.

26. Antonelli M, Penfold RS, Merino J, et al. Risk factors and disease profile of post-vaccination SARS-CoV-2 infection in UK users of the COVID Symptom Study app: a prospective, community-based, nested, case-control study. Lancet Infect Dis 2022;22(1):43–55. https://doi.org/10.1016/S1473-3099(21)00460-6.

27. Zhang J, Cao Y, Tan G, et al. Clinical, radiological, and laboratory characteristics and risk factors for severity and mortality of 289 hospitalized COVID-19 patients. Allergy 2021;76(2):533–50. https://doi.org/10.1111/all.14496.

28. Lampart M, Zellweger N, Bassetti S, et al. Clinical utility of inflammatory biomarkers in COVID-19 in direct comparison to other respiratory infections—a prospective cohort study. In: Faverio P, editor. PLoS One 2022;17(5):e0269005. https://doi.org/10.1371/journal.pone.0269005.

29. Huang G, Kovalic AJ, Graber CJ. Prognostic value of leukocytosis and lymphopenia for coronavirus disease severity. Emerg Infect Dis 2020;26(8):1839–41. https://doi.org/10.3201/eid2608.201160.

30. Tan L, Wang Q, Zhang D, et al. Lymphopenia predicts disease severity of COVID-19: a descriptive and predictive study. Signal Transduct Target Ther 2020;5(1):33. https://doi.org/10.1038/s41392-020-0148-4.

31. Liu J, Li S, Liu J, et al. Longitudinal characteristics of lymphocyte responses and cytokine profiles in the peripheral blood of SARS-CoV-2 infected patients. EBioMedicine 2020;55:102763. https://doi.org/10.1016/j.ebiom.2020.102763.

32. Liu M, Jiang H, Li Y, et al. Independent risk factors for the dynamic development of COVID-19: a retrospective study. Int J Gen Med 2021;14:4349–67. https://doi.org/10.2147/IJGM.S325112.

33. Lee J, Park SS, Kim TY, et al. Lymphopenia as a biological predictor of outcomes in COVID-19 patients: a nationwide cohort study. Cancers 2021;13(3):471. https://doi.org/10.3390/cancers13030471.

34. Amgalan A, Othman M. Hemostatic laboratory derangements in COVID-19 with a focus on platelet count. Platelets 2020;31(6):740–5. https://doi.org/10.1080/09537104.2020.1768523.

35. Lippi G, Plebani M, Henry BM. Thrombocytopenia is associated with severe coronavirus disease 2019 (COVID-19) infections: a meta-analysis. Clin Chim Acta 2020;506:145–8. https://doi.org/10.1016/j.cca.2020.03.022.

36. Liao D, Zhou F, Luo L, et al. Haematological characteristics and risk factors in the classification and prognosis evaluation of COVID-19: a retrospective cohort study. Lancet Haematol 2020;7(9):e671–8. https://doi.org/10.1016/S2352-3026(20)30217-9.

37. Wu C, Chen X, Cai Y, et al. Risk factors associated with acute respiratory distress syndrome and death in patients with coronavirus disease 2019 pneumonia in Wuhan, China. JAMA Intern Med 2020; 180(7):934. https://doi.org/10.1001/jamainternmed. 2020.0994.

38. Del Valle DM, Kim-Schulze S, Huang HH, et al. An inflammatory cytokine signature predicts COVID-19 severity and survival. Nat Med 2020;26(10): 1636–43. https://doi.org/10.1038/s41591-020-1051-9.

39. Xu XW, Wu XX, Jiang XG, et al. Clinical findings in a group of patients infected with the 2019 novel coronavirus (SARS-Cov-2) outside of Wuhan, China: retrospective case series. BMJ 2020;19:m606. https://doi.org/10.1136/bmj.m606. Published online February.

40. Hogan CA, Stevens BA, Sahoo MK, et al. High frequency of SARS-CoV-2 RNAemia and association with severe disease. Clin Infect Dis 2021;72(9): e291–5. https://doi.org/10.1093/cid/ciaa1054.

41. ACTIV-3/TICO Study Group*. The association of baseline plasma SARS-CoV-2 nucleocapsid antigen level and outcomes in patients hospitalized with COVID-19. Ann Intern Med 2022;175(10):1401–10. https://doi.org/10.7326/M22-0924. Published online August 30.

42. COVID-19 Treatment Guidelines Panel. Clinical spectrum of SARS-CoV-2 infection. National Institutes of Health. Available at: https://www. covid19treatmentguidelines.nih.gov/overview/ clinical-spectrum/. Accessed October 5, 2022.

43. Brandal LT, MacDonald E, Veneti L, et al. Outbreak caused by the SARS-CoV-2 omicron variant in Norway, november to december 2021. Eurosurveillance 2021;26(50). https://doi.org/10.2807/1560-7917.ES. 2021.26.50.2101147.

44. Wu Y, Kang L, Guo Z, et al. incubation period of COVID-19 caused by unique SARS-CoV-2 strains: a systematic review and meta-analysis. JAMA Netw Open 2022;5(8):e2228008. https://doi.org/10. 1001/jamanetworkopen.2022.28008.

45. Cohen PA, Hall LE, John JN, et al. The early natural history of SARS-CoV-2 infection. Mayo Clin Proc 2020; 95(6):1124–6. https://doi.org/10.1016/j.mayocp.2020. 04.010.

46. Huang C, Wang Y, Li X, et al. Clinical features of patients infected with 2019 novel coronavirus in Wuhan, China. The Lancet 2020;395(10223):497–506. https://doi.org/10.1016/S0140-6736(20)30183-5.

47. Blair PW, Brown DM, Jang M, et al. The clinical course of COVID-19 in the outpatient setting: a prospective cohort study. Open Forum Infect Dis 2021; 8(2):ofab007. https://doi.org/10.1093/ofid/ofab007.

48. Struyf T, Deeks JJ, Dinnes J, et al. Signs and symptoms to determine if a patient presenting in primary care or hospital outpatient settings has COVID-19. Cochrane Database Syst Rev 2022;2022(5). https://doi.org/10.1002/14651858.CD013665.pub3. Cochrane Infectious Diseases Group, ed.

49. Daher A, Balfanz P, Aetou M, et al. Clinical course of COVID-19 patients needing supplemental oxygen outside the intensive care unit. Sci Rep 2021;11(1): 2256. https://doi.org/10.1038/s41598-021-81444-9.

50. Tobin MJ, Laghi F, Jubran A. Why COVID-19 silent hypoxemia is baffling to physicians. Am J Respir Crit Care Med 2020;202(3):356–60. https://doi.org/ 10.1164/rccm.202006-2157CP.

51. Wilkerson RG, Adler JD, Shah NG, et al. Silent hypoxia: a harbinger of clinical deterioration in patients with COVID-19. Am J Emerg Med 2020;38(10):2243.e5–6. https://doi.org/10.1016/j.ajem.2020.05.044.

52. Jouffroy R, Jost D, Prunet B. Prehospital pulse oximetry: a red flag for early detection of silent hypoxemia in COVID-19 patients. Crit Care 2020;24(1): 313. https://doi.org/10.1186/s13054-020-03036-9.

53. Moosavi SH, Golestanian E, Binks AP, et al. Hypoxic and hypercapnic drives to breathe generate equivalent levels of air hunger in humans. J Appl Physiol 2003;94:14.

54. Jalili M, Payandemehr P, Saghaei A, et al. Characteristics and mortality of hospitalized patients with COVID-19 in Iran: a national retrospective cohort study. Ann Intern Med 2021;174(1):125–7. https:// doi.org/10.7326/M20-2911.

55. Chand S, Kapoor S, Orsi D, et al. COVID-19-Associated critical illness—report of the first 300 patients admitted to intensive care units at a New York city medical center. J Intensive Care Med 2020;35(10): 963–70. https://doi.org/10.1177/0885066620946692.

56. Argenziano MG, Bruce SL, Slater CL, et al. Characterization and clinical course of 1000 patients with coronavirus disease 2019 in New York: retrospective case series. BMJ 2020;369:m1996. https://doi.org/ 10.1136/bmj.m1996. Published online May 29.

57. Yang X, Yu Y, Xu J, et al. Clinical course and outcomes of critically ill patients with SARS-CoV-2 pneumonia in Wuhan, China: a single-centered, retrospective, observational study. Lancet Respir Med 2020;8(5):475–81. https://doi.org/10.1016/ S2213-2600(20)30079-5.

58. Wang D, Hu B, Hu C, et al. Clinical characteristics of 138 hospitalized patients with 2019 novel coronavirus–infected pneumonia in Wuhan, China. JAMA 2020;323(11):1061. https://doi.org/10.1001/ jama.2020.1585.

59. McGuinness G, Zhan C, Rosenberg N, et al. Increased incidence of barotrauma in patients with COVID-19 on invasive mechanical ventilation. Radiology 2020;297(2):E252–62. https://doi.org/10.1148/ radiol.2020202352.

60. Kahn MR, Watson RL, Thetford JT, et al. High incidence of barotrauma in patients with severe coronavirus disease 2019. J Intensive Care Med 2021;36(6):646–54. https://doi.org/10.1177/0885066621989959.

61. Rajdev K, Spanel AJ, McMillan S, et al. Pulmonary barotrauma in COVID-19 patients with ARDS on invasive and non-invasive positive pressure ventilation. J Intensive Care Med 2021;36(9):1013–7. https://doi.org/10.1177/08850666211019719.

62. Gabrielli M, Valletta F, Franceschi F. On behalf of Gemelli against COVID 2019. Barotrauma during non-invasive ventilation for acute respiratory distress syndrome caused by COVID-19: a balance between risks and benefits. Br J Hosp Med 2021;82(6):1–9. https://doi.org/10.12968/hmed.2021.0109.

63. Bain W, Yang H, Shah FA, et al. COVID-19 versus non–COVID-19 acute respiratory distress syndrome: comparison of demographics, physiologic parameters, inflammatory biomarkers, and clinical outcomes. Ann Am Thorac Soc 2021;18(7):1202–10. https://doi.org/10.1513/AnnalsATS.202008-1026OC.

64. Sjoding MW, Admon AJ, Saha AK, et al. Comparing clinical features and outcomes in mechanically ventilated patients with COVID-19 and acute respiratory distress syndrome. Ann Am Thorac Soc 2021; 18(11):1876–85. https://doi.org/10.1513/AnnalsATS.202008-1076OC.

65. Soriano JB, Murthy S, Marshall JC, et al. A clinical case definition of post-COVID-19 condition by a Delphi consensus. Lancet Infect Dis 2022;22(4):e102–7. https://doi.org/10.1016/S1473-3099(21)00703-9.

66. Seeßle J, Waterboer T, Hippchen T, et al. Persistent symptoms in adult patients 1 Year after coronavirus disease 2019 (COVID-19): a prospective cohort study. Clin Infect Dis 2022;74(7):1191–8. https://doi.org/10.1093/cid/ciab611.

67. Tran VT, Porcher R, Pane I, et al. Course of post COVID-19 disease symptoms over time in the ComPaRe long COVID prospective e-cohort. Nat Commun 2022;13(1):1812. https://doi.org/10.1038/s41467-022-29513-z.

68. Garcia-Vidal C, Sanjuan G, Moreno-García E, et al. Incidence of co-infections and superinfections in hospitalized patients with COVID-19: a retrospective cohort study. Clin Microbiol Infect 2021;27(1):83–8. https://doi.org/10.1016/j.cmi.2020.07.041.

69. Musuuza JS, Watson L, Parmasad V, et al. Prevalence and outcomes of co-infection and superinfection with SARS-CoV-2 and other pathogens: a systematic review and meta-analysis. In: Huber VC, editor. PLoS One 2021;16(5):e0251170. https://doi.org/10.1371/journal.pone.0251170.

70. Wong Ho YF, Hiu Yin SL, Ambrose Ho-Tung F, et al. Frequency and distribution of chest radiographic findings in COVID-19 positive patients. Radiology 2020;296:E72–8.

71. Pan F, Ye T, Sun P, et al. Time course of lung changes at chest CT during recovery from coronavirus disease 2019 (COVID-19). Radiology 2020;295(3):715–21. https://doi.org/10.1148/radiol.2020200370.

72. Kanne JP, Bai H, Bernheim A, et al. COVID-19 imaging: what We know now and what remains unknown. Radiology 2021;299(3):E262–79. https://doi.org/10.1148/radiol.2021204522.

73. for the Zhongnan Hospital of Wuhan University Novel Coronavirus Management and Research Team, Evidence-Based Medicine Chapter of China International Exchange and Promotive Association for Medical and Health Care (CPAM), Jin YH, Cai L, et al. A rapid advice guideline for the diagnosis and treatment of 2019 novel coronavirus (2019-nCoV) infected pneumonia (standard version). Mil Med Res 2020;7(1):4. https://doi.org/10.1186/s40779-020-0233-6.

74. Radiological Society of North America. Radiological society of North America expert consensus statement on reporting chest CT findings related to COVID-19. Endorsed by the society of thoracic radiology, the American college of radiology, and RSNA. J Thorac Imaging 2020. https://doi.org/10.1148/ryct.2020200152.podcast.

75. Lee JE, Hwang M, Kim YH, et al. Imaging and clinical features of COVID-19 breakthrough infections: a multicenter study. Radiology 2022;303(3):682–92. https://doi.org/10.1148/radiol.213072.

76. Yoon SH, Lee JH, Kim, Baek-Nam K. Chest CT findings in hospitalized patients with SARS-CoV-2: delta versus omicron variants. Radiology, 2022. doi: 10.1148/radiol.220676

77. Hui KPY, Ho JCW, Cheung M C, et al. SARS-CoV-2 Omicron variant replication in human bronchus and lung ex vivo. Nature 2022;603(7907):715–20. https://doi.org/10.1038/s41586-022-04479-6.

78. Morris MF, Pershad Y, Kang P, et al. Altered pulmonary blood volume distribution as a biomarker for predicting outcomes in COVID-19 disease. Eur Respir J 2021;58(3):2004133. https://doi.org/10.1183/13993003.04133-2020.

79. Center for Forecasting and Outbreak Analytics. Resources and publications of the center for forecasting and Outbreak Analytics. Available at: https://www.cdc.gov/forecast-outbreak-analysis/reources.html. Accessed October 6, 2022.

80. Health Resources & Services Administration. Ensuring equity in COVID-19 vaccine distribution. Available at: https://www.hrsa.gov/coronavirus/health-center-program. Accessed October 6, 2022.

Pathophysiology of Hypoxemia in COVID-19 Lung Disease

Kai E. Swenson, MD[a,b,*], Charles C. Hardin, MD, PhD[b]

KEYWORDS

- COVID-19 • SARS-CoV-2 • Hypoxemia • ARDS

KEY POINTS

- Hypoxemia is common in coronavirus disease 2019 (COVID-19) lung disease and a prognosticator of disease severity, although challenges exist with its measurement.
- Ventilation-perfusion mismatching is the predominant cause of hypoxemia in COVID-19.
- COVID-19 lung disease leads to a wide range of pulmonary compliances, poorly correlated with degree of hypoxemia.
- Incongruence among degree of parenchymal involvement, respiratory system compliance, and hypoxemia could be explained by a diffuse pulmonary vascular process, lack of appropriate vasoconstriction in diseased regions, or both.
- The phenomenon of silent hypoxemia is best considered a consequence of the limited dyspneogenic effect of hypoxemia in comparison to mild hypocapnia and relatively normal work of breathing.

INTRODUCTION

From the beginning of the pandemic, the diagnosis and management of hypoxemia has been an essential aspect of coronavirus disease 2019 (COVID-19) care. Within the first 2 weeks after symptom onset, patients may present with increasing respiratory complaints such as cough, difficulty breathing, and exertional intolerance, which may progress to a requirement for supplemental oxygen. These symptoms are often associated with abnormalities on lung imaging, most commonly bilateral, basilar predominant ground glass opacities that may progress to consolidations. This classic pattern of COVID-19 lung disease affected most patients in the earlier waves of the pandemic,[1] although that may be changing with higher rates of vaccination, greater herd immunity from prior infection, and possibly different viral strains. Nevertheless, it remains the pattern most commonly recognized by clinicians and likely the presentation with highest morbidity and mortality.

Hypoxemia is an important prognostic indicator for patient-centered outcomes such as hospital length of stay, ICU admission, intubation, and death[2]; additionally, it may be independently associated with prolonged delays in recovery of mental status.[3] Obesity, elderly age, and underlying renal and cardiac diseases are associated more severe degrees of hypoxemia and severe COVID-19.[4] However, early in the pandemic, it was observed that the degree of hypoxemia caused by COVID-19 lung disease was poorly associated with both the severity of parenchymal involvement on computed tomography (CT) and the presence of respiratory symptoms, especially dyspnea. Additionally, early reports of intubated, critically ill patients with COVID-19 suggested a subgroup of patients in which impaired gas exchange was associated with preserved compliance, a pattern

a Division of Thoracic Surgery and Interventional Pulmonology, Beth Israel Deaconess Medical Center, Boston, MA, USA; b Division of Pulmonary and Critical Care Medicine, Massachusetts General Hospital, Bulfinch 148, 55 Fruit Street, Boston, MA 02114, USA
* Corresponding author.
E-mail address: keswenson@mgh.harvard.edu

Clin Chest Med 44 (2023) 239–248
https://doi.org/10.1016/j.ccm.2022.11.007
0272-5231/23/© 2022 Elsevier Inc. All rights reserved.

purportedly unique to COVID-19.[5] These reported mismatches between degree of hypoxemia and other markers of severity spawned great confusion and a search for new pathophysiologic mechanisms unique to COVID-19 infection. However, as our understanding of COVID-19 epidemiology has grown, it has become clear that many of these paradoxic findings are likely the consequences of relevant but often-forgotten tenets of respiratory physiology, potentially magnified by specific features inherent to COVID-19 pathophysiology and epidemiology.

Challenges with Interpreting Hypoxemia in COVID-19

The challenge with interpretation of the severity of hypoxemia in COVID-19 lies firstly in the heterogeneity of the underlying patient population; many of the physiologic studies noted above included patients at varying time points in their disease course, with different underlying comorbidities and severity of disease, and especially on different respiratory support settings. This latter point becomes particularly important when using $P_{a}O_2$/F_iO_2 to describe hypoxemia. Although this ratio should ideally provide some comparable indication of disease severity, in actuality, it is strongly influenced by the degree of venous admixture and cardiac output in the individual patient, both of which are highly affected by positive end-expiratory pressure (PEEP); for example,[6] $P_{a}O_2$/F_iO_2 ratios are highly variable even in the same patient when compared before and after the use of mechanical ventilation, suggesting that its use to prognosticate in spontaneously ventilation in patients with COVID-19 (especially those on high-flow nasal cannula) is limited.[7]

Others have recommended the use of alternative (and less invasive) options for prognostication, such as the respiratory rate-oxygenation index, based in part of oxygen saturation rather than $P_{a}O_2$.[8] However, it is well known that pulse oximetry becomes quite inaccurate in comparison to arterial blood samples at saturations less than 75% to 80%, depending on device quality.[9] Moreover, perhaps more importantly, it has become clear during the course of the COVID-19 pandemic that pulse oximeters may also routinely overestimate oxygen saturation measurements in mild-moderate hypoxemia, especially in patients with darker skin tone. One study of paired samples of arterial oxygen ($S_{a}O_2$) and pulse oximetry ($S_{p}O_2$) saturations found an overall average difference of 1.4%; however, when restricted to the group with $S_{a}O_2$ 85% to 89%, the difference was 2.8%, and up to 3.9% in Black and 5.8% in Asian

patients.[10] Rates of occult hypoxemia from pulse oximetry (defined as $S_{a}O_2$ <88% despite $S_{p}O_2$ 92%–96%) may be as high as 30% in Asian, 29% in Black, and 30% of Hispanic patient populations, as compared with 17% in Caucasian patients.[11] These discrepancies in saturation data highlight the challenges associated with accurately measuring hypoxemia in COVID-19 lung injury, especially among certain ethnic groups at highest risk for severe disease.

Pathogenesis of Hypoxemia in COVID-19

COVID-19 infection is known to cause acute damage to the alveolar-capillary barrier, involving damage to both alveolar epithelium and capillary endothelium; this injury is directly viral-mediated or due to the consequent inflammatory response.[12] Lung histology in nonsurvivors suggest that COVID-19 pathologic condition generally mimics that of classic ARDS, with diffuse alveolar damage and consequent formation of hyaline membranes.[13] Less severe or prolonged cases of COVID-19 lung injury in survivors may suggest organizing pneumonia, which is thought to represent an aberrant parenchymal recovery process after acute injury.[14] Importantly, COVID-19 autopsy studies often reveal significant capillary endothelial injury and intracapillary thrombosis, similar to classic ARDS although perhaps at a greater prevalence.[15] The mechanisms by which viral-mediated and immune-mediated damage occurs to endothelial and epithelial membranes is beyond the scope of this article; nevertheless, there is likely an interplay between vascular effects from endothelialitis and thrombosis, and direct or indirect alveolar injury leading to alveolar filling.

Physiologically, the 5 causes of hypoxemia are (1) low partial pressure of inspired oxygen, (2) alveolar hypoventilation, (3) diffusion limitation, (4) ventilation-perfusion mismatching (and specifically low ratios of ventilation/perfusion, or V_A/Q), and (5) right-to-left shunt. Of these causes, only ventilation/perfusion mismatching and pure right-to-left shunt lead to hypoxemia in ARDS, as measured by the multiple inert gas elimination technique (MIGET).[16] Traditionally, pure right-to-left shunt through nonventilated lung regions has been considered the predominant cause of hypoxemia in classic ARDS, perhaps because those patients studied via MIGET had predominant findings of significant consolidation on lung imaging, with relative sparing of other lung regions (the overall reduced volume of normal parenchyma being known as "baby lung").[16] However, this pattern may not hold true for all cases of lung infection, especially early in the disease course when consolidations are often absent.[17] Additionally, the degree of venous admixture from low V_A/Q regions will increase in the context of a high cardiac output, often seen in both COVID-19 lung disease and non-COVID-19 ARDS.[18]

MIGET studies have not yet been performed in COVID-19 lung disease to our knowledge; however, in the absence of such direct testing, computational models of ventilation and perfusion associated with high-resolution CT have yielded interesting findings. In computational models of V_A/Q mismatch and shunt physiology, based on CT imaging and markers of gas exchange in severe COVID-19 lung disease, it has been suggested that the degree of hypoxemia cannot be solely due to shunt through nonaerated regions, such that low V_A/Q units are additionally responsible.[19] In such models with small fractions of nonaerated or poorly aerated lung parenchyma, significant hypoxemia could be explained by either significant hyperperfusion of nonaerated lung regions, or alternatively due to the presence of ventilation/perfusion mismatch in aerated lung regions through a diffuse vascular process such as endothelialitis or microthrombosis.[20]

Regional Ventilation-Perfusion Mismatch in COVID-19 Lung Disease

The 2 predominant theories that could explain the findings of the computational models described above are the presence of diffuse pulmonary vascular endothelialitis and thromboembolism (leading to hypoperfusion in relatively preserved lung regions) and vascular dilation not responsive to normal hypoxic pulmonary vasoconstriction (HPV, leading to hyperperfusion in poorly aerated or nonaerated lung regions). These theories are certainly not mutually exclusive; indeed, several cross-sectional imaging studies, including techniques for measuring regional perfusion, have provided support for both theories.

For example, subtraction CT angiography with iodine mapping demonstrates that hypoperfusion of apparently healthy lung parenchyma is common, with more severe perfusion abnormalities associated with lower P_aO_2/F_iO_2 ratios and more likely to require invasive mechanical ventilation.[21] Similarly, dual energy computed tomography (DECT) in COVID-19 lung disease has revealed mosaic perfusion patterns in the absence of macroscopic pulmonary embolism, and not clearly matched by pulmonary opacities, strongly arguing in favor of a diffuse pulmonary microvascular process.[22] Indeed, diffuse endothelialitis and microvascular thrombosis are commonly found on autopsy in COVID-19,[23] even in the setting of

therapeutic anticoagulation.[24] However, pulmonary vascular abnormalities and hypercoagulability are also well documented in non-COVID-19 ARDS.[25] Although some therapeutic trials have suggested improvements in oxygenation with empiric initiation of therapeutic anticoagulation in patients with COVID-19, especially those with increased dead space fraction,[26,27] this finding has not been reproduced in larger trials.[28–30]

Other imaging studies suggest abnormal hyperperfusion in areas of parenchymal involvement. Understandably, lung aeration loss is strongly associated with lower P_aO_2/F_iO_2 ratios, mostly due to gas–blood volume mismatch noted on DECT.[31] Peripheral vessel dilation is noted in almost two-thirds of mechanically ventilated patients undergoing DECT, involving almost half of the lung parenchyma,[23] with an interesting pattern of "vascular tree-in-bud" abnormalities correlating with increased dead space, prolonged hospitalization, and need for mechanical ventilation. Although some groups have noted abnormally dilated pulmonary vessels adjacent to areas of parenchymal involvement,[32] which could suggest a sort of locoregional perfusion abnormality, this has not been reported in other studies.[33] Therapeutic maneuvers to improve ventilation-perfusion matching, including inhaled pulmonary vasodilators and almitrine (which may act to augment HPV) have demonstrated improvements in oxygenation in patients with COVID-19,[34] although these same benefits have been described previously in non-COVID ARDS without a survival benefit.[35,36] Finally, ventilation-perfusion mismatching and hypoxemia may develop via abnormal intrapulmonary shunts in COVID-19. Physiologically, the presence of such shunts is suggested by the appearance of microbubbles in the systemic circulation based on transcranial Doppler imaging[37] and in up to 16% of patients on echocardiography.[38] They have also been demonstrated radiographically at the level of the secondary pulmonary lobule on CT reconstructions,[39] and on autopsy in severe COVID-19 lung disease.[40] However, it should be noted that the presence of such shunts has been reported in a subset of non-COVID ARDS undergoing echocardiography, suggesting that this process is likely not unique to COVID-19 lung injury.[41]

Are there specific pathophysiologic factors unique to COVID-19, which cause a greater degree of ventilation-perfusion mismatch, such as a virally-mediated impairment of HPV? One theory posits that binding of ACE-2 receptors by SARS coronaviruses in pulmonary vascular endothelium leads to downregulation of these receptors and abrogation of normal vasoregulation in these regions.[42] Indeed, ACE-2 inhibition by lisinopril has previously been shown to attenuate hypoxic pulmonary vasoconstriction.[43] Although this theory is intriguing, the renin-angiotensin-aldosterone system remains a minor contributor to pulmonary vasoregulation in comparison to the release of local mediators (endothelin, prostacyclin, and nitric oxide), which could be affected by direct viral injury to pulmonary artery endothelial cells.[15] At this time, there is no clear evidence supporting a direct impact of SARS-CoV-2 infection on local mechanisms of HPV.[44] However, even in the absence of direct modulation by viral infection, local and systemic inflammatory responses to infection can significantly attenuate HPV responses in animal models.[45] Finally, opening of preexisting intrapulmonary bronchopulmonary anastomoses could provide a unifying explanation for abnormal ventilation-perfusion matching, without invoking a direct effect on HPV.

Hypoxemia and Respiratory Mechanics in COVID-19 Lung Disease

Multiple large observational studies have demonstrated a broad unimodal distribution of respiratory system compliance (C_{RS}) in COVID-19 ARDS. The overall clinical data suggest that C_{RS} in COVID-19 lung injury has a wide range across studies (20–90 mL/cmH$_2$O),[46–50] not dissimilar to pre-COVID ARDS cohorts.[51,52] Based in part on these accumulated data, clinical practice guidelines[53] and most experts[54] agree that equivalent ventilatory strategies be used for both COVID-19 and non-COVID-19 forms of ARDS, especially the routine use of lung protective ventilation. One explanation for the high heterogeneity in compliance is the presence of a predominant vascular pathologic condition, as discussed previously. Proponents of this theory point to the high dead space fractions and ventilatory ratios calculated from many patients with COVID-19.[55,56] Indeed, high ventilatory ratios (a marker of increased dead space) are associated with elevated levels of D-dimer and areas of hypoperfusion on CT pulmonary angiograms.[57] However, it is important to mention that dead space ventilation does not directly contribute to hypoxemia, but rather can cause concomitant hyperperfusion and low V_A/Q in other regions, as is classically noted in pulmonary emboli.[58] Additionally, calculations of dead space fraction that rely on measurement of arterial CO$_2$ and estimation of alveolar CO$_2$ (the Enghoff modification to the Bohr equation for dead space fraction) will not correct for decreased CO$_2$ elimination in areas of shunt, and thereby overestimate dead space.[59] Ventilatory ratios have been variably associated with degree of hypoxemia in

COVID-19 lung disease, and this association can change during the course of disease.[4,57,60,61]

An alternative reason for the heterogeneity of compliance, which seems quite likely, is that compliance changes as COVID-19 lung disease progresses. For example, in cohorts of COVID-19 ARDS in which preserved compliance has been described, there is a clear negative correlation between compliance and number of days since symptom onset[62]; perhaps early intubation due to concerns with viral transmission played a large role in these findings. Indeed, in other groups, prolonged time to intubation[63,64] or prolonged duration of symptoms[49] are associated with worsened compliance, suggesting a later stage in the disease, although patient self-inflicted lung injury (hypothesized to occur during spontaneous ventilation in the setting of acute lung injury and impaired compliance) could conceivably be implicated.[65] The presence and severity of obesity has also been implicated as a potential explanation for the heterogeneous compliance values noted in COVID-19 lung disease. However, although it contributes to alveolar derecruitment, obesity does not seem to significantly affect overall respiratory system compliance. Esophageal balloon measurements demonstrate that elevated body mass index (BMI) is associated with elevated end-expiratory pleural pressures but normal chest wall compliance, and in these patients, lung compliance correlates poorly with P_aO_2/F_iO_2 ratios.[66]

How do respiratory mechanics correlate with degree of hypoxemia in COVID-19? A positive, although relatively weak, correlation has been noted between compliance and degree of hypoxemia,[50,67] although this is not universal.[57,66] In one study, compliance and oxygenation were not initially correlated on day 1 of intubation but there was a strong positive correlation by day 7,[61] suggesting progression of parenchymal injury and nonaerated lung regions; however, other longitudinal studies have not reproduced this finding.[4] Recruitability, or the ability of nonaerated or poorly aerated lung parenchyma to be reopened with additional PEEP, is similarly variably associated with the severity of hypoxemia before recruitment.[49,61] Surprisingly, even with significant interindividual variability, recruitability does not seem to predict oxygenation response to increases in PEEP.[50,68] This seems counterintuitive if considering that the mechanism of improved oxygenation with increased PEEP is by recruitment of previously nonventilated alveoli. However, increased PEEP may also cause a decrease in cardiac output and resultant pulmonary blood flow to nonrecruitable alveoli. Although this effect remains poorly understood in COVID-19 and ARDS in general, it may be related to partial correction of an underlying hyperdynamic pulmonary circulation in the setting of impaired hypoxic vasoconstriction.[16,69]

Similarly, prone positioning may improve oxygenation in COVID-19 not by improving overall compliance but through a mix of posterior recruitment and ventral derecruitment[70]; this allows for greater homogenization (and therefore matching) of ventilation and perfusion throughout.[71]

Most studies in intubated patients with COVID-19 have noted an average improvement in oxygenation with prone positioning even in the absence of a change in respiratory system compliance,[72–74] which seems to persist after resupination.[75] However, prone positioning does not always lead to better oxygenation, with one large study noting improved P_aO_2/F_iO_2 in only 45% of intubated patients with COVID-19 after proning.[76] Although prone positioning in nonintubated patients likely improves oxygenation transiently and may delay the need for intubation,[77] the effect seems to be mostly reversible on resuming supine positioning.[78,79]

Hypoxemia and Respiratory Symptoms in COVID-19 Lung Disease

From very early in the COVID-19 pandemic, clinicians reported a subset of patients presenting with COVID-19 lung disease causing hypoxemia but in the absence of concomitant respiratory symptoms such as dyspnea. This syndrome, most commonly referred to as "silent hypoxemia," was seemingly unique and not previously described in the medical literature. Indeed, it is difficult retrospectively to find evidence of silent hypoxemia in previous cohorts of acute lung injury, or to dissociate symptoms of acute lung injury from those of the underlying insult itself, such as pneumonia, sepsis, or trauma. There is likely a strong ascertainment bias at work when considering the prevalence of silent hypoxemia in COVID-19 infection, given the ability to accurately detect cases at early stages or even before lung disease develops, as compared with many other causes of acute lung injury. However, prior case series of virally-mediated causes of acute lung injury, notably infection by SARS-CoV-1, reported the absence of dyspnea in up to a quarter of patients, suggesting at least some degree of silent hypoxemia could have been present in earlier epidemics.[80,81]

Nevertheless, the absence of dyspnea is common at the time of hospitalization for COVID-19, occurring in up to 65% of patients in one study of hospitalized patients, most of whom had evidence of lung disease on CT.[82] The prevalence of silent hypoxemia specifically has varied widely

by study, ranging between 9% and 36%, in part, due to reporting biases and the lack of a universal definition.[46,48,83,84] In one large cohort of patients admitted with COVID-19 lung disease and acute respiratory failure (of whom 83% required either supplemental oxygen or ventilatory support on presentation), lack of dyspnea was reported in 36%.[84] In another cohort, dyspnea was absent in 13% of patients with COVID-19 presenting with arterial oxygenation saturation less than 90%.[85] The frequency of dyspnea at presentation in later strains of COVID-19 is not well described and difficult to estimate, in part, due to the high efficacy of vaccination; however, it has been noted that hospitalization rates in Delta and Omicron waves were not lower than the initial Alpha wave among unvaccinated patients.[86] It is also likely that the prevalence of silent hypoxemia varies significantly based on time of presentation, severity of illness, or presence of comorbidities known to be associated with severe disease such as elderly age, obesity, and diabetes mellitus.[87] Patients with silent hypoxemia may present earlier after symptom onset to medical attention, and often for nonrespiratory complaints, suggesting that this may represent an earlier time point in their disease course before the onset of respiratory symptoms.[88] Although it likely delays the use of respiratory support, it remains unclear to what extent silent hypoxemia leads to worse clinical outcomes, with studies suggesting equal, better, or worse outcomes as compared with symptomatic hypoxemia.[82,85,89]

There was considerable interest initially in the possibility of reduced hypoxic ventilatory response (HVR) in patients with COVID-19, in part due to the neurotropic manifestations commonly recognized in COVID-19 infection such as olfactory dysfunction and high rates altered mental status during severe disease. However, although HVR has never been formally tested in patients with COVID-19 and can vary widely in the healthy population,[90] the almost universal presence of hypocapnia in patients presenting with hypoxemia argues against the presence of a reduced ventilatory response. For example, in one series of patients with mildly symptomatic COVID-19 and hypoxemia, calculations of alveolar CO_2 correlated against arterial oxygen suggested that alveolar ventilation was increased between 1.1-fold and 1.7-fold as compared with known values for healthy controls undergoing formal HVR testing.[91] Indeed, elevated respiratory rates are often anecdotally noted in patients with COVID-19 not describing dyspnea, with one study describing a median respiratory rate of 31 breaths per minute in the 5% of its cohort with silent hypoxemia.[87] In another cohort of 45 patients admitted to a respiratory unit for COVID-19, the average Pa_{CO_2} was 32 mm Hg, with significantly lower Borg dyspnea scores in the COVID-19 population as compared with non-COVID patients admitted during the same time period (although the control group had a significantly increased rate of underlying lung disease and hypercapnia).[92] However, it must be noted that another group found a lower ratio of oxygen saturation to respiratory rate in patients with COVID-19 as compared with historical controls; without blood gas analysis, it is impossible to know if hypocapnia (which blunts HVR) could help to explain this finding.[93]

In the absence of demonstrable hypoventilation, the best explanation for silent hypoxemia invokes the common characteristics of COVID-19 lung disease described in this article correlated with the known physiologic basis for ventilatory drive. First, it must be noted that hypoxemia is a very weak stimulant for increased ventilation and for the onset of dyspnea, as compared with increased work of breathing or hypercapnia[94]; and in fact, increased ventilation may occur in mild-to-moderate hypoxemia even without patients noting dyspnea.[95] Early COVID-19 may otherwise lack strong dyspneogenic stimuli, such as increased work of breathing due to poor compliance or high airway resistance. Second, increased ventilation in an asymptomatic patient, in turn, will efficiently eliminate CO_2, given a presumed low-normal work of breathing and at least some regions of retained ventilation-perfusion matching. Thus, the mild stimulant effect of hypoxemia will be more than outweighed by hypocapnia, which significantly suppresses ventilation and which has been observed frequently in the silent hypoxemia cohorts described above. Furthermore, respiratory alkalosis per se is known to attenuate HPV responses.[45] Finally, hypoxemia caused by mismatches in ventilation and perfusion are not corrected by increased ventilation, such that hypoxemia will be persistent. Thus, silent hypoxemia is most probably the result of a combination of factors: poorly aerated, hyperperfused lung regions with retained compliance, the weak dyspneogenic effect of hypoxemia counterbalance by the resultant hypocapnia from mild hyperventilation, and the inability of increased ventilation to correct hypoxemia due to these low V_A/Q regions.

SUMMARY

A practical effect of the immense amount of research produced in describing gas exchange abnormalities in COVID-19 lung disease has been to reiterate the importance of basic respiratory physiology in making sense of novel causative agents

of lung injury. Impairment of ventilation-perfusion matching is the hallmark of any lung disease associated with gas exchange abnormalities, regardless of parenchymal or vascular predominance, and the range of mismatch does not seem to be unique to the effect of SARS-CoV-2. Although studies remain to be done, especially in terms of understanding the interplay between vascular and alveolar injury during the course of COVID-19 and the potential for direct viral mediation of hypoxic pulmonary vasoconstriction, the preponderance of the current evidence suggests that the effect of COVID-19 infection on gas exchange is well explained by established tenets of respiratory physiology and should not preclude the use of standard treatments for acute lung injury.

CLINICS CARE POINTS

- Hypoxemia is a prognosticator of disease severity in COVID-19 lung injury; however, inaccuracy in measurement through pulse oximetry (especially among non-Caucasian patients) is an important obstacle to early risk stratification and equitable treatment decisions.

- The predominant cause of hypoxemia in COVID-19 is the presence of lung regions with a low ventilation/perfusion ratio, although right-to-left shunting through consolidated lung regions also contributes, especially as the disease progresses.

- Theories to explain the degree of ventilation-perfusion mismatch include a diffuse pulmonary vascular process, which limits perfusion to normally aerated regions, and overperfusion of nonaerated areas, either due to loss of normal vasoconstrictory responses or potentially the effect of intrapulmonary bronchopulmonary anastomoses.

- Hypoxemia in COVID-19 lung disease is poorly correlated with both pulmonary compliance and recruitment responses to increased PEEP.

- Prone positioning may help to homogenize ventilation and perfusion and improve oxygenation in COVID-19, similar to its effect on gas exchange in non-COVID-19 ARDS.

- In the absence of any clear evidence of a virus-specific effect on ventilatory control, the phenomenon of silent hypoxemia is best understood because of the limited dyspneogenic effect of hypoxemia in comparison to the mild degree of hypocapnia and relatively normal work of breathing commonly noted in such patients.

DISCLOSURE

Dr Swenson and Hardin have no disclosures relevant to this article.

REFERENCES

1. Guan WJ, Ni ZY, Hu Y, et al. Clinical characteristics of coronavirus disease 2019 in China. N Engl J Med 2020;382(18):1708–20.
2. Xie J, Covassin N, Fan Z, et al. Association between hypoxemia and mortality in patients with COVID-19. Mayo Clin Proc 2020;95(6):1138–47.
3. Waldrop G, Safavynia SA, Barra ME, et al. Prolonged unconsciousness is common in COVID-19 and associated with hypoxemia. Ann Neurol 2022; 91(6):740–55.
4. Estenssoro E, Loudet CI, Dubin A, et al. Clinical characteristics, respiratory management, and determinants of oxygenation in COVID-19 ARDS: a prospective cohort study. J Crit Care 2022;71:154021.
5. Gattinoni L, Coppola S, Cressoni M, et al. COVID-19 does not lead to a "typical" acute respiratory distress syndrome. Am J Respir Crit Care Med 2020;201(10): 1299–300.
6. Gattinoni L, Vassalli F, Romitti F. Benefits and risks of the P/F approach. Intensive Care Med 2018;44(12): 2245–7.
7. Hultström M, Hellkvist O, Covaciu L, et al. Limitations of the ARDS criteria during high-flow oxygen or non-invasive ventilation: evidence from critically ill COVID-19 patients. Crit Care 2022;26(1):55.
8. Myers LC, Mark D, Ley B, et al. Validation of respiratory rate-oxygenation index in patients with COVID-19-related respiratory failure. Crit Care Med 2022. https://doi.org/10.1097/CCM.0000000000005474.
9. Luks AM, Swenson ER. Pulse oximetry for monitoring patients with COVID-19 at home. potential pitfalls and practical guidance. Ann Am Thorac Soc 2020;17(9):1040–6.
10. Crooks CJ, West J, Morling JR, et al. Pulse oximeter measurements vary across ethnic groups: an observational study in patients with COVID-19. Eur Respir J 2022;59(4):2103246.
11. Fawzy A, Wu TD, Wang K, et al. Racial and ethnic discrepancy in pulse oximetry and delayed identification of treatment eligibility among patients with COVID-19. JAMA Intern Med 2022;182(7):730–8.
12. Leisman DE, Mehta A, Thompson BT, et al. Alveolar, endothelial, and organ injury marker dynamics in severe COVID-19. Am J Respir Crit Care Med 2022; 205(5):507–19.
13. Hariri LP, North CM, Shih AR, et al. Lung histopathology in coronavirus disease 2019 as compared with severe acute respiratory sydrome and H1N1 influenza: a systematic review. CHEST 2021;159(1):73–84.

14. Myall KJ, Mukherjee B, Castanheira AM, et al. Persistent Post-COVID-19 interstitial lung disease. an observational study of corticosteroid treatment. Ann Am Thorac Soc 2021;18(5):799–806.
15. Ackermann M, Verleden SE, Kuehnel M, et al. Pulmonary vascular endothelialitis, thrombosis, and angiogenesis in Covid-19. N Engl J Med 2020; 383(2):120–8.
16. Dantzker DR, Brook CJ, Dehart P, et al. Ventilation-perfusion distributions in the adult respiratory distress syndrome. Am Rev Respir Dis 1979; 120(5):1039–52.
17. Salehi S, Abedi A, Balakrishnan S, et al. Coronavirus disease 2019 (COVID-19): a systematic review of imaging findings in 919 patients. AJR Am J Roentgenol 2020;215(1):87–93.
18. Caravita S, Baratto C, Di Marco F, et al. Haemodynamic characteristics of COVID-19 patients with acute respiratory distress syndrome requiring mechanical ventilation. An invasive assessment using right heart catheterization. Eur J Heart Fail 2020; 22(12):2228–37.
19. Busana M, Giosa L, Cressoni M, et al. The impact of ventilation-perfusion inequality in COVID-19: a computational model. J Appl Physiol (1985) 2021; 130(3):865–76.
20. Herrmann J, Mori V, Bates JHT, et al. Modeling lung perfusion abnormalities to explain early COVID-19 hypoxemia. Nat Commun 2020;11(1):4883.
21. Santamarina MG, Boisier Riscal D, Beddings I, et al. COVID-19: what iodine maps from perfusion CT can reveal-a prospective cohort study. Crit Care 2020; 24(1):619.
22. Afat S, Othman AE, Nikolaou K, et al. Dual-energy computed tomography of the lung in COVID-19 patients: mismatch of perfusion defects and pulmonary opacities. Diagnostics (Basel) 2020;10(11):870.
23. Patel BV, Arachchillage DJ, Ridge CA, et al. Pulmonary angiopathy in severe COVID-19: physiologic, imaging, and hematologic observations. Am J Respir Crit Care Med 2020;202(5):690–9.
24. Wichmann D, Sperhake JP, Lütgehetmann M, et al. Autopsy findings and venous thromboembolism in patients with COVID-19: a prospective cohort study. Ann Intern Med 2020;173(4):268–77.
25. Schultz MJ, Haitsma JJ, Zhang H, et al. Pulmonary coagulopathy as a new target in therapeutic studies of acute lung injury or pneumonia–a review. Crit Care Med 2006;34(3):871–7.
26. Lemos ACB, do Espírito Santo DA, Salvetti MC, et al. Therapeutic versus prophylactic anticoagulation for severe COVID-19: a randomized phase II clinical trial (HESACOVID). Thromb Res 2020;196: 359–66.
27. Poor HD, Ventetuolo CE, Tolbert T, et al. COVID-19 critical illness pathophysiology driven by diffuse pulmonary thrombi and pulmonary endothelial

dysfunction responsive to thrombolysis. Clin Transl Med 2020;10(2):e44.

28. Goligher EC, Bradbury CA, McVerry BJ, et al. Therapeutic anticoagulation with heparin in critically ill patients with Covid-19. N Engl J Med 2021;385(9):777–89.

29. Sadeghipour P, Talasaz AH, Rashidi F, et al. Effect of intermediate-dose vs standard-dose prophylactic anticoagulation on thrombotic events, extracorporeal membrane oxygenation treatment, or mortality among patients with COVID-19 admitted to the intensive care unit: the inspiration randomized clinical trial. JAMA 2021;325(16):1620–30.

30. Lawler PR, Goligher EC, Berger JS, et al. Therapeutic anticoagulation with heparin in noncritically ill patients with covid-19. N Engl J Med 2021;385(9):790–802.

31. Ball L, Robba C, Herrmann J, et al. Lung distribution of gas and blood volume in critically ill COVID-19 patients: a quantitative dual-energy computed tomography study. Crit Care 2021;25(1):214.

32. Lang M, Som A, Mendoza DP, et al. Hypoxaemia related to COVID-19: vascular and perfusion abnormalities on dual-energy CT. Lancet Infect Dis 2020;20(12):1365–6.

33. Arru CD, Digumarthy SR, Hansen JV, et al. Qualitative and quantitative DECT pulmonary angiography in COVID-19 pneumonia and pulmonary embolism. Clin Radiol 2021;76(5):392.e391–9.

34. Laghlam D, Rahoual G, Malvy J, et al. Use of almitrine and inhaled nitric oxide in ARDS due to COVID-19. Front Med (Lausanne) 2021;8:655763.

35. Gallart L, Lu Q, Puybasset L, et al. Intravenous almitrine combined with inhaled nitric oxide for acute respiratory distress syndrome. The NO Almitrine Study Group. Am J Respir Crit Care Med 1998;158(6):1770–7.

36. Adhikari NK, Dellinger RP, Lundin S, et al. Inhaled nitric oxide does not reduce mortality in patients with acute respiratory distress syndrome regardless of severity: systematic review and meta-analysis. Crit Care Med 2014;42(2):404–12.

37. Reynolds AS, Lee AG, Renz J, et al. Pulmonary vascular dilatation detected by automated transcranial Doppler in COVID-19 pneumonia. Am J Respir Crit Care Med 2020;202(7):1037–9.

38. Trifi A, Ouhibi A, Mahdi A, et al. Shunt in critically ill Covid-19 ARDS patients: prevalence and impact on outcome (cross-sectional study). J Crit Care 2022;70:154048.

39. Ackermann M, Tafforeau P, Wagner WL, et al. The bronchial circulation in COVID-19 pneumonia. Am J Respir Crit Care Med 2022;205(1):121–5.

40. Galambos C, Bush D, Abman SH. Intrapulmonary bronchopulmonary anastomoses in COVID-19 respiratory failure. Eur Respir J 2021;58(2):2004397.

41. Boissier F, Razazi K, Thille AW, et al. Echocardiographic detection of transpulmonary bubble transit during acute respiratory distress syndrome. Ann Intensive Care 2015;5:5.

42. Seltzer S. Linking ACE2 and angiotensin II to pulmonary immunovascular dysregulation in SARS-CoV-2 infection. Int J Infect Dis 2020;101:42–5.

43. Cargill RI, Lipworth BJ. Lisinopril attenuates acute hypoxic pulmonary vasoconstriction in humans. CHEST 1996;109(2):424–9.

44. Gierhardt M, Pak O, Walmrath D, et al. Impairment of hypoxic pulmonary vasoconstriction in acute respiratory distress syndrome. Eur Respir Rev 2021;30(161):210059.

45. Sylvester JT, Shimoda LA, Aaronson PI, et al. Hypoxic pulmonary vasoconstriction. Physiol Rev 2012;92(1):367–520.

46. Ziehr DR, Alladina J, Petri CR, et al. Respiratory pathophysiology of mechanically ventilated patients with COVID-19: a cohort study. Am J Respir Crit Care Med 2020;201(12):1560–4.

47. Bos LDJ, Paulus F, Vlaar APJ, et al. Subphenotyping acute respiratory distress syndrome in patients with COVID-19: consequences for ventilator management. Ann Am Thorac Soc 2020;17(9):1161–3.

48. Bhatraju PK, Ghassemieh BJ, Nichols M, et al. Covid-19 in critically ill patients in the seattle region - case series. N Engl J Med 2020;382(21):2012–22.

49. Haudebourg AF, Perier F, Tuffet S, et al. Respiratory mechanics of COVID-19- versus non-covid-19-associated acute respiratory distress syndrome. Am J Respir Crit Care Med 2020;202(2):287–90.

50. Grieco DL, Bongiovanni F, Chen L, et al. Respiratory physiology of COVID-19-induced respiratory failure compared to ARDS of other etiologies. Crit Care 2020;24(1):529.

51. Guérin C, Reignier J, Richard JC, et al. Prone positioning in severe acute respiratory distress syndrome. N Engl J Med 2013;368(23):2159–68.

52. Panwar R, Madotto F, Laffey JG, et al. Compliance phenotypes in early acute respiratory distress syndrome before the COVID-19 pandemic. Am J Respir Crit Care Med 2020;202(9):1244–52.

53. Alhazzani W, Evans L, Alshamsi F, et al. Surviving sepsis campaign guidelines on the management of adults with coronavirus disease 2019 (COVID-19) in the ICU: first Update. Crit Care Med 2021;49(3):e219–34.

54. Nasa P, Azoulay E, Khanna AK, et al. Expert consensus statements for the management of COVID-19-related acute respiratory failure using a Delphi method. Crit Care 2021;25(1):106.

55. Morales-Quinteros L, Neto AS, Artigas A, et al. Dead space estimates may not be independently associated with 28-day mortality in COVID-19 ARDS. Crit Care 2021;25(1):171.

56. Schenck EJ, Hoffman K, Goyal P, et al. Respiratory mechanics and gas exchange in Covid-19–

associated respiratory failure. Ann Am Thorac Soc 2020;17(9):1158–61.

57. Grasselli G, Tonetti T, Protti A, et al. Pathophysiology of COVID-19-associated acute respiratory distress syndrome: a multicentre prospective observational study. Lancet Respir Med 2020;8(12):1201–8.

58. Altemeier WA, Robertson HT, McKinney S, et al. Pulmonary embolization causes hypoxemia by redistributing regional blood flow without changing ventilation. J Appl Physiol (1985) 1998;85(6):2337–43.

59. Wagner PD. Causes of a high physiological dead space in critically ill patients. Crit Care 2008;12(3):148.

60. Liu X, Liu X, Xu Y, et al. Ventilatory ratio in hypercapnic mechanically ventilated patients with COVID-19-associated acute respiratory distress syndrome. Am J Respir Crit Care Med 2020;201(10):1297–9.

61. Beloncle F, Studer A, Seegers V, et al. Longitudinal changes in compliance, oxygenation and ventilatory ratio in COVID-19 versus non-COVID-19 pulmonary acute respiratory distress syndrome. Crit Care 2021;25(1):248.

62. Gattinoni L, Coppola S, Cressoni M, et al. Reply by Gattinoni et al. to Hedenstierna et al., to Maley et al., to Fowler et al., to Bhatia and Mohammed, to Bos, to Koumbourlis and Motoyama, and to Haouzi et al. Am J Respir Crit Care Med 2020;202(4):628–30.

63. Jafari D, Gandomi A, Makhnevich A, et al. Trajectories of hypoxemia and pulmonary mechanics of COVID-19 ARDS in the NorthCARDS dataset. BMC Pulm Med 2022;22(1):51.

64. Pandya A, Kaur NA, Sacher D, et al. Ventilatory mechanics in early vs late intubation in a cohort of coronavirus disease 2019 patients with ARDS: a single center's experience. CHEST 2021;159(2):653–6.

65. Brochard L, Slutsky A, Pesenti A. Mechanical ventilation to minimize progression of lung injury in acute respiratory failure. Am J Respir Crit Care Med 2017;195(4):438–42.

66. Baedorf Kassis E, Schaefer MS, Maley JH, et al. Transpulmonary pressure measurements and lung mechanics in patients with early ARDS and SARS-CoV-2. J Crit Care 2021;63:106–12.

67. Vandenbunder B, Ehrmann S, Piagnerelli M, et al. Static compliance of the respiratory system in COVID-19 related ARDS: an international multicenter study. Crit Care 2021;25(1):52.

68. Grasso S, Mirabella L, Murgolo F, et al. Effects of positive end-expiratory pressure in "high compliance" severe acute respiratory syndrome coronavirus 2 acute respiratory distress syndrome. Crit Care Med 2020;48(12):e1332–6.

69. Dell'Anna AM, Carelli S, Cicetti M, et al. Hemodynamic response to positive end-expiratory pressure and prone position in COVID-19 ARDS. Respir Physiol Neurobiol 2022;298:103844.

70. Fossali T, Pavlovsky B, Ottolina D, et al. Effects of prone position on lung recruitment and ventilation-perfusion matching in patients with COVID-19 acute respiratory distress syndrome: a combined CT scan/electrical impedance tomography study. Crit Care Med 2022;50(5):723–32.

71. Zarantonello F, Andreatta G, Sella N, et al. Prone position and lung ventilation and perfusion matching in acute respiratory failure due to COVID-19. Am J Respir Crit Care Med 2020;202(2):278–9.

72. Perier F, Tuffet S, Maraffi T, et al. Effect of positive end-expiratory pressure and proning on ventilation and perfusion in COVID-19 acute respiratory distress syndrome. Am J Respir Crit Care Med 2020;202(12):1713–7.

73. Abou-Arab O, Haye G, Beyls C, et al. Hypoxemia and prone position in mechanically ventilated COVID-19 patients: a prospective cohort study. Can J Anaesth 2021;68(2):262–3.

74. Langer T, Brioni M, Guzzardella A, et al. Prone position in intubated, mechanically ventilated patients with COVID-19: a multi-centric study of more than 1000 patients. Crit Care 2021;25(1):128.

75. Bell J, William Pike C, Kreisel C, et al. Predicting impact of prone position on oxygenation in mechanically ventilated patients with COVID-19. J Intensive Care Med 2022;37(7):883–9.

76. Patel BV, Haar S, Handslip R, et al. Natural history, trajectory, and management of mechanically ventilated COVID-19 patients in the United Kingdom. Intensive Care Med 2021;47(5):549–65.

77. Thompson AE, Ranard BL, Wei Y, et al. Prone positioning in awake, nonintubated patients with Covid-19 hypoxemic respiratory failure. JAMA Intern Med 2020;180(11):1537–9.

78. Retucci M, Aliberti S, Ceruti C, et al. Prone and lateral positioning in spontaneously breathing patients with COVID-19 pneumonia undergoing noninvasive helmet CPAP treatment. CHEST 2020;158(6):2431–5.

79. Coppo A, Bellani G, Winterton D, et al. Feasibility and physiological effects of prone positioning in non-intubated patients with acute respiratory failure due to COVID-19 (PRON-COVID): a prospective cohort study. Lancet Respir Med 2020;8(8):765–74.

80. Xiao Z, Li Y, Chen R, et al. A retrospective study of 78 patients with severe acute respiratory syndrome. Chin Med J (Engl) 2003;116(6):805–10.

81. Siau C, Law J, Tee A, et al. Severe refractory hypoxaemia in H1N1 (2009) intensive care patients: initial experience in an Asian regional hospital. Singapore Med J 2010;51(6):490–5.

82. Brouqui P, Amrane S, Million M, et al. Asymptomatic hypoxia in COVID-19 is associated with poor outcome. Int J Infect Dis 2021;102:233–8.

83. Yang X, Yu Y, Xu J, et al. Clinical course and outcomes of critically ill patients with SARS-CoV-2 pneumonia in Wuhan, China: a single-centered, retrospective, observational study. Lancet Respir Med 2020;8(5):475–81.

84. Novelli L, Raimondi F, Ghirardi A, et al. Frequency, characteristics, and outcome of patients with COVID-19 pneumonia and "silent hypoxemia" at admission: a severity-matched analysis. Panminerva Med 2022. https://doi.org/10.23736/S0031-0808.22.04609-2.

85. Alhusain F, Alromaih A, Alhajress G, et al. Predictors and clinical outcomes of silent hypoxia in COVID-19 patients, a single-center retrospective cohort study. J Infect Public Health 2021;14(11):1595–9.

86. Lauring AS, Tenforde MW, Chappell JD, et al. Clinical severity of, and effectiveness of mRNA vaccines against, covid-19 from omicron, delta, and alpha SARS-CoV-2 variants in the United States: prospective observational study. BMJ 2022;376:e069761.

87. Akiyama Y, Morioka S, Asai Y, et al. Risk factors associated with asymptomatic hypoxemia among COVID-19 patients: a retrospective study using the nationwide Japanese registry, COVIREGI-JP. J Infect Public Health 2022;15(3):312–4.

88. García-Grimshaw M, Flores-Silva FD, Chiquete E, et al. Characteristics and predictors for silent hypoxemia in a cohort of hospitalized COVID-19 patients. Auton Neurosci 2021;235:102855.

89. Santus P, Radovanovic D, Saderi L, et al. Severity of respiratory failure at admission and in-hospital mortality in patients with COVID-19: a prospective observational multicentre study. BMJ Open 2020;10(10):e043651.

90. Weil JV. Variation in human ventilatory control-genetic influence on the hypoxic ventilatory response. Respir Physiol Neurobiol 2003;135(2–3):239–46.

91. Kairaitis K, Harbut P, Hedenstierna G, et al. Ventilation is not depressed in patients with hypoxemia and acute COVID-19 infection. Am J Respir Crit Care Med 2022;205(9):1119–20.

92. Fuehner T, Renger I, Welte T, et al. Silent hypoxia in COVID-19: a case series. Respiration 2022;101(4):376–80.

93. Jouffroy R, Jost D, Prunet B. Prehospital pulse oximetry: a red flag for early detection of silent hypoxemia in COVID-19 patients. Crit Care 2020;24(1):313.

94. Kobayashi S, Nishimura M, Yamomoto M, et al. Relationship between breathlessness and hypoxic and hypercapnic ventilatory response in patients with COPD. Eur Respir J 1996;9(11):2340–5.

95. Sato M, Severinghaus JW, Bickler P. Time course of augmentation and depression of hypoxic ventilatory responses at altitude. J Appl Physiol (1985) 1994;77(1):313–6.

Impact of COVID-19 on Nonpulmonary Critical Illness
Prevalence, Clinical Manifestations, Management, and Outcomes

Mina Pirzadeh, MD[a,b],*, Hallie C. Prescott, MD, MSc[a,b,c]

KEYWORDS

- COVID-19 • Organ failure • Critical illness • Sepsis

KEY POINTS

- SARS-CoV-2 infection has a significant influence on multiple organ systems in the body, a distinctive feature compared with past viral epidemics.
- It is uncommon for hospitalized patients to need nonpulmonary organ support without respiratory failure.
- Nearly every organ failure is independently associated with poorer outcomes in COVID-19 infection.
- Long-term outcomes of isolated and multiorgan failure are underway.

INTRODUCTION

During the past 2 years, SARS-CoV-2 has infected millions of patients worldwide, contributing to 513 million cases and 6.2 million deaths[1] as of May 1, 2022. Although respiratory manifestations are the most common driver of hospitalization, SARS-CoV-2 infection has a wide range of manifestations, including multisystem organ failure in severe cases (**Fig. 1**, **Table 1**). In this review, we discuss the prevalence, pathophysiology, clinical manifestations, treatment, and outcomes of nonpulmonary organ dysfunction from SARS-CoV-2.

Sepsis and Multiorgan Failure

Prevalence

Before the COVID-19 pandemic, viral sepsis was an underrecognized cause of sepsis in adults.[2] However, sepsis may result from any type of infection, including viruses such as influenza, MERS, SARS, and SARS-CoV-2.[3,4] In a meta-analysis by Karakike *and colleagues* of 151 studies published between August 2020 and March 2021 including 218,184 patients hospitalized with COVID-19 (mostly in Asia, Europe, and North America), the prevalence of sepsis (inferred by SOFA scoring, acute organ dysfunction, or organ support) was 33% among ward-treated patients, 78% among intensive care unit (ICU)-treated patients, and 52% overall (**Table 2**).[2] Among ICU-treated patients, the most common organ supports were mechanical ventilation (60%), vasopressor therapy (50%), and renal replacement therapy (RRT; 20%).[2] Overall, although respiratory support was most common, a large proportion of ICU hospitalizations for COVID-19 required nonpulmonary organ support.

In the Society of Critical Care Medicine (SCCM) VIRUS cohort of 20,608 adult hospitalizations for COVID-19 in 16 countries during February to November 2020, 15,001 (72.3%) patients required

a Division of Pulmonary and Critical Care Medicine, University of Michigan, Ann Arbor, MI 48109, USA;
b Veterans Affairs Ann Arbor Healthcare System, Ann Arbor, MI 48105, USA; c VA Center for Clinical Management Research, University of Michigan, Ann Arbor, MI 48109, USA
* Corresponding author. 2215 Fuller Road (111G), Ann Arbor, MI 48105.
E-mail address: mpirzad@med.umich.edu

Clin Chest Med 44 (2023) 249–262
https://doi.org/10.1016/j.ccm.2022.11.011
0272-5231/23/Published by Elsevier Inc.

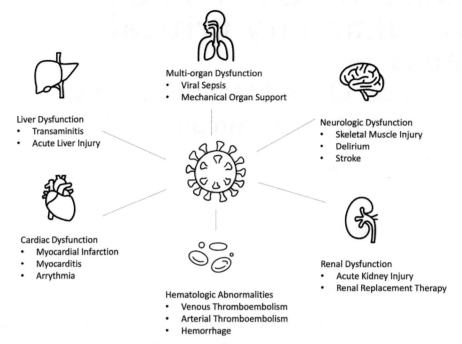

Fig. 1. Nonpulmonary critical organ dysfunctions due to COVID-19 infection.

no organ support, 5005 (24.3%) required invasive mechanical ventilation (IMV), and 602 (2.9%) required vasopressor therapy and/or acute RRT without IMV. Of the 5005 who required IMV, 1749 (34.9%) required IMV only; 2032 (40.6%) required IMV and vasopressors; 655 (13.1%) required IMV, vasopressors, and RRT; 180 (3.6%) required IMV and RRT; and 389 (7.8%) underwent extracorporeal membrane oxygenation.[5] Among 5837 patients in the Health Outcome Predictive Evaluation (HOPE) COVID-19 registry, an international registry of patients hospitalized from March to June 2020 in 8 countries, patients with COVID-19 who developed viral sepsis were older, admitted sooner after symptom onset, and had higher burden of comorbid disease.[6]

Pathophysiology

SARS-COV-2 enters the human host by inhalation. Once viral particles are inhaled, a spike protein on the virus surface attaches to the angiotensin 1 converting enzyme 2 (ACE-2) receptor, then relies on transmembrane protease serine 2 (TMPRSS2) expressed on the surface of respiratory epithelium to enter the cell.[7,8] Once inside the host cell, the virus can replicate. The ACE-2 receptor and TMPRSS2 have been identified in lung alveolar epithelial cells, but also on many other cell types, suggesting that direct viral invasion may be a common mechanism of injury across organs. Beyond direct viral invasion, several other mechanisms may be implicated, including endothelial damage

with thrombo-inflammation,[9] dysregulation of the immune response via high serum level of proinflammatory cytokines such as interleukin (IL) 6 and IL-1 beta, and tumor necrosis factor,[8,10] viral sepsis-induced immune paralysis,[6] and dysregulation of the renin-angiotensin-aldosterone system.[9] Mechanisms of specific organ dysfunctions are discussed further in sections specific to each organ.

Clinical Manifestations

Respiratory failure is the most common organ dysfunction in COVID-19, and other organ dysfunctions rarely occur without respiratory dysfunction. In the HOPE-COVID-19 registry, patients with COVID-19-related sepsis had higher levels of D-dimer, procalcitonin, CRP, troponin, transaminases, ferritin, LDH, and creatinine.[6] Prevalence of leukocytopenia and lymphocytopenia, however, were similar among patients with versus without sepsis.[6] The parsimonious HOPE Sepsis Score identified the following risk factors for sepsis during COVID-19 hospitalization: current smoking, respiratory rate, SpO_2, blood pressure, Glasgow Coma Scale, procalcitonin, troponin I, creatinine, and hemoptysis.[6]

Outcomes

Hospital mortality for COVID-19 is strongly associated with the severity and number of acute organ dysfunctions. In the SCCM VIRUS cohort,

Table 1
Prevalence of organ dysfunction by hospitalization status and association with mortality

Organ Dysfunction	General Prevalence in Hospitalized Patients	ICU Prevalence	Association with Mortality
Sepsis[2]	5% (pooled)	Septic shock 36.4%; Lactate elevated (>2 mmol/L) 47.2%	Mortality could not be assessed separately for patients with and without sepsis because none of the studies reported such outcomes
Cardiac[42,43,89]	21%–45% with troponin elevation; 10%–20% with symptomatic dysfunction	Troponin elevation more common in patients requiring >50% Fraction of inspired oxygen support	Troponin elevation has 2.7× risk in-hospital mortality and associated with 2× increase in major complications, including sepsis, acute kidney failure, multiorgan failure, pulmonary embolism, and major bleeding
Renal[2,30,31,39]	37% to 46% with AKI defined by KDIGO[29] criteria	28.6% to 76% with AKI; 19% received renal replacement therapy	3.4× risk in-hospital mortality; 50% with AKI vs 8% without AKI
Liver[2,51,56]	14% (>2–3 UNL transaminitis); 58%–62% (>ULN)	20.3%	Elevation in AST and direct bilirubin on admission associated with 2× increase in hospital mortality
Neurologic[57]	Fatigue (31%) and myalgia (30%) more common in hospitalized COVID-19 cases; stroke 2%	Skeletal muscle injury (5%) and disturbances of consciousness more likely in severe than nonsevere COVID-19 infection; 50% delirium	In patients ≥60 y of age, the presence of any neurologic manifestations was significantly associated with increased mortality (OR 1.80, 95% CI 1.11–2.91); nonsignificant higher odds of mortality in all patients with neurologic manifestations compared with those without them (OR 1.39)
Coagulopathy[71,81,90]	8%–21%	Pooled prevalence of VTE 24%–31%	Pooled odds mortality 74% higher (OR 1.74) for patients with VTE

in-hospital mortality among 5005 IMV-treated patients was 50% versus 8% among 15,001 patients without organ support.[5] In-hospital mortality increased with additional organ supports from 41% among IMV-treated patients to 71.6% among patient receiving IMV, vasopressors, and RRT (n = 655).[5] In the meta-analysis by Karakike *and colleagues*, in-hospital mortality was 33% among ICU-treated patients, and 42% among IMV-treated patients.[2]

Table 2
Multiorgan dysfunction studies in detail

Study Author	Study Characteristics; Patient No.	Dates of Study	Findings	Conclusion
Karakike et al[2] 2021(Meta-analysis)	151 studies; 218,184 patients Forty-seven studies reported results from Asia, mainly China (21 studies), 21 from North America, 7 from Central and South America, 73 across Europe, one from Australia, and 2 were international	104 studies published in 2020 and 47 published in 2021	Sepsis prevalence was 77.9% (95% CI, 75.9–79.8; I2 = 91%; 57 studies) in the ICU, and 33.3% (95% CI, 30.3–36.4; I2 = 99%; 86 studies) in the general ward Pooled prevalence of organ support: vasopressor use 9.5%; Noninvasive ventilation (NIV) 20.9%; IMV 62.4%; Extracorporeal membrane oxygenation 6.2%; Continuous renal replacement therapy/dialysis 19.9% Pooled prevalence of organ dysfunction: Septic shock 36.4%; lactate elevated (>2 mmol/L) 47.2%; renal dysfunction 28.6%; coagulopathy 17.7%, liver dysfunction 20.3%, CNS dysfunction 8.8%, acute respiratory distress syndrome (ARDS) 87.5%, mild ARDS 21.5%, moderate ARDS 43.7%, severe ARDS 32.1%	The majority COVID-19 patients hospitalized in the ICU meet Sepsis-3 criteria and present with infection-associated organ dysfunction. Awareness and systematic reporting of COVID 19 viral sepsis is crucial to understand prognostic and treatment implications
Domecq et al.[5] 2021(Registry)	16 countries; 168 hospitals (150 from the United States); 20,608 patients	Patient hospitalized from February 15, 2020, to November 30, 2020	Mean age 60.5 y, 54.3% men; 42.4% were admitted to the ICU Organ Support and Mortality: IMV Only 40.8%; IMV + vasopressors 53%; IMV + vasopressors + RRT 71.6%; ECMO 35%; No organ support 8.2%; All patients 19%	Prognosis varies by age and level of organ support. Interhospital variation in mortality of mechanically ventilated patients was not explained by patient characteristics and requires further evaluation

Management

Treatment of COVID-19-related sepsis focuses on resuscitation and supportive therapy, as with other causes of sepsis.[11] Although antibacterial therapy is crucial to the treatment of bacterial sepsis, anti-SARS-CoV-2 therapies such as antivirals and monoclonal antibodies are most effective in earlier phases of SARS-CoV-2 infection, before the onset of acute organ dysfunction.

There has been particular interest in regulating the hyperinflammatory response to SARS-CoV-2 and subsequent viral-induced immunosuppression.[11] High-quality evidence indicate that corticosteroids,[12] IL-6 inhibition,[13] and JAK inhibition[14] reduce mortality, and these therapies are broadly recommended in COVID-19 treatment guidelines.[15] However, timing of initiation is important, and patients should be initiated on these therapies promptly on meeting illness severity criteria. Research is ongoing to clarify the optimal dosing regimens and patient populations for these therapies.

Beyond corticosteroids and IL-6 inhibitors, many other therapies under investigation for treatment/mitigation of disease, including stem cell therapy,[16] short-chain fatty acids,[17] anakinra,[18] infliximab,[19] cytokine therapy (ie, IL-17 inhibitors),[20] vitamin D,[21] vitamin C,[22,23] fecal microbiota transplantation,[24] blood filters,[25] convalescent plasma,[26] plasma exchange,[27] and CRP-apheresis.[28]

Acute Renal Dysfunction

Prevalence

RRT for acute renal failure is the third most common organ support among patients with COVID-19. In a cohort of 3993 patients hospitalized with COVID-19 at 5 hospitals in New York during March to May 2020, 46% had acute kidney injury (AKI, defined by Kidney Disease Improving Global Outcomes criteria[29]), including 76% of ICU-treated patients.[30] About 19% of patients with AKI received RRT.[30] In a separate cohort of 5449 patients hospitalized with COVID-19 at 13 hospitals in New York during March to May 2020, 37% had AKI, including 90% of IMV-treated patients. Renal failure and RRT were largely limited to patients with respiratory failure. Indeed, in the 13-hospital New York cohort, nearly all patients treated with RRT were also receiving IMV.[31] In the meta-analysis by Karakike *and colleagues*, the pooled prevalence of RRT among ICU patients with COVID-19 was 20%.

Histology and pathophysiology

The hypothesized mechanisms of COVID-19-related AKI are largely drawn from biopsy and autopsy studies. In a series of 10 patients with COVID-19-related renal failure requiring RRT, the most common histologic finding was acute tubular injury,[32] with ACE2 highly expressed on proximal tubular cells.[33] In a series of 63 decedents with COVID-19 respiratory infection, SARS-CoV-2 RNA was detected in 60%, including 72% of decedents with AKI.[34] Other findings included thrombotic microangiopathy, pauci-immune crescent glomerulonephritis, widespread myoglobin casts.[32] Several studies found evidence of live virus, suggesting direct kidney tropism through angiotensin-converting enzyme-2 receptors expressed on proximal tubule cells and podocytes.[34] Additionally, microthrombi formation of the capillaries around the renal tubulars was seen on autopsy, suggesting a hypercoagulable effect.[33,35] Whether from direct viral invasion, hypoxia, or hypercoagulability, there may be indirect causes for renal injury including hemodynamic instability, mitochondrial dysfunction,[36] excessive diuresis, nephrotoxic exposure, cytokine storm, and rhabdomyolysis.[34]

Clinical manifestations

COVID-19-related AKI manifests as decreased glomerular filtration, elevated serum creatinine and BUN, frequent proteinuria,[30,33,37] and occasional hematuria and leukocyturia.[30] In a cohort of 182 patients hospitalized with COVID-19-associated AKI, serum creatine was similar, proteinuria was more common, and dialysis was more common than in non–COVID-19-related AKI.[38]

Outcomes

The development of COVID-19-related AKI is associated with worse outcomes, particularly among patients requiring RRT. Although AKI is a marker of worse disease, the association persists after adjustment for illness severity, suggesting that renal injury may also directly contribute to worse outcomes. In the 13-hospital New York cohort, the development of AKI was associated with a 3.4-fold increased risk of in-hospital mortality in adjusted analysis, whereas RRT was associated with 6.4-fold increased risk.[39] In the 5-hospital New York cohort, in-hospital mortality was 50% among patients with COVID-19 and AKI versus 8% among patients without renal injury.[30] Furthermore, among 832 patients with AKI who survived to hospital discharge, 35% had not returned to baseline renal function by discharge.[30] In a single-center telephone follow-up of 300 patients who survived ICU hospitalization for COVID-19 during March to April of 2020 in New York, only 42% survived to 6 months postdischarge. At 6 months postdischarge, AKI recovered in 74% of survivors, including 77% who liberated from dialysis.[40]

Management

Treatment strategies for COVID-19-related AKI are similar to standard management of AKI from other causes. Management focuses on mitigating further renal injury through avoidance of nephrotoxic medications, renally dosing medications, and maintaining perfusion to the kidney. The threshold for initiating RRT is similar to non–COVID-19-related renal failure. Clotting of continuous renal replacement therapy (CRRT) filters has led to significant resource utilization. In a case series of 65 patients who received CRRT for COVID-19-related renal failure at a single U.S. hospital, 85% lost at least one filter, with a median filter life of only 6.5 hours.[41] Studies are underway testing interventions to mitigate progression of renal disease, including oral medications targeting inflammatory pathways (NCT05038488) and treatments such as CRP-apheresis (NCT04898062) (**Table 3**).

Cardiac Dysfunction

Prevalence

The spectrum of cardiac manifestations of COVID-19 includes asymptomatic cardiac biomarker elevation and symptomatic cardiac dysfunction such as heart failure, arrhythmia, and sudden cardiac arrest. Biomarker elevation occurs in approximately 20% to 35% of patients hospitalized with COVID-19. In a meta-analysis of 35 studies of 22,473 patients hospitalized in 2020 with COVID-19, troponin was elevated in 21% of patients tested on admission.[42] In a cohort of 2736 patients hospitalized in single system in New York, troponin was elevated in 36%.[43] Symptomatic cardiac dysfunction is present in approximately 10% to 20% of hospitalized patients. In a study of 748 patients hospitalized in Europe and Australia during January-October 2020, 141 (19%) had an acute cardiac complication, including cardiovascular death (7%), heart failure (5%), pulmonary embolism (5%), sustained supraventricular tachycardia or ventricular arrhythmia (4%), cardiac arrest (2%), myocarditis (2%), and acute coronary syndrome (1%).[44]

Pathophysiology/mechanisms

SARS-COV-2 is hypothesized to cause cardiac injury via endothelial inflammation, immune activation, direct myocardial injury, acute right heart strain secondary to acute respiratory distress syndrome and/or pulmonary embolism, and hypoxic injury.[45]

Clinical manifestations

Cardiac biomarkers, including troponin and BNP, may be elevated in up to one-third of patients hospitalized with COVID-19. Cardiac arrhythmias, including atrial fibrillation, bradyarrhythmias, and ventricular arrhythmias, occur in a minority of patients. The extent to which arrhythmias are directly mediated by SARS-CoV-2 versus general acute illness is unclear. Myocarditis may be triggered by a variety of viral infections including SARS-CoV-2, but the prevalence of this manifestation is unknown.[46] Most myocarditis occurs simultaneous to acute respiratory disease, but case reports of delayed myocarditis have been reported.[46] Although not common, cardiac manifestations can be the presenting symptom of COVID-19. In a series of 28 patients hospitalized in Italy during February-March 2020 with COVID-19 and ST segment elevation myocardial infarction (STEMI), 24 of 28 patients had the STEMI as the first manifestation of SARS-CoV-2 infection.[47] Seventeen had a culprit lesion and underwent revascularization.[47]

Outcomes

Troponin elevation indicates myocardial injury and is consistently associated with worse outcomes.[44,48] In a meta-analysis of 11 studies of patients hospitalized with COVID-19 during 2020, troponin elevation was associated with 2.7-fold increased risk of in-hospital mortality[42] in adjusted analysis. In a study of 416 patients hospitalized with COVID-19 in China in 2020, cardiac biomarker elevation was associated with increased need for IMV.[49] In a meta-analysis of 3 studies of in-hospital cardiac arrest, SARS-CoV-2 infection was associated with lower rates of shockable rhythm (9.6% vs 19.8%, $P < .001$), lower rates of ROSC (33.9% vs 52.1%, $P < .001$), and higher 30-day mortality (77.2% vs 59.7%, $P = .003$).[50]

Management/treatment

Treatment of COVID-19-related cardiac injury is similar to the management of cardiac injury from other causes. As of May 1, 2022, 253 phase 2 to 4 interventional clinical trials were registered in clinicaltrials.gov to test interventions, prevent or mitigate cardiac complications, including trials of colchicine (NCT04510038), antiplatelet and anticoagulant triple therapy (NCT04333407), angiotensin receptor neprilysin inhibitors (NCT04883528) and anti-IL1b (NCT04365153) antibody therapy.

Table 3
Organ-specific randomized control trials of therapeutics in COVID-19 infections[a]

Organ Function	NCT Number	Name of Study
Cardiac	NCT04883528 NCT04365153	Protecting with ARNI against cardiac consequences of Coronavirus Disease 2019 with Drug: Sacubitril/Valsartan Oral Tablet [Entresto] Canakinumab to Reduce Deterioration of Cardiac and Respiratory Function in SARSCoV2 Associated Acute Myocardial Injury with Heightened Inflammation (completed)
Renal	NCT04402957 NCT04818216	LSALT Peptide vs Placebo to Prevent ARDS and Acute Kidney Injury in Patients Infected With SARS-CoV-2(COVID-19) Nicotinamide Riboside in SARS-CoV-2 (COVID-19) Patients for Renal Protection (NIRVANA)
Liver	NCT04816682	Silymarin, phase 4, Does Silymarin Mitigate Clinical Course of COVID-19 in Patients Admitted to an Internal Medicine Ward with Elevated Liver Enzymes?
Neuro	NCT04904536	An International, Investigator Initiated and Conducted, Pragmatic Clinical Trial to Determine Whether 40 mg Atorvastatin Daily Can Improve Neurocognitive Function in Adults With Long COVID Neurologic Symptoms; Statin TReatment for COVID-19 to OptimiseNeuroloGical recovERy (STRONGER)
Coagulopathy	NCT04650087 NCT04508023	COVID-19 Post-hospital Thrombosis Prevention Trial: An Adaptive, Multicenter, Prospective, Randomized Platform Trial Evaluating the Efficacy and Safety of Antithrombotic Strategies in Patients With COVID-19 Following Hospital Discharge A Study of Rivaroxaban to Reduce the Risk of Major Venous and Arterial Thrombotic Events, Hospitalization and Death in Medically Ill Outpatients With Acute, Symptomatic Coronavirus Disease 2019 (COVID-19) Infection (PREVENT-HD)

[a] Partial list of active interventional phase 2–4 randomized control trials.

Liver Dysfunction

Prevalence

Liver enzymes elevations are common in patients requiring hospitalization for COVID-19 but severe liver dysfunction is a rare manifestation of COVID-19. In a study of 2073 patients hospitalized with COVID-19 in China during January to April 2020, 62% of patients had liver enzymes greater than the upper limit of normal (ULN), including 46% on admission. Liver dysfunction was hepatocellular in 40%, cholestatic in 3%, mixed in 12%, and other in 8%. However, liver injury (>2–3× ULN) occurred in only 14%, including 5% on admission.[51] In a US cohort of 834 patients hospitalized with COVID-19 during April 2020, 12% had significant liver injury (5× ULN) during hospitalization.[52] Acute liver failure (defined as acute liver injury with hepatic encephalopathy) is a rare complication of COVID-19.[51]

Pathophysiology/mechanisms

Similar to other solid organs, the liver is susceptible to hypoxic, ischemic, thrombotic, congestive, and direct viral injury. Several therapies for COVID-19, such as remdesivir and tocilizumab can be hepatotoxic, making drug-induced liver injury a potential cause of liver injury during hospitalization. The ACE2 receptor, where the SARS CoV-2 enters the host is expressed in higher amounts on cholangiocytes than hepatocytes.[53] In series of 40 decedents, macrovesicular steatosis was the most common finding (75%), followed by lobular necroinflammation (50%), portal inflammation (50%), and cholestasis (38%).[54]

Clinical manifestations

Liver enzyme abnormalities in COVID-19 include hepatocellular, cholestatic, and mixed patterns of injury, with most cases being mild (1–2× the ULN). The 834-patient US cohort found that the most common liver abnormalities were AST (63%), ALT (34%), alkaline phosphatase (12%), and total bilirubin (3%).[52] The median time to peak of AST level was 3 days (IQR 1–6 days) postadmission.[52]

Outcomes

Liver injury due to COVID-19 is associated with worse outcomes. In a meta-analysis of 26 studies of patients hospitalized with COVID-19 in China, baseline AST greater than ULN was associated with increased mortality (odds ratio [OR] = 3.82, P = .05), ICU admission (OR = 2.98, P = .06), and nonfatal complications (OR = 2.95, P = .08).[55] In study of 565 patients hospitalized with COVID-19 on general medicine wards in Italy during 2020, 58% had abnormal liver function, which was associated with higher rates of ICU transfer (20% vs 8%), AKI (22% vs 13%), need for IMV (14% vs 6%), and mortality (21% vs 11%).[56] Abnormal liver function was independently associated with death and/or transfer to the ICU (aOR = 3.5).[56]

Management/treatment

The management of acute liver injury in COVID-19—including hepatocellular, cholestatic, and mixed liver injury—is consistent with current strategies for management of non–COVID-19-related liver injury, including maintaining perfusion, minimizing hepatotoxic medications, optimizing volume status, and ruling out of other causes of hepatic injury. As of May 1, 2022, there was one interventional clinical trial registered on clinicaltrials.gov targeted specifically at patients with elevated liver enzymes in the setting of COVID-19 (NCT04816682).

Neurologic Dysfunction

Prevalence and clinical manifestations

The neurologic manifestations of COVID-19 are varied but can cause severe debility.

A meta-analysis of 48 studies published in the 2020, including 2839 patients with severe/critical COVID and 7493 with nonsevere COVID-19, analyzed neurologic manifestations and their association with COVID-19 severity.[57] Severe COVID-19 was associated with skeletal muscle injury, delirium or impaired consciousness, and fatigue, and less alteration in smell or taste. Myopathy was associated with prolonged hospitalization,[58] and critical illness neuropathy was more prevalent in COVID-19 cohorts than non-COVID-19 cohorts.[59] In a retrospective cohort of 277 patients admitted with a stroke to a large NYC hospital in March to April 2020, 38% were SARS-CoV-2 positive. The COVID-19-positive patients were more likely to have a cryptogenic stroke cause, lobar stroke location, admission to the ICU, and in-hospital mortality.[60] The majority (68%) of COVID-19-positive patients with stroke had parenchymal abnormalities on chest imaging, although stroke has been reported as the presenting sign of COVID-19 in patients without respiratory symptoms.[61] A meta-analysis of 29 studies published in 2020 with 43,024 patients found a 2% pooled prevalence of stroke, which is higher than the prevalence in influenza (0.2%).[62]

Delirium is a common manifestation in critical COVID-19 and known to be associated long-term cognitive impairment.[63] In an international cohort of 2088 ICU-treated patients during January to April 2020, 82% were comatose, for a median of 10 days, and 54.9% experienced delirium, for a median of 3 days.[64]

Pathophysiology/mechanisms

The expression of ACE2 receptor is significantly lower in the central and peripheral nervous system compared with other organs but is found in glial cells in the brain and spinal neurons. In vitro models of the human blood–brain barrier showed a negative impact of SARS CoV-2 spike protein, and brain endothelial cells showed a distinct proinflammatory response.[65,66] Endothelial dysfunction, coagulation abnormalities, direct viral transmission through olfactory nerve, hypoxic brain injury, and disruption of the blood–brain barrier[65] are all postulated to play a role in neurologic manifestation of patients.[8] Loss of taste/smell, meningitis, encephalitis, cerebral vasculitis, and myalgia may all result from direct viral invasion of the nervous system.[16] Encephalopathy from hypoxia, hyperinflammatory response, and hypercoagulability (leading to stroke) are indirect manifestations of COVID-19 infection on the central nervous system.

Outcomes

Similar to other acute organ dysfunction, neurologic dysfunction is associated with increased mortality. In a meta-analysis of 21 studies, 770 of 2982 patients with neurologic manifestations died. The pooled prevalence of mortality among patients with neurologic manifestations was 27% (95% CI 19%–35%).[57] For patients aged older than 60 years, any neurologic manifestation was associated with mortality (OR 1.80, 95% CI 1.11–2.91).[57] Nearly 1 in 50 patients developed a stroke, which has been associated with marked increase in risk of mortality.[67] COVID-19 infection is also associated with significant morbidity in ICU survivors. A multicenter Dutch prospective cohort with follow-up to 1 year post-ICU, physical symptoms were reported in 74.3%, mental symptoms in 26.2%, and cognitive symptoms in 16.2%.[68] The most symptoms were weakened condition (38.9%), joint stiffness (26.3%), joint pain (25.5%), muscle weakness (24.8%), and myalgia (21.3%).[68]

Management/treatment

The management and treatment of neurologic manifestations of COVID-19 mirror strategies used for non–COVID-19-associated symptoms/diseases. Given the known association of delirium

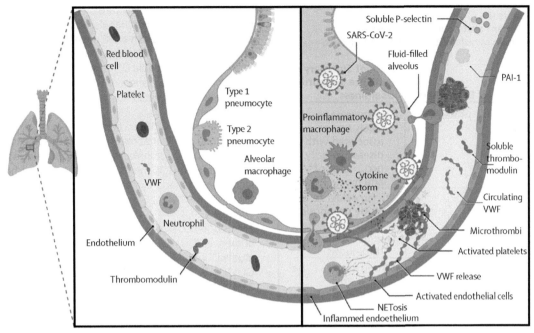

Fig. 2. Endotheliopathy in COVID-19 coagulopathy. (Reprinted with permission from Elsevier, The Lancet, August 2020, 7(8), e553-e555.)

and poor outcomes,[69] strategies to reduce delirium in mechanically ventilated patients is extremely important. In a large international cohort of 2088 ICU patients, of which 87.5% undergoing mechanical ventilation at some point in their hospitalization, benzodiazepine use was identified as a modifiable risk factor for the development of delirium while the family visitation was associated with decreased risk for delirium. This information should be considered for sedations protocols as well as hospital policies regarding visitation. The treatment of stroke follows guidelines for non–COVID-19 stroke but studies are underway to assess the safety, feasibility, and efficacy of thrombectomy for the management of acute ischemia strokes in patients with COVID-19 (NCT04406090). Early mobility and rehabilitation are crucial to reduce the morbidity associated with COVID-19 disease.

Hematologic Abnormalities (Coagulopathy)

Prevalence
Coagulation abnormalities are a common manifestation of severe and critical COVID-19. In a meta-analysis of 24 studies including 2570 patients with critical COVID-19, the pooled prevalence of clinically detected venous thromboembolism (VTE) was 31% and increased to 48% if using systematic screening (eg, for extremity swelling and/or

elevated D-dimer).[70] A subsequent meta-analysis of 19 studies with 1599 patients receiving prophylactic anticoagulation reported pooled prevalences of VTE, deep vein thrombosis (DVT), and PE in 30.1%, 27.2% and 18.3%, respectively.[71] Among studies with routine screening, DVT was identified in 48% versus in 15% with symptom-driven testing ($P < .0001$).[71] The frequent occurrence of VTE when not clinically suspected is corroborated on postmortem studies.[72] Although rare, aortic thrombosis, occlusion of large vessels, and solid organ infarct have been reported.[73] In the abdomen and pelvis, hemorrhagic complications were more common than thrombotic complications, including hematomas of retroperitoneum and abdominal wall.[73] Overall, rates of VTE among patients hospitalized with COVID-19 are approximately 3-fold higher than among historical matched controls,[74] whereas rates of arterial thromboembolism (ATE) are lower.[75]

Pathophysiology and clinical manifestations
The balance of coagulation and fibrinolysis is deranged in SARS-CoV-2 infection (**Fig. 2**). Abnormal laboratories associated with coagulopathy in COVID-19 are summarized in **Table 4**. Although the exact mechanism is incompletely understood, endothelial dysfunction is widely regarded as the major driver of the prothrombotic state in COVID-19.[73,76] Most patients hospitalized

Table 4
Current and novel biomarkers of hypercoagulability in COVID-19 disease

Serologic Biomarkers	Current Summary of Evidence Supporting Usefulness
C-reactive protein	Strong evidence that levels are associated with disease severity, occurrence of VTE and mortality
IL-6	Strong evidence to guide prognosis but not for prediction of thrombosis
D-dimer	Strong evidence that levels are associated with disease severity and adverse outcomes, including mortality
aPTT/Anti-Xa	Not useful as a marker of COVID-19 severity or prognosis
Neuroendocrine tumors	Potential use in detecting severe vs nonsevere COVID-19 but not in predicting thrombotic risk
Complement factors	Potentially of use in detecting severe COVID-19, longer-term prognostic utility unknown
ACE2	Discrimination of COVID-19 severity not shown
Calprotectin	Potentially of use in detecting severe COVID-19 and assessing the risk of thrombosis

From Gorog DA, Storey RF, Gurbel PA, et al. Current and novel biomarkers of thrombotic risk in COVID-19: a Consensus Statement from the International COVID-19 Thrombosis Biomarkers Colloquium. Nat Rev Cardiol. 2022;19(7):475-495.

with COVID-19 have elevated D-dimer, mild prolongation of aPTT and/or PT, and mild thrombocytopenia.[77] It is unclear whether these abnormalities indicate hypercoagulability or consumptive disseminated intravascular coagulation (DIC).[77]

Hypofibrinogenemia is rare[77] and peripheral smears support a hypercoagulable state.[78] However, in prospective cohort of 98 patients hospitalized in ICU with COVID-19 in the United States during 2020 to 2021 at a single US center, thromboelastographic parameters and conventional coagulation parameters suggested a relative consumptive coagulopathy.[79]

Overall, COVID-19 is associated with a prothrombotic profile that may be driven by excessive inflammation, endothelial activation, platelet activation, impaired fibrinolysis, immune-related molecular events, and systemic hypercoagulability.[80]

Outcomes
Thromboembolism is associated with worse outcomes in COVID-19. In a meta-analysis of 42 studies with 8217 patients hospitalized with COVID-19, the pooled VTE rate in-hospital was 21% (31% among ICU-treated patients).[81] Pooled in-hospital mortality was 23% vs 13% among patients with versus without thromboembolism. The pooled odds of mortality were 74% higher for patients diagnosed with a thromboembolism (OR 1.74, $P = .04$).[81]

Treatment
Several high-quality randomized control trials (RCT)s have addressed the prevention of thrombotic complications in COVID-19. The current evidence supports prophylactic anticoagulation in critically ill patients but therapeutic anticoagulation in ward patients. An open-label trial[82] that randomized 1207 patients to therapeutic heparin anticoagulation versus heparin thromboprophylaxis was stopped for futility. Patients randomized to therapeutic anticoagulation had fewer organ-support free days (median 1 vs 4 days) and similar survival to discharge (62.7% vs 64.5%).[82] However, among noncritically patients, full-dose anticoagulation decreased the need for IMV and other organ supports (aOR = 1.27), without increasing major bleeding (1.9% vs 0.9%).[83] Similarly, a multicenter US trial evaluated the impact of therapeutic anticoagulation for patients hospitalized with COVID-19 with elevated D-dimer levels (>4× ULN) or sepsis-induced coagulopathy score of 4 or more. The study found that—among noncritically ill patients—the combined outcome of VTE, ATE, or mortality was lower (16.7% vs 36.1%, $P = .004$) among patients randomized to therapeutic-dose anticoagulation.[75] However, among critically patients, outcomes were similar between arms (51.1 vs 55.3%, $P = .71$).[75] A multicenter RCT in Iran randomized 562 patients with critical COVID to intermediate-dose thromboprophylaxis (enoxaparin 1 mg/kg daily) vs standard thromboprophylaxis (enoxaparin

40 mg daily).[84] Outcomes, including composite outcome of VTE or ATE, ECMO treatment, and 30-day mortality, were similar among patients randomized to intermediate versus standard enoxaparin dosing. At this time, it is unclear whether continuing anticoagulation after hospital discharge affects short-term or long-term outcomes. However, studies are underway evaluating posthospitalization direct oral anticoagulants to prevent or reduce long-term symptoms associated with COVID-19 infection (NCT04801940).

New biomarkers for tests of coagulation, fibrinolysis, and platelet activation are being studied to support its usefulness for prognostic, diagnostic and management decisions in COVID-19-related thrombosis[80] (**Table 4**). Many advocate for the use of personalized protocol-based titration of heparin anticoagulation,[85,86] as studies consistently show heparin resistance manifested by subtherapeutic anti-Xa levels compared with standard dosing protocols[87,88]; however, the exact biomarker of choice has yet to be determined. In all, the prevalence and severe prognostic implications of thromboembolism should make thrombotic risk assessment and VTE prevention a priority.

SUMMARY

Although SARS-CoV-2 infection most commonly causes respiratory symptoms and impairment, it can also cause nonpulmonary organ dysfunction, most commonly shock, AKI, and hypercoagulability. Neurologic, cardiac, and, to a lesser degree, liver injury may also occur from SARS-CoV-2. Management of extrapulmonary organ dysfunction largely focuses on supportive care practices that are applicable regardless of the cause of organ injury. However, there is emerging evidence to support therapeutic anticoagulation in noncritically ill patients to mitigate risk for VTE.

CLINICS CARE POINTS

- Severe COVID-19 respiratory infection is often accompanied with other organ injuries, which are independently associated with poor outcomes.
- It is important for providers to assess for multi-organ involvement of COVID-19 infection, as each organ injury impacts patient morbidity and mortality.
- At this time, non-pulmonary organ injury is managed with supportive care and follows best practices that are applicable regardless of the cause of injury.

- There is emerging data that supports therapeutic over prophylactic anticoagulation in non-critically ill patients admitted to the general hospital ward.

DISCLOSURE

The authors have no commercial or financial conflicts of interest. H.C. Prescott has grant funding from VA, United States, AHRQ, United States, and BCBSM, unrelated to this article.

REFERENCES

1. Coronavirus World Map: tracking the global outbreak. the New York times. Available at: https://www.nytimes.com/interactive/2021/world/covid-cases.html?smid=url-share. Updated May 1, 2022. Accessed May 1, 2022, 2022.
2. Karakike E, Giamarellos-Bourboulis EJ, Kyprianou M, et al. Coronavirus disease 2019 as cause of viral sepsis: a systematic review and meta-analysis. Crit Care Med 2021;49(12):2042–57.
3. Shappell CN, Klompas M, Rhee C. Quantifying the burden of viral sepsis during the coronavirus disease 2019 pandemic and beyond. Crit Care Med 2021;49(12):2140–3.
4. Lopes-Pacheco M, Silva PL, Cruz FF, et al. Pathogenesis of multiple organ injury in covid-19 and potential therapeutic strategies. review. Front Physiol 2021;12. https://doi.org/10.3389/fphys.2021.593223.
5. Domecq JP, Lal A, Sheldrick CR, et al. Outcomes of patients with coronavirus disease 2019 receiving organ support therapies: the international viral infection and respiratory illness universal study registry. Crit Care Med 2021;49(3):437–48.
6. Abumayyaleh M, Nunez-Gil IJ, El-Battrawy I, et al. Sepsis of patients infected by SARS-CoV-2: real-World experience from the international HOPE-COVID-19-registry and validation of hope sepsis score. Front Med (Lausanne) 2021;8:728102.
7. Loganathan S, Kuppusamy M, Wankhar W, et al. Angiotensin-converting enzyme 2 (ACE2): COVID 19 gate way to multiple organ failure syndromes. Respir Physiol Neurobiol 2021;283:103548.
8. Mokhtari T, Hassani F, Ghaffari N, et al. COVID-19 and multiorgan failure: a narrative review on potential mechanisms. J Mol Histol 2020;51(6):613–28.
9. Gupta A, Madhavan MV, Sehgal K, et al. Extrapulmonary manifestations of COVID-19. Nat Med 2020;26(7):1017–32.
10. Xu Z, Shi L, Wang Y, et al. Pathological findings of COVID-19 associated with acute respiratory distress syndrome. Lancet Respir Med 2020;8(4):420–2.

11. Olwal CO, Nganyewo NN, Tapela K, et al. Parallels in sepsis and COVID-19 conditions: implications for managing severe COVID-19. Front Immunol 2021; 12:602848.
12. Group RC, Horby P, Lim WS, et al. Dexamethasone in hospitalized patients with covid-19. N Engl J Med 2021;384(8):693–704.
13. Group RC. Tocilizumab in patients admitted to hospital with COVID-19 (RECOVERY): a randomised, controlled, open-label, platform trial. Lancet 2021; 397(10285):1637–45.
14. Kramer A, Prinz C, Fichtner F, et al. Janus kinase inhibitors for the treatment of COVID-19. Cochrane Database Syst Rev 2022;6:CD015209.
15. COVID-19 Treatment Guidelines Panel. Coronavirus disease 2019 (COVID-19) treatment guidelines. national institutes of health. Available at. https://www.covid19treatmentguidelines.nih.gov/. Accessed August 28th, 2022.
16. Bhalerao A, Raut S, Noorani B, et al. Molecular mechanisms of multi-organ failure in COVID-19 and potential of stem cell therapy. Cells 2021; 10(11). https://doi.org/10.3390/cells10112878.
17. Jardou M, Lawson R. Supportive therapy during COVID-19: the proposed mechanism of short-chain fatty acids to prevent cytokine storm and multi-organ failure. Med Hypotheses 2021;154:110661.
18. Hellenic Institute for the Study of S. suPAR-Guided Anakinra Treatment for Management of Severe Respiratory Failure by COVID-19. https://clinicaltrials.gov/ct2/show/NCT04680949.
19. Jena University H, German Federal Ministry of E. Celltrion. Infliximab in the Treatment of Patients With Severe COVID-19 Disease. 2022. https://clinicaltrials.gov/ct2/show/NCT04922827.
20. University of Sao P, Conselho Nacional de Desenvolvimento Científico eT, Science Valley Research I. Survival TRial using CytoKines in COVID-19 (STRUCK trial). Updated March 31. https://ClinicalTrials.gov/show/NCT04724629.
21. Prof. Dr. Jörg L, Cantonal Hosptal B. High Dose Vitamin-D Substitution in Patients With COVID-19: a Randomized Controlled, Multi Center Study. 2021. https://clinicaltrials.gov/ct2/show/NCT04525820
22. Hunter Holmes Mcguire Veteran Affairs Medical C, McGuire Research I. Administration of Intravenous Vitamin C in Novel Coronavirus Infection (COVID-19) and Decreased Oxygenation. 2020. https://clinicaltrials.gov/ct2/show/NCT04357782.
23. Université de S, Lotte, John Hecht Memorial F. Lessening organ dysfunction with VITamin C. Updated August 15. https://ClinicalTrials.gov/show/NCT03680274.
24. Medical University of W, Human Biome Institute P. The Impact of Fecal Microbiota Transplantation as an Immunomodulation on the Risk Reduction of COVID-19 Disease Progression With Escalating Cytokine Storm and Inflammatory Parameters. 2022. https://clinicaltrials.gov/ct2/show/NCT04824222.
25. ExThera Medical Europe BV, ExThera Medical C, Vivantes Klinikum N. Safety & Effectiveness Evaluation of Seraph 100 in Treatment of Pts With COVID-19. 2022. https://clinicaltrials.gov/ct2/show/NCT04547257
26. Helsinki University Central H. Finnish Red C. Convalescent Plasma in the Treatment of Covid-19. https://clinicaltrials.gov/ct2/show/NCT04730401.
27. Unicef, Pak Emirates Military Hospital R. Therapeutic Plasma Exchange for Coronavirus Disease-2019 Triggered Cytokine Release. Storm 2020;. https://clinicaltrials.gov/ct2/show/NCT04485169.
28. Bechman K, Yates M, Mann K, et al. Inpatient COVID-19 mortality has reduced over time: results from an observational cohort. PLoS One 2022; 17(1):e0261142.
29. 2012 kidney disease: improving global outcomes (KDIGO) Clinical practice guideline for acute kidney injury (AKI). Available at: https://kdigo.org/guidelines/acute-kidney-injury/. Accessed May 1, 2022.
30. Chan L, Chaudhary K, Saha A, et al. AKI in hospitalized patients with COVID-19. J Am Soc Nephrol 2021;32(1):151–60.
31. Hirsch JS, Ng JH, Ross DW, et al. Acute kidney injury in patients hospitalized with COVID-19. Kidney Int 2020;98(1):209–18.
32. Sharma P, Uppal NN, Wanchoo R, et al. COVID-19-Associated kidney injury: a case series of kidney biopsy findings. J Am Soc Nephrol 2020;31(9):1948–58.
33. Yang X, Jin Y, Li R, et al. Prevalence and impact of acute renal impairment on COVID-19: a systematic review and meta-analysis. Crit Care 2020;24(1):356.
34. Braun F, Lutgehetmann M, Pfefferle S, et al. SARS-CoV-2 renal tropism associates with acute kidney injury. Lancet 2020;396(10251):597–8.
35. Wang D, Hu B, Hu C, et al. Clinical characteristics of 138 hospitalized patients with 2019 novel coronavirus-infected pneumonia in Wuhan, China. JAMA 2020;323(11):1061–9.
36. Alexander MP, Mangalaparthi KK, Madugundu AK, et al. Acute kidney injury in severe covid-19 has similarities to sepsis-associated kidney injury: a multiomics study. Mayo Clin Proc 2021;96(10):2561–75.
37. Cheng Y, Luo R, Wang K, et al. Kidney disease is associated with in-hospital death of patients with COVID-19. Kidney Int 2020;97(5):829–38.
38. Nugent J, Aklilu A, Yamamoto Y, et al. Assessment of acute kidney injury and longitudinal kidney function after hospital discharge among patients with and without COVID-19. JAMA Netw Open 2021;4(3): e211095.
39. Ng JH, Hirsch JS, Hazzan A, et al. Outcomes Among patients hospitalized with COVID-19 and

acute kidney injury. Am J Kidney Dis 2021;77(2): 204–15.e1.

40. Chand S, Kapoor S, Naqvi A, et al. Long-term follow up of renal and other acute organ failure in survivors of critical illness due to covid-19. J Intensive Care Med 2021;37(6):736–42.

41. Endres P, Rosovsky R, Zhao S, et al. Filter clotting with continuous renal replacement therapy in COVID-19. J Thromb Thrombolysis 2021;51(4): 966–70.

42. Zhao B-C, Liu W-F, Lei S-H, et al. Prevalence and prognostic value of elevated troponins in patients hospitalised for coronavirus disease 2019: a systematic review and meta-analysis. J Intensive Care 2020;8(1):88.

43. Lala A, Johnson KW, Januzzi JL, et al. Prevalence and impact of myocardial injury in patients hospitalized with COVID-19 infection. J Am Coll Cardiol 2020;76(5):533–46.

44. Henein MY, Mandoli GE, Pastore MC, et al. Biomarkers predict in-hospital major adverse cardiac events in COVID-19 patients: a multicenter international study. J Clin Med 2021;10(24). https://doi.org/10.3390/jcm10245863.

45. Tanacli R, Doeblin P, Gotze C, et al. COVID-19 vs. classical myocarditis associated myocardial injury evaluated by cardiac magnetic resonance and endomyocardial biopsy. Front Cardiovasc Med 2021; 8:737257.

46. Farshidfar F, Koleini N, Ardehali H. Cardiovascular complications of COVID-19. JCI Insight 2021;6(13). https://doi.org/10.1172/jci.insight.148980.

47. Stefanini GG, Montorfano M, Trabattoni D, et al. ST-elevation myocardial infarction in patients with COVID-19: clinical and angiographic outcomes. Circulation 2020;141(25):2113–6.

48. Guo T, Fan Y, Chen M, et al. Cardiovascular implications of fatal outcomes of patients with coronavirus disease 2019 (COVID-19). JAMA Cardiol 2020; 5(7):811–8.

49. Shi S, Qin M, Shen B, et al. Association of cardiac injury with mortality in hospitalized patients with COVID-19 in Wuhan, China. JAMA Cardiol 2020; 5(7):802–10.

50. Bielski K, Makowska K, Makowski A, et al. Impact of COVID-19 on in-hospital cardiac arrest outcomes: an updated meta-analysis. Cardiol J 2021;28(6): 816–24.

51. Ding ZY, Li GX, Chen L, et al. Association of liver abnormalities with in-hospital mortality in patients with COVID-19. J Hepatol 2021;74(6):1295–302.

52. Chew M, Tang Z, Radcliffe C, et al. Significant liver injury during hospitalization for COVID-19 is not associated with liver insufficiency or death. Clin Gastroenterol Hepatol 2021;19(10):2182–91. e7.

53. Chai X, Hu L, Zhang Y, et al. Specific ACE2 expression in cholangiocytes may cause liver damage after 2019-nCoV infection. bioRxiv 2020;2020. https://doi.org/10.1101/2020.02.03.931766.

54. Lagana SM, Kudose S, Iuga AC, et al. Hepatic pathology in patients dying of COVID-19: a series of 40 cases including clinical, histologic, and virologic data. Mod Pathol 2020;33(11):2147–55.

55. Ampuero J, Sanchez Y, Garcia-Lozano MR, et al. Impact of liver injury on the severity of COVID-19: a systematic review with meta-analysis. Rev Esp Enferm Dig 2021;113(2):125–35.

56. Piano S, Dalbeni A, Vettore E, et al. Abnormal liver function tests predict transfer to intensive care unit and death in COVID-19. Liver Int 2020;40(10): 2394–406.

57. Misra S, Kolappa K, Prasad M, et al. Frequency of neurologic manifestations in COVID-19: a systematic review and meta-analysis. Neurology 2021; 97(23):e2269–81.

58. Romero-Sánchez CM, Díaz-Maroto I, Fernández-Díaz E, et al. Neurologic manifestations in hospitalized patients with COVID-19. ALBACOVID registry 2020;95(8):e1060–70.

59. Bocci T, Campiglio L, Zardoni M, et al. Critical illness neuropathy in severe COVID-19: a case series. Neurol Sci 2021;42(12):4893–8.

60. Dhamoon MS, Thaler A, Gururangan K, et al. Acute cerebrovascular events with COVID-19 infection. Stroke 2021;52(1):48–56.

61. Morassi M, Bagatto D, Cobelli M, et al. Stroke in patients with SARS-CoV-2 infection: case series. J Neurol 2020;267(8):2185–92.

62. Merkler AE, Parikh NS, Mir S, et al. Risk of ischemic stroke in patients with coronavirus disease 2019 (COVID-19) vs patients with influenza. JAMA Neurol 2020. https://doi.org/10.1001/jamaneurol.2020.2730.

63. Jackson JC, Pandharipande PP, Girard TD, et al. Depression, post-traumatic stress disorder, and functional disability in survivors of critical illness in the BRAIN-ICU study: a longitudinal cohort study. Lancet Respir Med 2014;2(5):369–79.

64. Pun BT, Badenes R, Heras La Calle G, et al. Prevalence and risk factors for delirium in critically ill patients with COVID-19 (COVID-D): a multicentre cohort study. Lancet Respir Med 2021;9(3): 239–50.

65. Buzhdygan TP, DeOre BJ, Baldwin-Leclair A, et al. The SARS-CoV-2 spike protein alters barrier function in 2D static and 3D microfluidic in-vitro models of the human blood–brain barrier. Neurobiol Dis 2020;146: 105131.

66. Whitmore HAB, Kim LA. Understanding the role of blood vessels in the neurologic manifestations of coronavirus disease 2019 (COVID-19). Am J Pathol 2021;191(11):1946–54.

67. Yaghi S, Ishida K, Torres J, et al. SARS-CoV-2 and stroke in a New York healthcare system. Stroke 2020;51(7):2002–11.

68. Heesakkers H, van der Hoeven JG, Corsten S, et al. Clinical outcomes among patients with 1-year survival following intensive care unit treatment for COVID-19. JAMA 2022;327(6):559–65.

69. Ely EW, Shintani A, Truman B, et al. Delirium as a predictor of mortality in mechanically ventilated patients in the intensive care unit. JAMA 2004; 291(14):1753–62.

70. Mohamed MFH, Al-Shokri SD, Shunnar KM, et al. Prevalence of venous thromboembolism in critically ill Covid-19 patients: systematic review and meta-analysis. systematic Review. Front Cardiovasc Med 2021;7. https://doi.org/10.3389/fcvm.2020.598846.

71. Wu C, Liu Y, Cai X, et al. Prevalence of venous thromboembolism in critically ill patients with coronavirus disease 2019: a meta-analysis. systematic review. Front Med 2021;8. https://doi.org/10.3389/fmed.2021.603558.

72. Wichmann DS, Lütgehetmann M, Steurer S, et al. Autopsy findings and venous thromboembolism in patients with COVID-19. Ann Intern Med 2020; 173(4):268–77.

73. Lee EE, Gong AJ, Gawande RS, et al. Vascular findings in CTA body and extremity of critically ill COVID-19 patients: commonly encountered vascular complications with review of literature. Emerg Radiol 2022. https://doi.org/10.1007/s10140-021-02013-1.

74. Malato A, Dentali F, Siragusa S, et al. The impact of deep vein thrombosis in critically ill patients: a meta-analysis of major clinical outcomes. Blood Transfus 2015;13(4):559–68.

75. Spyropoulos AC, Goldin M, Giannis D, et al. Efficacy and safety of therapeutic-dose heparin vs standard prophylactic or intermediate-dose heparins for thromboprophylaxis in high-risk hospitalized patients with COVID-19: the HEP-COVID randomized clinical trial. JAMA Intern Med 2021;181(12):1612–20.

76. Connors JM, Levy JH. COVID-19 and its implications for thrombosis and anticoagulation. Blood 2020;135(23):2033–40.

77. Wool GD, Miller JL. The impact of COVID-19 disease on platelets and coagulation. Pathobiology 2021; 88(1):15–27.

78. Abou-Ismail MY, Diamond A, Kapoor S, et al. The hypercoagulable state in COVID-19: incidence, pathophysiology, and management. Thromb Res 2020; 194:101–15.

79. Marvi TK, Stubblefield WB, Tillman BF, et al. Serial thromboelastography and the development of venous thromboembolism in critically ill patients with COVID-19. Crit Care Explor 2022;4(1):e0618.

80. Gorog DA, Storey RF, Gurbel PA, et al. Current and novel biomarkers of thrombotic risk in COVID-19: a Consensus statement from the international COVID-19 thrombosis biomarkers colloquium. Nat Rev Cardiol 2022. https://doi.org/10.1038/s41569-021-00665-7.

81. Malas MB, Naazie IN, Elsayed N, et al. Thromboembolism risk of COVID-19 is high and associated with a higher risk of mortality: a systematic review and meta-analysis. EClinicalMedicine 2020;29:100639.

82. Investigators R-C, Investigators AC-a, Investigators A, et al. Therapeutic anticoagulation with heparin in critically ill patients with covid-19. N Engl J Med 2021;385(9):777–89.

83. Therapeutic anticoagulation with heparin in noncritically ill patients with covid-19. N Engl J Med 2021; 385(9):790–802.

84. Investigators I. Effect of intermediate-dose vs standard-dose prophylactic anticoagulation on thrombotic events, extracorporeal membrane oxygenation treatment, or mortality among patients with covid-19 admitted to the intensive care unit: the inspiration randomized clinical trial. JAMA 2021;325(16):1620–30.

85. Flaczyk A, Rosovsky RP, Reed CT, et al. Comparison of published guidelines for management of coagulopathy and thrombosis in critically ill patients with COVID 19: implications for clinical practice and future investigations. Crit Care 2020;24(1):559.

86. Farrar JE, Trujillo TC, Mueller SW, et al. Evaluation of a patient specific, targeted-intensity pharmacologic thromboprophylaxis protocol in hospitalized patients with COVID-19. J Thromb Thrombolysis 2021. https://doi.org/10.1007/s11239-021-02552-x.

87. Trunfio M, Salvador E, Cabodi D, et al. Anti-Xa monitoring improves low-molecular-weight heparin effectiveness in patients with SARS-CoV-2 infection. Thromb Res 2020;196:432–4.

88. White D, MacDonald S, Bull T, et al. Heparin resistance in COVID-19 patients in the intensive care unit. J Thromb Thrombolysis 2020;50(2):287–91.

89. Lombardi CM, Carubelli V, Iorio A, et al. Association of troponin levels with mortality in Italian patients hospitalized with coronavirus disease 2019: results of a multicenter study. JAMA Cardiol 2020;5(11):1274–80.

90. Mansory EM, Srigunapalan S, Lazo-Langner A. Venous thromboembolism in hospitalized critical and noncritical COVID-19 patients: a systematic review and meta-analysis. TH Open 2021;5(3):e286–94.

Post-COVID Interstitial Lung Disease and Other Lung Sequelae

Mark Barash, DO[a],*, Vijaya Ramalingam, MD, FCCP[a,b]

KEYWORDS

- COVID-19 • Pulmonary function test • Computed tomography • Biopsy • Sequelae • PASC
- Pulmonary fibrosis

KEY POINTS

- Post-acute sequelae of SARS-COV-2 or post-COVID conditions are a poorly defined syndrome, possibly with long-lasting effects.
- Respiratory failure is one of the most serious complications of COVID-19 infection and contributes to major morbidity and mortality.
- Several studies have demonstrated abnormal lung function tests and radiological findings in patients who recovered from COVID-19 infection.
- Evidence on post-COVID pulmonary fibrosis is evolving.

INTRODUCTION

Respiratory failure is one of the most serious complications of COVID-19 infection and contributes to significant morbidity and mortality. Illness severity ranges from mild/asymptomatic disease to critical illness requiring mechanical ventilation. There has been increasing concern about pulmonary sequelae, including symptoms, pulmonary function testing (PFT) abnormalities, and pulmonary fibrosis.[1] Our knowledge about the natural history of recovery after COVID-19 infection is limited.

This article focuses on two concepts. First, the authors seek to describe available knowledge of post-COVID lung disease including pulmonary physiologic changes, imaging characteristics, fibrotic lung disease, and other complications. Next, the authors discuss the post-acute sequelae of SARS-CoV-2 (PASC): a poorly understood syndrome comprising a conglomerate of "head-to-toe" symptoms that afflicts a subset of patients recovering from COVID-19.

POST-COVID LUNG DISEASE
Abnormal Pulmonary Function Tests

Survivors of COVID-19 demonstrate heterogenous abnormalities in PFT (**Table 1**) and decrements in exercise capacity/diffusion of oxygen (**Table 2**). To this end, PFT abnormalities in survivors of severe lung injury are not a wholly new concept. For example, 5-year survivors of acute respiratory distress syndrome (ARDS) were found to be functionally impaired with a median 6 minute walk distance (6MWD) 76% predicted.[2] A meta-analysis of long-term outcomes after severe acute respiratory syndrome (SARS) and Middle Eastern respiratory syndrome (MERS) identified a reduced 6MWD and diffusing capacity for carbon monoxide (DLCO) compared with healthy individuals.[3]

Several studies from across the world have demonstrated reduced diffusion capacity, lung volumes (total lung capacity [TLC]), 6MWD, and exertional desaturation in COVID-19 patients during follow-up. Reduction in DLCO is the most

---

[a] Division of Pulmonary, Critical Care and Sleep Medicine, Medical College of Wisconsin, HUB for Collaborative Medicine, 8701 Watertown Plank Road, 8th Floor, Milwaukee, WI 53226, USA; [b] Department of Pulmonary, Critical Care Medicine, Northeast Georgia Health System, 1439 Jesse Jewell Parkway, Gainesville, GA 30501, USA
* Corresponding author.
E-mail address: mbarash@mcw.edu

Clin Chest Med 44 (2023) 263–277
https://doi.org/10.1016/j.ccm.2022.11.019

Table 1
Pulmonary function testing sequelae in patients recovering from COVID-19

Study	N	Timing	Obstructive Pattern (FEV1/FVC < 70 or < LLN)	Restrictive Pattern (FVC < LLN or 80% TLC < LLN or 80%)	DLCO < 80%
Van Gassel et al,[10] 2021	43	3 mo after discharge	0	16 (37.2%) 23 (53.5%)	36 (87.8%)
Van den Borst et al,[7] 2021	124	10 wk after discharge	12 (10%)	15 (13%)	41 (34%)
Gonzalez et al,[8] 2021	62	3 mo after discharge	1 (2%)	23 (37.1%)	50 (82%)
Liang et al,[9] 2020	76	3 mo after discharge	5 (6.6%)	0	15 (19.7%)
Lerum et al,[6] 2021	103	3 mo after admission	NA	7 (7%)	24 (24%)
You et al,[97] 2020	18	40 ± 11.6 d in cases with nonsevere illness, and 34.7 ± 16.5 d in cases with severe illness	3 (33%)	3 (33%)	NA
Huang et al,[70] 2021	349	6 mo after symptom onset	22 (6.3%)	56 (16%)	114 (32.7%)
Huang et al,[98] 2020	57	30 d after discharge	1 (1.8%)	6 (10.5%)	30 (52.6%)
Bellan et al,[5] 2021	224	3–4 mo after discharge	NA	NA	113 (50.4%)
Smet et al,[99] 2021	220	74 ± 12 d after diagnosis	NA	84 (38%)	48 (22%)
Shah et al,[100] 2021	60	3 mo after symptom onset	11.7% (7)	23.3% (14)	51.7% (31)
Zhao et al,[12] 2020	55	3 mo after discharge	NA	4 (7.25%)	9 (16.4%)
Mo et al,[101] 2020	110	On discharge	5 (4.5%)	27 (25%)	51 (47.2%)
Chen et al,[4] 2021	41	1 y after discharge	3 (7.3%)	5 (12.2%)	3 (7.3%)

Abbreviations: DLCO, diffusing capacity for carbon monoxide; FEV1, forced expiratory volume in 1 s; FVC, forced vital capacity; LLN, lower limit of normal; NA, not available; TLC, total lung capacity.
Adapted from So M, Kabata H, Fukunaga K, Takagi H, Kuno T. Radiological and functional lung sequelae of COVID-19: a systematic review and meta-analysis. BMC Pulm Med. 2021;21(1):97. Published 2021 Mar 22.

common PFT abnormality.[4] In a large Italian study,[5] female sex, chronic kidney disease, and the modality of oxygen delivery during hospital stay were shown to be risk factors for DLCO less than 80% at follow-up and female sex, COPD, and intensive care unit (ICU) admission were shown to be risk factors associated with DLCO less than 60% at follow-up. However, in another study, the prevalence of reduced lung function was similar between ICU and non-ICU participants.[6] High-Resolution computed tomography (HRCT) score during acute illness and residual pulmonary parenchymal opacities at discharge also correlated with the lower diffusion capacity after 3 months.[7–9] A European study that assessed respiratory sequelae of mechanically ventilated patients with COVID-19 showed high prevalence of

abnormal lung function testing; 53.5% patients had reduced TLC, whereas 87% had reduced DLCO at 3 months post-discharge. The median 6MWD was 482 m (82% predicted).[10] A prospective cohort study showed a significant reduction in the 6MWD in COVID-19 patients compared with the healthy population (median difference −128.43 m).[8]

The Swiss COVID-19 lung study reported PFT findings 4 months after initial symptoms in 113 patients. Patients with prior severe or critical disease had lower lung volumes than patients with mild or moderate disease and had abnormally reduced diffusion capacity, reduced functional capacity, and demonstrated exertional oxygen desaturation.[11] Zhao and colleagues[12] showed that elevated D-dimer was associated with decreased

Table 2
Exercise capacity and oxygenation in patients recovering from COVID-19 infection

	Timing	Dyspnea mMRC N (%)	6 MW Test (Distance in Mean or Median)	6 MWD <80% or < LLN	Significant Desaturation
Van Gassel et al,[10] 2021	3 mo after discharge	16 (37.2%) with score ≥ 1	482 m (82% p)	NA	2 (4.7%)
Van der Borst et al,[7] 2021	10 wk after discharge	Median 1	Normal	25 (22%)	20 (16%)
Gonzalez et al,[8] 2021	3 mo after discharge	NA	400 m	NA	NA
Lerum et al,[6] 2021	3 mo after admission	37 (54%) with score ≥ 1	580 m	NA	NA
Huang et al,[70] 2021	6 mo after symptom onset	419/1615 (26%)	495 m (87.7% p)	392 (23%)	NA
Shah et al,[100] 2021	3 mo after symptom onset	NA	NA	NA	4 (7%)
Huang et al,[98] 2020	30 d after discharge	NA	561 m (94% p)	NA	NA
Guler et al,[11] 2021	4 mo after discharge	NA	456 m (severe/critical disease) 576 (mild/moderate disease)	NA	NA

Abbreviation: NA, not available.

diffusion capacity in follow-up PFTs, possibly indicative of microthrombus formation.

In a 1-year follow-up study, only a small number of patients had DLCO less than 80% suggesting improvement in lung function from 6 months to 12 months.[4] Similar observations were made in a 2-year follow-up study. The proportion of COVID-19 survivors with an mMRC score of at least 1 was 168 (14%) of 1191 patients at 2 years, significantly lower than the 288 (26%) of 1104 at 6 months ($P < 0.0001$). The proportion of individuals with a 6MWD less than the lower limit of the normal range declined continuously in COVID-19 survivors overall and in the three subgroups of varying initial disease severity. However, critically ill patients had a significantly higher burden of restrictive ventilatory impairment and lung diffusion impairment than controls at the 2-year follow-up.[13]

Radiological Sequelae

The development of pulmonary fibrosis is a known complication after severe respiratory tract infection and such changes have been reported in survivors of SARS and MERS.[14] Residual radiographic abnormalities are seen in a large proportion of COVID-19 survivors at the time of discharge and subsequent follow-up.[15,16] In one study, the predominant pattern on CT scan changed over time with consolidative changes peaking 3 weeks after onset of symptoms and decreasing thereafter. Ground-glass opacification (GGO) or GGO with reticular pattern was the most common abnormal patterns from onset of symptoms until 12 months after hospital discharge.[4]

van Gassel and colleagues[10] reported normal pulmonary findings in only 2/46 patients at 3 month follow-up and GGO was noted in 89% of cases. Patients admitted to ICU showed interlobular septal thickening and bronchiectasis as the most frequent changes seen on CT chest at 3 months.[8] Patients admitted to ICU had higher prevalence of persistent CT abnormalities at 3 month follow-up. The distribution of GGO was mainly subpleural and similar in appearance to a nonspecific interstitial pneumonia (NSIP) pattern. Participants with limited residual changes mainly showed subpleural parenchymal bands or small plate atelectasis.[6]

More than one-third of severe COVID-19 survivors demonstrated fibrotic-like changes (traction bronchiectasis, parenchymal bands, and honeycombing) at 6 months after illness onset, and two-thirds of participants showed either complete radiographic resolution or residual GGO or interstitial thickening.[15] A 12-month follow-up CT in a subset of patients who had fibrotic interstitial lung abnormalities (ILAs) at 6-month period demonstrated stable fibrotic ILAs in more than two-thirds and slight improvement in the rest. Age greater than 50 years, ARDS, and higher baseline CT lung involvement score were predictors of fibrotic-like changes in the lung. The need for noninvasive mechanical ventilation was also a predictor of fibrotic-like changes.[17] Of note, progression of ILAs was not apparent. In another 1-year follow-up study, investigators found that age, smoking, hypertension, lower SaO_2, and secondary bacterial infections during acute phase were significantly associated with residual radiological abnormalities. Lung volume parameters of TLC and residual volume were significantly lower in patients with residual CT abnormalities than those without abnormalities at 1 year after hospital discharge.[4]

In the Swiss lung study, mosaic attenuation was the most common radiological change at 4-month follow-up. More than 50% of patients with severe or critical disease had mosaic attenuation, reticular changes, and architectural distortion at 4-month follow-up. Risk factors for post-SARS and MERS fibrosis were also older age and likelihood of having been in the ICU[14,18,19]

Fibrotic Lung Disease: The Proof Is in the Pudding

It is possible that various insults such as ventilator-induced lung injury,[20–22] bacterial infection, and hyperoxia[23–25] contribute to post-COVID fibrosis. Most of the patients with persistent inflammatory interstitial lung disease (ILD) require supplemental oxygen, ICU stay, and mechanical ventilation during their hospital stay.[26]

A spectrum of lung injury patterns has been found in patients with COVID-19 and vary with time from initial illness. Transbronchial lung cryobiopsy performed in 12 patients within 20 days of symptom onset showed epithelial and endothelial cell abnormalities different from either classical interstitial lung diseases or diffuse alveolar damage (DAD). Alveolar type II cell hyperplasia was a prominent finding in most of the cases. No evidence of hyaline membranes was noticed.[27] Several other reports have shown acute and organizing DAD in postmortem tissue samples from patients who died of severe disease.[28–30] There is histologic evidence of diffuse fibrotic ILD in patients recovering from COVID-19 infection. NSIP-like fibrosis accompanied by acute lung injury has been described in lung explant specimens.[31–33]

In a large study of 50 patients who underwent transbronchial cryobiopsy at a mean duration of 87 days from discharge, organizing pneumonia was the most common pathologic finding (32%) followed by diffuse lymphoplasmacytic interstitial infiltrate. Patchy fibrosis was observed in only four patients. There was no evidence of hyaline membranes, fibroblastic enlargement of the interstitium. Classic UIP or NSIP was not identified.[34] In another study, surgical lung biopsy showed UIP as the most common pathologic finding in patients undergoing evaluation for post-COVID-19 ILD. The investigators proposed these patients had lung disease before developing COVID infection.[35]

Role of Steroids and Antifibrotics in Post-COVID Lung Disease

Unfortunately, a paucity of data exists regarding what (if any) intervention should be undertaken in patients with persistent/residual pulmonary abnormalities.

An observational study of corticosteroid treatment in post-COVID ILD patients showed improvement in dyspnea, physical functioning, chest imaging, and lung function. Seven percentage (or 4% of the entire cohort) of patients had persistent interstitial changes on chest CT 6 weeks after discharge and most of them had an organizing pneumonia pattern.[26] In a Swiss national survey of pulmonologists, moderate recommendation was given in favor of an empiric steroid trial for patients with interstitial abnormalities after COVID-19.[36] Corticosteroid treatment may shorten the time to recovery and return to functioning for patients recovering from organizing pneumonia-like pattern associated with COVID-19.[37] However, evidence supporting corticosteroid use in post- COVID ILD is limited, and physicians should be cautious when prescribing steroids until robust data are available for their use. For reference, a 15-year follow-up study of SARS survivors showed most pulmonary lesions recovered within 1 year, and high-dose steroid exposure was associated with femoral head necrosis.[38]

Evidence on incidence of post-COVID pulmonary fibrosis is evolving. Currently, there is no evidence for or against the use of antifibrotic agents in post-COVID ILD. The natural history of post-COVID ILD is unclear. There are few reports on the use of nintedanib and pirfenidone in patients with COVID.[39–41] In an interventional study of patients with COVID-19 requiring mechanical ventilation, the use of nintedanib was associated with shorter length of mechanical ventilation and lower percentages of high-attenuation areas on CT volumetry, suggesting lung-protective effects.[42] **Table 3** shows the completed and ongoing trials evaluating the use of antifibrotic medications in COVID-19, though randomized controlled trials are lacking.

Not surprisingly, pulmonary rehabilitation could improve physical and psychological conditions, including exercise training, muscle strength, walking, and functional ability in patients with post-COVID ILD.[43,44]

Post-Acute Sequelae of SARS-CoV-2

Colloquially called "long COVID" or "Long hauler's syndrome," the PASC or post-COVID conditions, is a poorly defined syndrome that includes a range of new, recurrent, or ongoing health problems that can last weeks, months, or years after infection with COVID-19.[45] Indeed, due to a lack of consensus on the underlying physiology, symptom burden and timeline for symptom onset and resolution, a formal definition remains elusive. Symptoms may include severe fatigue and post-exertional malaise, onset of neuropsychiatric symptoms and difficulty with memory/concentration, persistent loss of taste and smell, dyspnea, cough, palpitations and postural orthostasis and various gastrointestinal (GI) symptoms, to name a few. A meta-analysis of studies that included at least 100 patients describing PASC symptoms, 55 long-term effects were identified (**Fig. 1**).[46] In a large survey, 640 patients recovering from COVID-19 were given the opportunity to write in symptoms they attributed to PASC; over 200 additional symptoms were reported beyond the 62 choices provided by the researchers.[47] These studies illustrate, if nothing else, the profound sense of unwellness that many patients experience.

Post-Viral Syndromes

PASC seems to represent a post-viral syndrome. It is important to acknowledge that PASC is not the first (nor likely the last) syndrome of its kind. After

---

Table 3
Current studies investigating corticosteroid and antifibrotic therapy in patients with post-COVID (as of June 30, 2022)

ClinicalTrials.gov Identifier	Study	Status
NCT04657484	Comparison of Two Corticosteroid Regimens for Post-COVID-19 Diffuse Lung Disease (COLDSTER)	Completed
NCT04551781	Short-Term Low-Dose Corticosteroids for Management of Post-COVID-19 Pulmonary Fibrosis	Completed
NCT04988282	Systemic Corticosteroids in Treatment of Post-COVID-19 Interstitial Lung Disease (STERCOV-ILD)	Recruiting
NCT04534478	Oral Prednisone Regimens to Optimize the Therapeutic Strategy in Patients With Organizing Pneumonia Post-COVID-19 (NORCOVID)	Not yet recruiting
NCT04541680	Nintedanib for the Treatment of SARS-Cov-2 Induced Pulmonary Fibrosis (NINTECOR)	Recruiting
NCT04338802	Efficacy and Safety of Nintedanib in the Treatment of Pulmonary Fibrosis in Patients With Moderate to Severe COVID-19	Unknown
NCT04619680	The Study of the Use of Nintedanib in Slowing Lung Disease in Patients With Fibrotic or Non-Fibrotic Interstitial Lung Disease Related to COVID-19 (ENDCOV-I)	Recruiting
NCT04856111	Pirfenidone vs Nintedanib for Fibrotic Lung Disease After Coronavirus Disease-19 Pneumonia (PINCER)	Recruiting
NCT04653831	Treatment With Pirfenidone for COVID-19-Related Severe ARDS	Recruiting
NCT04607928	Pirfenidone Compared to Placebo in Post-COVID19 Pulmonary Fibrosis COVID-19 (FIBRO-COVID)	Recruiting

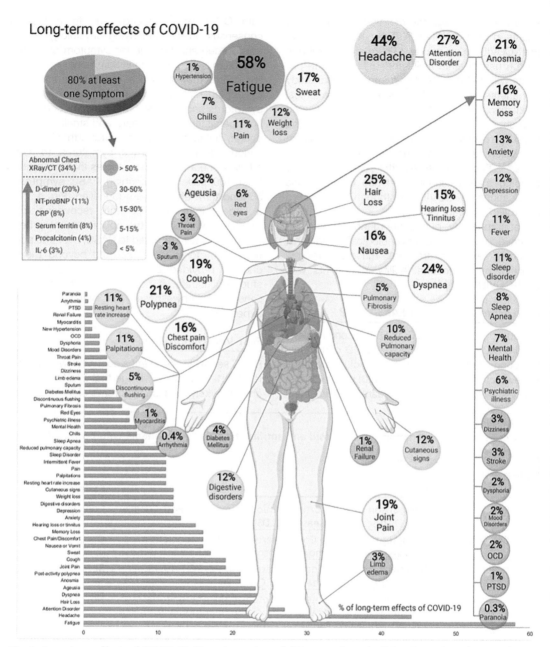

Fig. 1. Long-term effects of COVID-19. (*From* Lopez-Leon S, Wegman-Ostrosky T, Perelman C, et al. More than 50 long-term effects of COVID-19: a systematic review and meta-analysis. Sci Rep. 2021;11(1):16144. Published 2021 Aug 9.)

an outbreak of Russian Flu (1889 and 1892), observers noted a subset of survivors to develop symptoms of neuralgia, neurasthenia, neuritis, nerve exhaustion, grippe catalepsy, psychosis, anxiety, and paranoia.[48] After the Spanish Flu (1918–1919), patients displayed symptoms of parkinsonism and catatonia.[48] The term "encephalitis lethargica" gained prominence, though was first described a year earlier in 1917 after an outbreak of meningitis with delirium in Vienna.[49]

A 1935 outbreak of atypical poliomyelitis (atypical because 53 of 59 reported cases had normal cerebrospinal fluid [CSF] analysis) in a Los Angeles hospital led to prolonged symptoms of mental dullness and decreased ability to concentrate painful oculomotor and gastrointestinal symptoms.[50] During the 1950s and onward, several epidemics in London, Iceland, Australia, and Florida preferentially affected women and recovery was prolonged by fatigue and recurring myalgia, though no mortality was recorded.[51] From these outbreaks emerged the term myalgic encephalomyelitis (ME).[51] Following several mononucleosis-like outbreaks in the 1980s similarly characterized by prolonged symptoms, the first definition of chronic fatigue syndrome (CFS) was published.[52] An update on diagnostic criteria was published by the centers for disease control (CDC) in 1994, putting forth the term CFS/ME.[53–55] **Box 1** displays the criteria for CFS/ME.

More recent nonseasonal coronavirus outbreaks provide lessons as well. The 2003 SARS outbreak spread to 29 countries in Asia, Europe, and North America leading to 8422 cases recorded and 916 deaths (11% case fatality); Toronto, Ontario, had the highest concentration. Of 117 survivors surveyed 1 year from illness, 60% continued to experience fatigue, 45% complained of shortness of breath, 18% had reduced 6MWD, and 51 of 117 continued to require mental health visits; only 13% remained asymptomatic.[56] Long-term survivors from China continued to experience active psychiatric illness (40%), chronic fatigue (40.3%), and 27.1% met criteria for CFS/ME at a mean follow period of 41.3 months.[57] In 2012, the MERS infected 2519 people and led to 866 deaths (35% case fatality).

Similar to SARS, at 1 year, 48% of survivors demonstrated chronic fatigue and 42% complained of post-traumatic stress disorder (PTSD).[58,59] A large meta-analysis of SARS and MERS survivors found that 27.1% met criteria for CFS/ME and had reduced exercise capacity with lung function abnormalities.[3]

Incidence

The incidence of PASC is currently estimated to be between 10% and 35% of all infected individuals.[60,61] Morbidity can be so severe that as of July 2021, disability related to long-term symptoms from COVID-19 is covered under the Americans with Disabilities Act.[62] As of June 2022, the UK Office for National Statistics estimates that approximately 2 million people are experiencing symptoms of PASC. Of those surveyed, 405,000 (21%) were less than 12 weeks from onset of symptoms, 1.4 million (74%) remained symptomatic at greater than 12 weeks from symptom onset, 807,000 (41%) at 1 year, and 403,000 (21%) at 2 years.[63]

The impact of vaccination, current, and future viral variants on the development of PASC is also of great interest. A large study evaluated the effect of timing of vaccination along with variant of infection (Delta vs Omicron) on the development of PASC; the incidence of PASC was 4.5% (2501 of 56,003 people) among Omicron infections and 10.8% (4469 of 41,361 people) among Delta infections. In all age groups, the odds ratio (OR) of PASC ranged from 0.24 (0.20–0.32) to 0.50 (0.43–0.59) with Omicron compared with Delta. Vaccination status of less than 3 months had the highest OR of 0.5 (0.43–0.59), but there were insufficient data to determine PASC incidence in the unvaccinated population.[64] A survey of self-reported PASC symptoms in the United Kingdom found a 49.7% lower incidence of PASC from Omicron BA.1 variant compared with Delta in those who were double vaccinated. Interestingly, triple vaccination seemed to confer no difference in PASC risk between Delta and Omicron BA.1/BA.2, whereas infection compatible with Omicron BA.2 increased the odds of PASC symptoms by 21.8% compared with Omicron BA.1.[65] These findings may imply that a two-dose vaccination series could be sufficient to reduce PASC risk with Omicron but not with Delta. Last, there is some suggestion that vaccination itself may decrease the odds of PASC in those previously infected. A study of 28,356 adults infected before vaccination found that one dose of vaccine led to an initial 12.8% decrease in odds of PASC and a second dose led to an initial 8.8% decrease of PASC,

---

Box 1
Criteria for myalgic encephalomyelitis/chronic fatigue syndrome

Diagnosis requires that the patient has the following three symptoms:

1. A substantial reduction or impairment in the ability to engage in pre-illness levels of occupational, education, social, or personal activities that persist for more than 6 months and are accompanied by fatigue, which is often profound, is of new or definite onset (not lifelong), is not the result of ongoing excessive exertion, and is not substantially alleviated by rest

2. Post-exertional malaise

3. Unrefreshing sleep

At least one of the following manifestations is also required:

1. Cognitive impairment or

2. Orthostatic intolerance

From Herrera JE, Niehaus WN, Whiteson J, et al. Multidisciplinary collaborative consensus guidance statement on the assessment and treatment of fatigue in postacute sequelae of SARS-CoV-2 infection (PASC) patients [published correction appears in PM R. 2022 Jan;14(1):164]. PM R. 2021;13(9):1027-1043.

sustained at 67 days follow-up.[66] The evolution of viral variants, vaccine types, and community rates of herd immunity and vaccination make it difficult to generalize, though these observations raise fascinating questions about ways to decrease the incidence of PASC.

Hospitalized Patients

PASC affects people along the entire disease spectrum—from minimal/mild symptoms to critical illness. Among hospitalized patients, a telephone interview of 488 survivors, 60 days after symptom onset, found that 32% had persistent symptoms defined as a conglomerate of shortness of breath, cough, chest tightness, wheezing, difficulty ambulating, breathlessness with stairs, oxygen use, and continuous positive airway pressure (CPAP) use, with only 16% being able to return to work.[67] Another survey of 143 hospitalized patients performed at 60 days after initial diagnosis found that 87% had at least one persistent symptom and 55% had three or more; only 12% stated that they were completely free of symptoms.[68] Halpin and colleagues[69] performed a cross-sectional evaluation of 100 hospitalized patients at 4 to 8 weeks post-symptom onset; 70% continued to experience fatigue and 50% endorsed dyspnea. Huang and colleagues[70] performed an analysis of 17 different symptoms in 1733 hospitalized patients at 6 months post-admission, dividing the cohort into severity scales; 76% of the total cohort had at least one symptom, and symptom burden increased with severity of illness. Muscle weakness (63%), sleeping difficulties (26%), and anxiety or depression (23%) were the most common reported symptoms. Of note, 23% of the patients had a decreased age-adjusted 6MWD and diffusion defects which correlated with illness severity.

Nonhospitalized Patients

Similar observations have been made in nonhospitalized patients. Jacobsen and colleagues[71] found that in survey of 118 patients (96 outpatients), symptom burden was statistically similar between inpatient versus outpatient status and 67% of patients continued to experience symptoms, including a mean 6MWD of 59% of expected. Likewise, at a median follow-up of 169 days Logue and colleagues[72] found similar burden of persistence of at least one symptom (33 vs 31%) in outpatients versus inpatients, respectively. Patients are also more likely to use health system resources including outpatient primary care and outpatient hospital visits[73]

Risk Factors

The risk factors for PASC remain unknown, and data remain discordant. Wynberg and colleagues[74] found that female gender (adjusted hazard ration [aHR] 0.65, CI 0.47–0.92) and body mass index (BMI) greater than 30 (aHR 0.62 CI 0.39–0.97) were associated with slower recovery and symptoms beyond 6 months correlated with decreased chance of resolution. A large study of 2,149 health care professionals identified 323 participants who had no or mild symptoms and were found to be seropositive; 83% were women and 15% reported at least one persistent symptom at 8 months, as compared with seronegative participants (relative risk [RR] 4.4 [95 CI, 2.9–6.7]), causing significant disruption in work life, home life, and in any Sheehan Disability Scale category.[75] Among patients who survived hospitalization, the presence of ICU admission, need for respiratory support, premorbid lung problems, higher age, higher BMI, and BAME (Black, Asian, and Minority Ethnic) predicted breathlessness post-discharge.[69] Another study suggested that women were more likely to develop fatigue and anxiety/depression and presenting symptoms of palpitations, rhinitis, dysgeusia, insomnia, hyperhidrosis, anxiety, sore throat, and headache predicted PASC.[76] Sudre[77] and colleagues found that PASC was more likely with increasing age, female gender, higher BMI, and having five or more symptoms within the first week of onset A cohort study of 189 people similarly found that only female gender and preexisting anxiety disorder predicted PASC compared with controls; in this group of patients with predominantly mild/moderate initial infection, there was no association between developing PASC and any modality of diagnostic testing (PFTs, echocardiogram, serologic testing/ inflammatory markers, and cognitive testing), though participants with PASC had significantly lower scores on the SF-36 Health Survey. There was no evidence of abnormal systemic immune activation, autoimmune disease, or persistent viral infection.[78]

Post-Acute Sequelae of SARS-CoV-2 Phenotypes

Various phenotypes of PASC may exist. Defining them is complex due to the dynamic nature of both the initial illness and subsequent sequelae across illness severities. For example, a survivor of ARDS and ICU admission may develop dyspnea and abnormal PFTs that correlate with residual postinfectious fibrosis and overlap with the post-intensive care syndrome (PICS). A patient with only a mild illness without known history of pneumonia or hospitalization may also develop dyspnea out of proportion to imaging abnormalities and PFT derangements. Anecdotally, the latter is a remarkably common finding seen in our PASC clinic where most of the referrals are patients with no history of hospitalization and, generally, no known history of prior pneumonia. Several classifications systems have been proposed. Becker proposed a system based on the severity and evolution of symptoms over time.[79] Yong proposed subtypes based on long-term clinical and physiologic sequelae.[80] **Tables 4** and **5** summarize these two different schemas of subtyping PASC phenotypes. These descriptions will likely change over time and other schema will likely emerge, illustrating the complex nature of PASC that will undoubtedly continue to evolve along with our understanding. Newer schema would, ideally, group patients into phenotypes that also correlate with clinically relevant outcomes. No formal guidelines currently exist to define PASC phenotypes.

Mechanism(s) of Post-Acute Sequelae of SARS-CoV-2

A unifying mechanism for the variety and variability of symptoms of PASC remains elusive. Several studies have sought to clarify the causes of exercise intolerance as this is both common and debilitating symptoms. Studies using cardiopulmonary exercise testing (CPET) at various time points from illness and recovery have demonstrated predominantly circulatory and anaerobic threshold limitations when compared with matched controls[81–83]; however, ventilatory inefficiency has also been suggested.[82] Cassar and colleagues[83] performed a longitudinal evaluation of 58 survivors and 30 matched controls via symptom questionnaires, cardiac and lung magnetic resonance imaging (CMR) and CPET at 3 and 6 months. By 6 months, survivors demonstrated normalization of cardiac abnormalities noted on previous CMR imaging, though persistent (and improved) low-grade abnormalities of parenchymal abnormalities and peak V_{O_2} persisted in 52% of participants; importantly (and congruent with our real-world experience), these abnormalities did not correlate with cardiopulmonary symptoms. These impairments could be related to direct damage to muscle tissue, impaired oxygen extraction/utilization, or simple deconditioning from prolonged hospital stay and critical illness. To this end, the shear breadth of physical, neuropathic, and neuropsychiatric symptoms is likely not explained by these mechanisms alone and certainly not all patients will experience dyspnea or exercise intolerance.

Other proposed mechanisms include ACE-2/Ang 1 to 7 receptor down regulation with deleterious upstream effects,[84] autoantibody production targeting cytokines, chemokines, complement system, or cell surface proteins[85] and pro-inflammatory cytokines.[86,87] The nature of the initial immune response may also have bearing on both the clinical disease course and the long-lasting sequelae.[88]

Triage, Workup, and Treatment

Owing to the massive influx of patients with multitudes of symptoms, many centers around the United States and abroad have initiated multispecialty COVID clinics to help triage, treat, and address paucity of knowledge and expertise in this disease process. Clinics may have providers representing various medical specialties including neurology, neuropsychiatry and psychology, ear, nose and throat, cardiology, pulmonary, physical medicine and rehab, and physical and occupational therapy, among many others. No standardized approach has yet been validated but it is generally recommended that patients are approached in a holistic manner based on the severity of illness and symptom burden.[55,89,90] Basic laboratory testing such as

Table 4
Proposed COVID-19 sequelae subtype criteria

	Type 1	Type 2	Type 3		Type 4		Type 5
Initial symptoms	Variable[a]	Mild	A	B	A	B	None
		Mild	Mild	Mild	None	None	
Duration of symptoms	Variable[a]	>6 wk	3–6 mo	>6 mo	Variable	Variable	N/A
Period of quiescence	No	No	Yes	Yes	No	No	N/A
Delayed onset of symptoms	No	No	No	No	Yes	Yes	Yes

[a] Correlate with severity of initial infection, number of organ system injured and preexisting medical conditions.
From Becker RC. COVID-19 and its sequelae: a platform for optimal patient care, discovery and training. J Thromb Thrombolysis. 2021;51(3):587-594.

Table 5
Symptoms and the proposed pathophysiology of subtypes of post-acute sequelae of SARS-CoV-2

Subtype	Proposed Diagnostic Guide	Main Pathophysiology
NSC-MOS	Multi-organ symptoms lasting for ≥ 3 mo after acute COVID-19 (regardless of disease severity), especially fatigue, dyspnea, and cognitive impairment.	Tissue damage across multiple organs or system-wide dysregulation
PFS	Pulmonary fibrosis and other pulmonary sequelae (ie, impaired lung function or respiratory symptoms) lasting for ≥ 3 mo after acute COVID-19, especially severe COVID-19.	Extensive tissue damage, especially in the lungs
ME/CFS	Disabling fatigue, unrefreshing sleep, PEM, and either cognitive impairment or orthostatic intolerance lasting for ≥ 6 mo after acute COVID-19.	Dysfunction of the immune and nervous systems
POTS	Increased heart rate of >30 beats per minute within 5–10 min of standing or upright tilt without orthostatic hypotension. May occur with dizziness, palpitations, blurred vision, headache, generalized weakness, exercise intolerance, and fatigue.	Dysfunction of the autonomic nervous system
PICS	Physical (eg, muscular weakness, weakened handgrip, poor mobility), cognitive (eg, memory and concentration) and mental (eg, anxiety, depression and PTSD) sequelae lasting for ≥ 3 mo after acute COVID-19 of ICU level of severity.	Severe-to-critical illnesses in need of ICU level of care, from which full recovery is difficult
MCS	Acute or chronic diseases or other clinical sequelae that require medical care. Examples include respiratory, cardiovascular, gastrointestinal, kidney, liver and neurologic diseases, diabetes, infectious diseases, and mental health disorders.	Health deterioration or unmasking of chronic diseases

Abbreviations: MCS, medical or clinical sequelae; ME/CFS, myalgic encephalomyelitis or chronic fatigue syndrome; NSC-MOS, nonsevere COVID-19 multi-organ sequelae; PEM, post exertional malaise; PFS, pulmonary fibrosis sequelae; PICS, post-intensive care syndrome; POTS, postural orthostatic tachycardia syndrome.

Adapted from Yong SJ, Liu S. Proposed subtypes of post-COVID-19 syndrome (or long-COVID) and their respective potential therapies. Rev Med Virol. 2022;32(4):e2315.

complete blood count, basic metabolic panels, liver function, thyroid function is likely reasonable. More specialized testing, for example, looking for evidence of vitamin deficiencies, inflammatory markers, rheumatological conditions, or myocardial injury, and so forth, should be guided by symptoms and clinical gestalt. Advanced testing may include chest and cardiac imaging, electrocardiograms, and invasive testing such as heart catheterization or CPET if a high clinical suspicion exists. It should be noted that a "shot-gun" approach to testing is not recommended given dubious clinical utility, increasing cost and emotional burden on the patient.

In the author's experience (MB), patients often have trouble navigating their new symptoms and finding understanding from both their families, peers, and even other health care providers. In fact, a survey of 114 mostly female (80/114) medical professionals (51/114) with PASC in the United Kingdom described a heavy sense of loss and stigma, trouble accessing and navigating services, and difficulty being taken seriously.[91] The clinician should consider then, the extra burden placed on their nonmedical patients. Acknowledging symptoms is very important, as are validating statements like "what you are going through is very real" and "there are many others just like you, learning to navigate this new illness"; for example, after a thorough history and examination, we focus heavily on first, setting expectations that the time course of illness and recovery is unknown. Once both patient and provider are ready to move forward, appropriate testing is ordered to diagnose both preexisting and new conditions. Emphasis should be placed on symptomatic and supportive therapy.[60] Our practice is skewed heavily toward physical and occupational therapy as fatigue and sensation of dyspnea are often quite prevalent and debilitating. Patients should be counseled on paying particular attention to "post-exertional malaise," a debilitating state of fatigue onset from both physical and/or mental overexertion which has been well characterized in the setting of CFS/ME.[92] Healthy dietary habits, sleep hygiene, and modification of daily routines to prioritize certain activities over others are encouraged. Individualized reconditioning protocols should be implemented by experienced physical and occupational therapists with experience treating PASC patients.[55] The triage, evaluation, and treatment of patients suffering from PASC remains dynamic, and a holistic approach is paramount.[60,93–96]

SUMMARY

Post-COVID sequelae including lung injury and PASC are complex and poorly understood, representing heterogenous manifestations, mechanisms, and short- and long-term outcomes. The mainstay of therapy remains mostly supportive, though robust research is underway to better understand and characterize pathways for intervention. Historical insight remains important to clarify whether current observations are truly novel or representative of previously ignored or misunderstood syndromes.

CLINICS CARE POINTS

- Post-acute sequelae of SARS-CoV-2 (PASC) are a syndrome of nonspecific "head-to-toe" symptoms of unclear cause, mechanism, and duration. Supportive and holistic care is paramount.
- Abnormalities in lung function testing and chest imaging are fairly common in patients recovering from COVID-19. These abnormalities are heterogenous, often improve with time (though may not always normalize), and may not correlate with symptoms.

- Reduced diffusion capacity is the most common abnormality in pulmonary function testing.
- Patients who recover from COVID-19 may develop interstitial lung disease/pulmonary fibrosis. So far, data do not suggest that this represents a progressive fibrotic phenotype. The role of antifibrotic agents in the treatment of post-COVID fibrosis is being studied.

DISCLOSURE

The authors have nothing to disclose.

REFERENCES

1. So M, Kabata H, Fukunaga K, et al. Radiological and functional lung sequelae of COVID-19: a systematic review and meta-analysis. BMC Pulm Med 2021;21(1):97.
2. Herridge MS, Tansey CM, Matte A, et al. Functional disability 5 years after acute respiratory distress syndrome. N Engl J Med 2011;364(14):1293–304.
3. Ahmed H, Patel K, Greenwood DC, et al. Long-term clinical outcomes in survivors of severe acute respiratory syndrome and Middle East respiratory syndrome coronavirus outbreaks after hospitalisation or ICU admission: a systematic review and meta-analysis. J Rehabil Med 2020;52(5): jrm00063.
4. Chen Y, Ding C, Yu L, et al. One-year follow-up of chest CT findings in patients after SARS-CoV-2 infection. BMC Med 2021;19(1):191.
5. Bellan M, Soddu D, Balbo PE, et al. Respiratory and psychophysical sequelae among patients with COVID-19 four months after hospital discharge. JAMA Netw Open 2021;4(1):e2036142.
6. Lerum TV, Aalokken TM, Bronstad E, et al. Dyspnoea, lung function and CT findings 3 months after hospital admission for COVID-19. Eur Respir J 2021;57(4).
7. van den Borst B, Peters JB, Brink M, et al. Comprehensive health assessment 3 Months after recovery from acute coronavirus disease 2019 (COVID-19). Clin Infect Dis 2021;73(5):e1089–98.
8. Gonzalez J, Benitez ID, Carmona P, et al. Pulmonary function and radiologic features in survivors of critical COVID-19: a 3-month prospective cohort. Chest 2021;160(1):187–98.
9. Liang L, Yang B, Jiang N, et al. Three-month follow-up study of survivors of coronavirus disease 2019 after discharge. J Korean Med Sci 2020;35(47): e418.
10. van Gassel RJJ, Bels JLM, Raafs A, et al. High prevalence of pulmonary sequelae at 3 Months after hospital discharge in mechanically ventilated

survivors of COVID-19. Am J Respir Crit Care Med 2021;203(3):371–4.

11. Guler SA, Ebner L, Aubry-Beigelman C, et al. Pulmonary function and radiological features 4 months after COVID-19: first results from the national prospective observational Swiss COVID-19 lung study. Eur Respir J 2021;57(4):2003690.

12. Zhao YM, Shang YM, Song WB, et al. Follow-up study of the pulmonary function and related physiological characteristics of COVID-19 survivors three months after recovery. EClinicalMedicine 2020;25:100463.

13. Huang L, Li X, Gu X, et al. Health outcomes in people 2 years after surviving hospitalisation with COVID-19: a longitudinal cohort study. Lancet Respir Med 2022;10(9):863–76.

14. Ambardar SR, Hightower SL, Huprikar NA, et al. Post-COVID-19 pulmonary fibrosis: novel sequelae of the current pandemic. J Clin Med 2021;10(11):2452.

15. Han X, Fan Y, Alwalid O, et al. Six-month follow-up chest CT findings after severe COVID-19 pneumonia. Radiology 2021;299(1):E177–e186.

16. Wang Y, Dong C, Hu Y, et al. Temporal changes of CT findings in 90 patients with COVID-19 pneumonia: a longitudinal study. Radiology 2020;296(2):E55–e64.

17. Han X, Fan Y, Alwalid O, et al. Fibrotic interstitial lung abnormalities at 1-year follow-up CT after severe COVID-19. Radiology 2021;301(3):E438–e440.

18. Antonio GE, Wong KT, Hui DS, et al. Thin-section CT in patients with severe acute respiratory syndrome following hospital discharge: preliminary experience. Radiology 2003;228(3):810–5.

19. Das KM, Lee EY, Singh R, et al. Follow-up chest radiographic findings in patients with MERS-CoV after recovery. Indian J Radiol Imaging 2017;27(3):342–9.

20. Albert RK, Smith B, Perlman CE, et al. Is progression of pulmonary fibrosis due to ventilation-induced lung injury? Am J Respir Crit Care Med 2019;200(2):140–51.

21. Cabrera-Benitez NE, Laffey JG, Parotto M, et al. Mechanical ventilation-associated lung fibrosis in acute respiratory distress syndrome: a significant contributor to poor outcome. Anesthesiology 2014;121(1):189–98.

22. Cabrera-Benítez NE, Parotto M, Post M, et al. Mechanical stress induces lung fibrosis by epithelial-mesenchymal transition. Crit Care Med 2012;40(2):510–7.

23. Tzouvelekis A, Harokopos V, Paparountas T, et al. Comparative expression profiling in pulmonary fibrosis suggests a role of hypoxia-inducible factor-1alpha in disease pathogenesis. Am J Respir Crit Care Med 2007;176(11):1108–19.

24. Higgins DF, Kimura K, Bernhardt WM, et al. Hypoxia promotes fibrogenesis in vivo via HIF-1 stimulation of epithelial-to-mesenchymal transition. J Clin Invest 2007;117(12):3810–20.

25. Manresa MC, Godson C, Taylor CT. Hypoxia-sensitive pathways in inflammation-driven fibrosis. Am J Physiol Regul Integr Comp Physiol 2014;307(12):R1369–80.

26. Myall KJ, Mukherjee B, Castanheira AM, et al. Persistent post-COVID-19 interstitial lung disease. An observational study of corticosteroid treatment. Ann Am Thorac Soc 2021;18(5):799–806.

27. Doglioni C, Ravaglia C, Chilosi M, et al. Covid-19 interstitial pneumonia: histological and immunohistochemical features on cryobiopsies. Respiration 2021;100(6):488–98.

28. Menter T, Haslbauer JD, Nienhold R, et al. Postmortem examination of COVID-19 patients reveals diffuse alveolar damage with severe capillary congestion and variegated findings in lungs and other organs suggesting vascular dysfunction. Histopathology 2020;77(2):198–209.

29. Barisione E, Grillo F, Ball L, et al. Fibrotic progression and radiologic correlation in matched lung samples from COVID-19 post-mortems. Virchows Arch 2021;478(3):471–85.

30. Li Y, Wu J, Wang S, et al. Progression to fibrosing diffuse alveolar damage in a series of 30 minimally invasive autopsies with COVID-19 pneumonia in Wuhan, China. Histopathology 2021;78(4):542–55.

31. Bharat A, Querrey M, Markov NS, et al. Lung transplantation for patients with severe COVID-19. Sci Transl Med 2020;12(574):eabe4282.

32. Aesif SW, Bribriesco AC, Yadav R, et al. Pulmonary pathology of COVID-19 following 8 Weeks to 4 Months of severe disease: a report of three cases, including one with bilateral lung transplantation. Am J Clin Pathol 2021;155(4):506–14.

33. Bharat A, Machuca TN, Querrey M, et al. Early outcomes after lung transplantation for severe COVID-19: a series of the first consecutive cases from four countries. Lancet Respir Med 2021;9(5):487–97.

34. Culebras M, Loor K, Sansano I, et al. Histological findings in transbronchial cryobiopsies obtained from patients after COVID-19. Chest 2022;161(3):647–50.

35. Konopka KE, Perry W, Huang T, et al. Usual interstitial pneumonia is the most common finding in surgical lung biopsies from patients with persistent interstitial lung disease following infection with SARS-CoV-2. EClinicalMedicine 2021;42:101209.

36. Funke-Chambour M, Bridevaux PO, Clarenbach CF, et al. Swiss recommendations for the follow-up and treatment of pulmonary long COVID. Respiration 2021;100(8):826–41.

37. Kostorz-Nosal S, Jastrzębski D, Chyra M, et al. A prolonged steroid therapy may be beneficial in

some patients after the COVID-19 pneumonia. Eur Clin Respir J 2021;8(1):1945186.

38. Zhang P, Li J, Liu H, et al. Long-term bone and lung consequences associated with hospital-acquired severe acute respiratory syndrome: a 15-year follow-up from a prospective cohort study. Bone Res 2020;8:8.

39. Ogata H, Nakagawa T, Sakoda S, et al. Nintedanib treatment for pulmonary fibrosis after coronavirus disease 2019. Respirol Case Rep 2021;9(5): e00744.

40. Bussolari C, Palumbo D, Fominsky E, et al. Case report: nintedaninb may accelerate lung recovery in critical coronavirus disease 2019. Front Med (Lausanne) 2021;8:766486.

41. Zhang F, Wei Y, He L, et al. A trial of pirfenidone in hospitalized adult patients with severe coronavirus disease 2019. Chin Med J (Engl) 2021;135(3): 368-70.

42. Umemura Y, Mitsuyama Y, Minami K, et al. Efficacy and safety of nintedanib for pulmonary fibrosis in severe pneumonia induced by COVID-19: an interventional study. Int J Infect Dis 2021;108:454-60.

43. Reina-Gutiérrez S, Torres-Costoso A, Martínez-Vizcaíno V, et al. Effectiveness of pulmonary rehabilitation in interstitial lung disease, including coronavirus diseases: a systematic review and meta-analysis. Arch Phys Med Rehabil 2021;102(10): 1989-97. e1983.

44. Goodwin VA, Allan L, Bethel A, et al. Rehabilitation to enable recovery from COVID-19: a rapid systematic review. Physiotherapy 2021;111:4-22.

45. Post-COVID conditions: overview for healthcare providers. 2022. Available at: https://www.cdc.gov/coronavirus/2019-ncov/hcp/clinical-care/post-covid-conditions.html. Accessed June 1, 2022.

46. Lopez-Leon S, Wegman-Ostrosky T, Perelman C, et al. More than 50 long-term effects of COVID-19: a systematic review and meta-analysis. Sci Rep 2021;11(1):16144.

47. Assaf G.D.H., McCorkell L., Louise T., et al., What does COVID-19 recovery actually look like? An analysis of the prolonged COVID-19 symptoms survey by patient-led research team. Available at: https://patientresearchcovid19.com/research/report-1/ Accessed May 15, 2022 2020.

48. Honigsbaum M, Krishnan L. Taking pandemic sequelae seriously: from the Russian influenza to COVID-19 long-haulers. Lancet 2020;396(10260): 1389-91.

49. Reid AH, McCall S, Henry JM, et al. Experimenting on the past: the enigma of von Economo's encephalitis lethargica. J Neuropathol Exp Neurol 2001; 60(7):663-70.

50. Meals RW, Hauser VF, Bower AG. Poliomyelitis-the Los Angeles epidemic of 1934 : Part I. Cal West Med 1935;43(2):123-5.

51. Acheson ED. The clinical syndrome variously called benign myalgic encephalomyelitis, Iceland disease and epidemic neuromyasthenia. Am J Med 1959;26(4):569-95.

52. Holmes GP, Kaplan JE, Gantz NM, et al. Chronic fatigue syndrome: a working case definition. Ann Intern Med 1988;108(3):387-9.

53. Brurberg KG, Fønhus MS, Larun L, et al. Case definitions for chronic fatigue syndrome/myalgic encephalomyelitis (CFS/ME): a systematic review. BMJ Open 2014;4(2):e003973.

54. Fukuda K, Straus SE, Hickie I, et al. The chronic fatigue syndrome: a comprehensive approach to its definition and study. International Chronic Fatigue Syndrome Study Group. Ann Intern Med 1994; 121(12):953-9.

55. Herrera JE, Niehaus WN, Whiteson J, et al. Multidisciplinary collaborative consensus guidance statement on the assessment and treatment of fatigue in postacute sequelae of SARS-CoV-2 infection (PASC) patients. Pm r 2021;13(9): 1027-43.

56. Tansey CM, Louie M, Loeb M, et al. One-year outcomes and health care utilization in survivors of severe acute respiratory syndrome. Arch Intern Med 2007;167(12):1312-20.

57. Lam MH-B, Wing Y-K, Yu MW-M, et al. Mental morbidities and chronic fatigue in severe acute respiratory syndrome survivors: long-term follow-up. Arch Intern Med 2009;169(22):2142-7.

58. Batawi S, Tarazan N, Al-Raddadi R, et al. Quality of life reported by survivors after hospitalization for Middle East respiratory syndrome (MERS). Health Qual Life Outcomes 2019; 17(1):101.

59. Lee SH, Shin HS, Park HY, et al. Depression as a mediator of chronic fatigue and post-traumatic stress symptoms in Middle East respiratory syndrome survivors. Psychiatry Investig 2019;16(1): 59-64.

60. Greenhalgh T, Knight M, A'Court C, et al. Management of post-acute covid-19 in primary care. Bmj 2020;370:m3026.

61. Tenforde MW, Kim SS, Lindsell CJ, et al. Symptom duration and risk factors for delayed return to usual health among outpatients with COVID-19 in a multistate health care systems network - United States, march-june 2020. MMWR Morb Mortal Wkly Rep 2020;69(30):993-8.

62. Guidance on "long COVID" as a disability under the ADA, section 504, and section 1557. 2022. Available at: https://www.hhs.gov/civil-rights/for-providers/civil-rights-covid19/guidance-long-covid-disability/index.html#footnote3_m3r0yg1. Accessed June 1, 2022.

63. Prevalence of ongoing symptoms following coronavirus (COVID-19) infection in the UK. 2022. Available

at: https://www.ons.gov.uk/peoplepopulationand community/healthandsocialcare/conditionsanddiseases/bulletins/prevalenceofongoingsymptoms followingcoronaviruscovid19infectionintheuk/7july2022. Accessed July 7, 2022.

64. Antonelli M, Pujol JC, Spector TD, et al. Risk of long COVID associated with delta versus omicron variants of SARS-CoV-2. Lancet 2022;399(10343):2263–4.

65. Self-reported long COVID after infection with the Omicron variant in the UK: 6 May 2022. Available at: https://www.ons.gov.uk/peoplepopulationand community/healthandsocialcare/conditionsand diseases/bulletins/selfreportedlongcovid afterinfectionwiththeomicronvariant/6may2022. Accessed August 10, 2022.

66. Ayoubkhani D, Bermingham C, Pouwels KB, et al. Trajectory of long covid symptoms after covid-19 vaccination: community based cohort study. Bmj 2022;377:e069676.

67. Chopra V, Flanders SA, O'Malley M, et al. Sixty-day outcomes among patients hospitalized with COVID-19. Ann Intern Med 2021;174(4):576–8.

68. Carfi A, Bernabei R, Landi F. Persistent symptoms in patients after acute COVID-19. JAMA 2020;324(6):603–5.

69. Halpin SJ, McIvor C, Whyatt G, et al. Postdischarge symptoms and rehabilitation needs in survivors of COVID-19 infection: a cross-sectional evaluation. J Med Virol 2021;93(2):1013–22.

70. Huang C, Huang L, Wang Y, et al. 6-month consequences of COVID-19 in patients discharged from hospital: a cohort study. Lancet 2021;397(10270):220–32.

71. Jacobson KB, Rao M, Bonilla H, et al. Patients with uncomplicated coronavirus disease 2019 (COVID-19) have long-term persistent symptoms and functional impairment similar to patients with severe COVID-19: a cautionary tale during a global pandemic. Clin Infect Dis 2021;73(3):e826–9.

72. Logue JK, Franko NM, McCulloch DJ, et al. Sequelae in adults at 6 Months after COVID-19 infection. JAMA Netw Open 2021;4(2):e210830.

73. Lund LC, Hallas J, Nielsen H, et al. Post-acute effects of SARS-CoV-2 infection in individuals not requiring hospital admission: a Danish population-based cohort study. Lancet Infect Dis 2021;21(10):1373–82.

74. Wynberg E, van Willigen HDG, Dijkstra M, et al. Evolution of COVID-19 symptoms during the first 12 months after illness onset. Clin Infect Dis 2021;75(1):e482–90.

75. Haverwall S, Rosell A, Phillipson M, et al. Symptoms and functional impairment assessed 8 Months after mild COVID-19 among health care workers. JAMA 2021;325(19):2015–6.

76. Huang Y, Pinto MD, Borelli JL, et al. COVID symptoms, symptom clusters, and predictors for becoming a long-hauler: looking for clarity in the haze of the pandemic. medRxiv 2021;03(03):21252086.

77. Sudre CH, Murray B, Varsavsky T, et al. Attributes and predictors of long COVID. Nat Med 2021;27(4):626–31.

78. Sneller MC, Liang CJ, Marques AR, et al. A longitudinal study of COVID-19 Sequelae and immunity: baseline findings. Ann Intern Med 2022;175(7):969–79.

79. Becker RC. COVID-19 and its sequelae: a platform for optimal patient care, discovery and training. J Thromb Thrombolysis 2021;51(3):587–94.

80. Yong SJ, Liu S. Proposed subtypes of post-COVID-19 syndrome (or long-COVID) and their respective potential therapies. Rev Med Virol 2022;32(4):e2315.

81. Rinaldo RF, Mondoni M, Parazzini EM, et al. Deconditioning as main mechanism of impaired exercise response in COVID-19 survivors. Eur Respir J 2021;58(2):2100870.

82. Singh I, Joseph P, Heerdt PM, et al. Persistent exertional intolerance after COVID-19: insights from invasive cardiopulmonary exercise testing. Chest 2022;161(1):54–63.

83. Cassar MP, Tunnicliffe EM, Petousi N, et al. Symptom persistence despite improvement in cardiopulmonary health - insights from longitudinal CMR, CPET and lung function testing post-COVID-19. EClinicalMedicine 2021;41:101159.

84. Bolay H, Gul A, Baykan B. COVID-19 is a real headache. Headache 2020;60(7):1415–21.

85. Wang EY, Mao T, Klein J, et al. Diverse functional autoantibodies in patients with COVID-19. Nature 2021;595(7866):283–8.

86. Bhavana V, Thakor P, Singh SB, et al. COVID-19: pathophysiology, treatment options, nanotechnology approaches, and research agenda to combating the SARS-CoV2 pandemic. Life Sci Life Sci 2020;261:118336.

87. Alpert O, Begun L, Garren P, et al. Cytokine storm induced new onset depression in patients with COVID-19. A new look into the association between depression and cytokines -two case reports. Brain Behav Immun - Health 2020;9:100173.

88. Carvalho T, Krammer F, Iwasaki A. The first 12 months of COVID-19: a timeline of immunological insights. Nat Rev Immunol 2021;21(4):245–56.

89. Nalbandian A, Sehgal K, Gupta A, et al. Post-acute COVID-19 syndrome. Nat Med 2021;27(4):601–15.

90. Lutchmansingh DD, Knauert MP, Antin-Ozerkis DE, et al. A Clinic blueprint for post-coronavirus disease 2019 recovery: learning from the past, looking to the future. Chest 2021;159(3):949–58.

91. Ladds E, Rushforth A, Wieringa S, et al. Persistent symptoms after Covid-19: qualitative study of 114 "long Covid" patients and draft quality principles for services. BMC Health Serv Res 2020;20(1): 1144.

92. Chu L, Valencia IJ, Garvert DW, et al. Deconstructing post-exertional malaise in myalgic encephalomyelitis/chronic fatigue syndrome: a patient-centered, cross-sectional survey. PLoS One 2018;13(6): e0197811.

93. Pavli ATMMHC. Post-COVID syndrome: incidence, clinical spectrum, and challenges for primary healthcare professionals. ARCMED Arch Med Res 2021;52(6):575–81.

94. COVID-19 rapid guideline: managing the long-term effects of COVID-19. Available at: https://www.nice.org.uk/guidance/ng188/resources/covid19-rapid-guideline-managing-the-longterm-effects-of-covid19-pdf-51035515742. Accessed June 6, 2022.

95. Siso Almirall A, Brito Zeron P, Conangla Ferrin L, et al. Long Covid-19: proposed primary care clinical guidelines for diagnosis and disease management. Int J Environ Res Public Health 2021;18(8):4350.

96. Parkin A, Davison J, Tarrant R, et al. A Multidisciplinary NHS COVID-19 service to manage post-COVID-19 syndrome in the community. J Prim Care Community Health 2021;12. 21501327211010994.

97. You J, Zhang L, Ni-Jia-Ti MY, et al. Anormal pulmonary function and residual CT abnormalities in rehabilitating COVID-19 patients after discharge. J Infect 2020;81(2):e150–2.

98. Huang Y, Tan C, Wu J, et al. Impact of coronavirus disease 2019 on pulmonary function in early convalescence phase. Respir Res 2020;21(1):163.

99. Smet J, Stylemans D, Hanon S, et al. Clinical status and lung function 10 weeks after severe SARS-CoV-2 infection. Respir Med 2021;176:106276.

100. Shah AS, Wong AW, Hague CJ, et al. A prospective study of 12-week respiratory outcomes in COVID-19-related hospitalisations. Thorax 2021;76(4): 402–4.

101. Mo X, Jian W, Su Z, et al. Abnormal pulmonary function in COVID-19 patients at time of hospital discharge. Eur Respir J 2020;55(6):2001217.

Antiviral Treatment of Coronavirus Disease-2019 Pneumonia

Christopher Radcliffe, MD[a], Maricar Malinis, MD[a], Marwan M. Azar, MD[a,b],*

KEYWORDS

- COVID-19 • SARS-CoV-2 • Remdesivir • Molnupiravir • Nirmatrelvir • Bebtelovimab
- Tixagevimab/cilgavimab

KEY POINTS

- Coronavirus disease-2019 (COVID-19) therapies are most effective when administered early in the disease course.
- Standard of care for hospitalized persons with moderate-to-severe COVID-19 remains remdesivir with immunomodulatory therapy.
- Oral antiviral agents and monoclonal antibodies are cornerstones of outpatient COVID-19 treatment.

INTRODUCTION

With 614 million cumulative cases and over 6.3 million deaths worldwide as of September 30, 2022, the severe acute respiratory syndrome coronavirus 2 (SARS-CoV-2) pandemic persists.[1] The periodic emergence of novel variants produces a changing landscape, making the development of novel mitigation strategies to reduce coronavirus disease-2019 (COVID-19) associated morbidity and mortality increasingly important. Vaccination and other public health measures (eg, masking and social distancing) are vital for reducing infection rates, but disparities related to distribution and uptake of vaccines remain.[2,3]

For persons who develop SARS-CoV-2 infection, clinical manifestations are highly variable, and illness severity can range from asymptomatic to life-threatening.[4,5] In addition to supportive care, treatment is indicated for outpatient persons at risk for disease progression or inpatient persons with moderate-to-severe disease. A diverse assemblage of COVID-19 management strategies has been evaluated, and several evidence-based treatment options are now available (**Fig. 1, Table 1**).

In light of the pathophysiology of COVID-19, treatment options aim to reduce viral replication, block viral entry into host cells, and/or modulate the host immune response. In this review, we focus on the body of evidence supporting the use of direct antiviral agents and monoclonal antibodies for the treatment of COVID-19. We aim to enumerate treatment options and summarize management approaches in relevant patient populations.

DIRECT ANTIVIRAL AGENTS

Remdesivir

Remdesivir is an adenosine analog with in vitro activity against SARS-CoV-2.[6] Its spectrum of antiviral activity extends to other RNA viruses (eg, Ebola virus).[7] After intracellular processing, remdesivir's active triphosphate form interferes with RNA-dependent RNA polymerase and causes termination of RNA transcripts.[7] **Fig. 2** displays an overview of the SARS-CoV-2 replication cycle and

[a] Section of Infectious Diseases, Yale University School of Medicine, 333 Cedar Street, New Haven, CT 06520, USA; [b] Department of Laboratory Medicine, Yale University School of Medicine, New Haven, CT, USA
* Corresponding author. Section of Infectious Diseases, Yale University School of Medicine, 333 Cedar Street, New Haven, CT 06520.
E-mail address: marwan.azar@yale.edu

Clin Chest Med 44 (2023) 279–297
https://doi.org/10.1016/j.ccm.2022.11.008

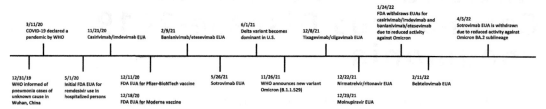

Fig. 1. Timeline for SARS-CoV-2 antiviral therapies in the United States. FDA, US Food and Drug Administration; EUA, emergency use authorization; WHO, World Health Organization.

the stage at which remdesivir exerts its antiviral activity. Remdesivir, administered intravenously, is US Food and Drug Administration (FDA) approved for the treatment of moderate-to-severe SARS-CoV-2 infection; oral formulations are not available due to poor bioavailability in humans.[8]

For hospitalized adult patients with COVID-19 who have evidence of lower respiratory tract involvement, the use of remdesivir is supported by ACTT-1, a double-blind, randomized control trial (RCT) comparing remdesivir ($n = 541$) with placebo ($n = 521$).[9] The median recovery time for patients who received remdesivir was 10 days compared with 15 days in those who received placebo (rate ratio for recovery, 1.29; 95% confidence interval [CI] 1.12–1.49; $p < 0.001$). In addition, Kaplan–Meier mortality estimates were lower for remdesivir compared with placebo at day 15 (6.7% vs 11.9%; hazard ratio [HR] 0.55, 95% CI 0.36–0.83), but differences in mortality estimates were not statistically significant at day 29 (11.4% vs 15.2%; HR 0.73, 95% CI 0.52–1.03).

Patients in the ACTT-1 trial received remdesivir for up to 10 days,[9] with a duration of therapy extrapolated from data on remdesivir's use in the treatment of other viral infections.[10,11] A randomized, open-label, phase 3 trial evaluated a 5-day course of remdesivir ($n = 200$) compared with a 10-day course ($n = 197$) in hospitalized adult patients with SARS-CoV-2 infection, oxygen saturation ≤94% on room air and evidence of pneumonia on imaging studies.[10] The investigators used a 7-point ordinal scale to evaluate clinical status at day 14 and did not find a significant difference between treatment groups after adjusting for differences in baseline clinical status. Results from this RCT are the basis for the 5-day treatment duration currently recommended by National Institutes of Health (NIH) and Infectious Diseases Society of America (IDSA) guidelines.[12,13]

The use of remdesivir in combination with baricitinib, a Janus kinase inhibitor with anti-inflammatory activity, has also been studied in hospitalized adult patients with COVID-19. The ACTT-2 trial was a double-blind, RCT comparing

remdesivir and baricitinib ($n = 515$) with remdesivir and placebo ($n = 518$).[14] The median time to recovery was 7 days in patients receiving remdesivir and baricitinib compared with 8 days in patients receiving remdesivir and placebo (rate ratio for recovery 1.16; 95% CI 1.01–1.32; $p = 0.03$). The benefit of combination therapy was more pronounced for patients receiving high-flow oxygen or noninvasive ventilation at time of enrollment. Overall, there was no significant difference in 28-day mortality (5.1% remdesivir and baricitinib vs 7.8% remdesivir and placebo; HR 0.65; 95% CI 0.39–1.09).

More recently, the ACTT-4 trial, a double-blind, double-placebo RCT, compared remdesivir plus baricitinib plus placebo ($n = 516$) with remdesivir plus dexamethasone plus placebo ($n = 494$) in hospitalized adults with COVID-19 who required supplemental oxygen by low flow, high flow, or noninvasive ventilation.[15] The primary outcome of mechanical ventilation-free survival at day 29 was not significantly different between treatment groups (87.0% vs 87.6%); however, more adverse events ($p = 0.014$), treatment-related adverse events ($p = 0.00041$), and severe or life-threatening grade 3 or 4 adverse events ($p = 0.012$) impacted the remdesivir plus dexamethasone plus placebo group. In addition to its combination with dexamethasone or baricitinib, remdesivir's use has been investigated in combination with tocilizumab,[16] and several tocilizumab RCTs included notable percentages of patients who received co-administered remdesivir (33% to 55%).[17,18] A single RCT has compared remdesivir plus tocilizumab ($n = 434$) with remdesivir plus placebo ($n = 215$) in hospitalized patients with severe COVID-19 requiring >6 L/min of supplemental oxygen.[16] The primary outcome of time elapsed between randomization and discharge or "ready for discharge" (evaluated using a 7-category ordinal scale) to day 28 was not different between treatment groups (median time 14 days in both groups).[16] However, based on other evidence, tocilizumab is recommended as an immunomodulatory alternative to baricitinib in combination with remdesivir and dexamethasone.[12,13]

Table 1
Direct acting antivirals and monoclonal antibodies for SARS-COV-2

Therapeutic Agent	Mechanism of Action	Indication(s) for Use	Drug-Drug Interaction(s)	Contraindication(s)	Adverse Event(s)
Remdesivir	Adenosine analog whose active form interferes with RNA-dependent RNA polymerase	5-day course for inpatient persons with moderate-to-severe COVID-19; 3-day course for outpatient persons with COVID-19 at-risk for disease progression	No significant interactions	Advanced hepatic or renal impairment	Constipation, nausea, possible transaminitis or AKI
Nirmatrelvir/ ritonavir	Nirmatrelvir is an inhibitor of SARS-CoV-2 3CL protease; ritonavir is an HIV protease inhibitor co-administered to inhibit CYP3A4 and achieve therapeutic nirmatrelvir levels	5-day course for outpatient persons with COVID-19 at-risk for disease progression	Co-administered medications with CYP3A4 metabolism (eg, phenytoin, tacrolimus, and warfarin) may impair antiviral activity or cause toxicity	Avoid co-administered medications with significant CYP3A4 interactions; avoid use in pregnant individuals	Diarrhea, dysgeusia
Molnupiravir	Ribonucleoside analog of N-hydroxycytidine whose active form interferes with RNA-dependent RNA polymerase	5-day course for outpatient persons with COVID-19 at-risk for disease progression	No significant interactions	Risk-benefit discussion advised for pregnant individuals	Diarrhea, nausea, dizziness
Casirivimab/ imdevimab	Monoclonal antibody which binds SARS-CoV-2 Spike protein	Single-dose infusion for outpatient persons with COVID-19 at-risk for disease progression (EUA withdrawn January 24, 2022)	No significant interactions	No absolute contraindications	Infusion-related reaction

(continued on next page)

Table 1
(continued)

Therapeutic Agent	Mechanism of Action	Indication(s) for Use	Drug-Drug Interaction(s)	Contraindication(s)	Adverse Event(s)
Bamlanivimab/ etesevimab	Monoclonal antibody which binds SARS-CoV-2 Spike protein	Single-dose infusion for outpatient persons with COVID-19 at-risk for disease progression (EUA withdrawn January 24, 2022)	No significant interactions	No absolute contraindications	Infusion-related reaction
Sotrovimab	Monoclonal antibody which binds SARS-CoV-2 Spike protein	Single-dose infusion for outpatient persons with COVID-19 at-risk for disease progression (EUA withdrawn April 5, 2022)	No significant interactions	No absolute contraindications	Infusion-related reaction
Bebtelovimab	Monoclonal antibody which binds SARS-CoV-2 Spike protein	Single-dose infusion for outpatient persons with COVID-19 at-risk for disease progression	No significant interactions	No absolute contraindications	Infusion-related reaction
Tixagevimab/ cilgavimab	Monoclonal antibody which binds SARS-CoV-2 Spike protein	Preexposure prophylaxis (two 600 mg doses) for persons who are not anticipated to respond to vaccine series and/or unable to complete vaccine series due to hypersensitivity reaction	No significant interactions	No absolute contraindications	Injection site reaction

Abbreviations: AKI, acute kidney injury; EUA, emergency use authorization; HIV, human immunodeficiency virus; RNA, ribonucleic acid.

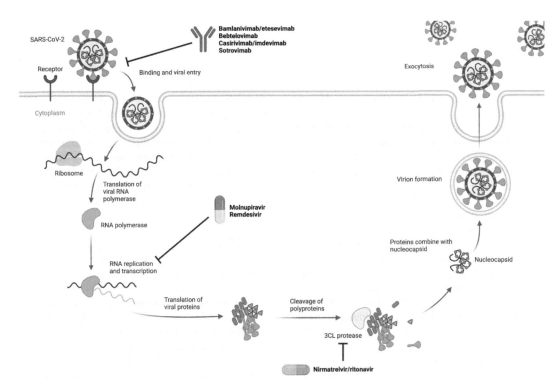

Fig. 2. Mechanism of SARS-CoV-2 antiviral therapies. (Created with BioRender.com.)

Remdesivir has also been evaluated as an agent to prevent disease progression in the outpatient setting.[19] The PINETREE trial was a double-blind, RCT that compared a 3-day course of remdesivir (n = 279) to placebo (n = 283) for outpatients with COVID-19 who had ≥ 1 risk factor for disease progression and ≤ 7 days of symptoms. COVID-19-related hospitalization or all-cause mortality at day 28 was lower for patients who received remdesivir (0.7%) compared with placebo (5.3%) (HR 0.13; 95% CI 0.03–0.59; p = 0.008). Notably, no deaths had occurred in either group by day 28. However, there are logistical challenges to setting up outpatient infusions of remdesivir.

In clinical trials, commonly reported adverse events associated with remdesivir include nausea, constipation, elevated aminotransferase levels, and acute kidney injury.[9,10] Reports of significant hepatic injury are rare, and most serum aminotransferase elevations associated with remdesivir's use are self-resolving.[20] It is unclear if nephrotoxicity observed in the setting of remdesivir use is a result of the drug or of end-organ damage in the setting of COVID-19 infection. There is concern that different formulations of remdesivir may be more nephrotoxic due to increased amounts of sulfobutylether-β-cyclodextrin, but a retrospective analysis did not support this

concern,[21] whereas another suggests that remdesivir is not nephrotoxic.[22] Nonetheless, it is prudent to participate in shared decision making with patients who qualify for remdesivir and have significant renal impairment.

Overall, the current body of evidence continues to support remdesivir's use in hospitalized patients with moderate-to-severe COVID-19. Although remdesivir resistance mutations have been reported in immunocompromised patients with delayed viral clearance,[23] widespread resistance to remdesivir has not emerged during the SARS-CoV-2 pandemic.[24] Newer evidence supports remdesivir's role in preventing disease progression in the outpatient setting, and further data exploring its real-world effectiveness in outpatient populations at-risk for disease progression are needed. Importantly, logistical challenges to its outpatient administration will require creative solutions, and oral antiviral therapies remain more convenient in the interim.

Nirmatrelvir/Ritonavir

Nirmatrelvir is an inhibitor of the SARS-CoV-2 3CL protease (also known as M^pro) and results in disruption of polyprotein cleavage during viral replication.[25] It is co-administered with ritonavir, an HIV protease inhibitor that inhibits CYP3A4 metabolism to achieve therapeutic plasma levels.[26] In contrast to remdesivir's intravenous route of administration, nirmatrelvir/ritonavir is orally administered as a twice daily combination of two tablets (300 mg of nirmatrelvir and 150 mg of ritonavir).

Nirmatrelvir/ritonavir is currently available under FDA emergency use authorization (EUA) for early treatment (within 5 days symptom onset) of outpatients with COVID-19 who are at risk for disease progression. In the EPIC-HR double-blind RCT, a 5-day course of nirmatrelvir/ritonavir ($n = 1120$) was compared with placebo ($n = 1126$) in symptomatic, non-hospitalized adults with COVID-19 within 5 days of symptom onset who were at risk for disease progression.[26] In the final analysis for the modified intention to treat population ($n = 1379$), the estimated event rate of COVID-19 related hospitalization or all-cause mortality at day 28 was 5.81 percentage points lower for those who received nirmatrelvir/ritonavir (0.72%) compared with placebo (6.53%) (relative risk reduction 88.9%; 95% CI -7.78 to -3.84; $p < 0.001$). No deaths were reported in the nirmatrelvir/ritonavir group compared with thirteen deaths in the placebo group. Nirmatrelvir/ritonavir has also been evaluated as post-exposure prophylaxis in the Phase 2/3 EPIC-PEP trial, but the differences in risk reduction offered by 5-day and 10-day courses of nirmatrelvir/ritonavir were not significant relative to placebo.[27]

In the EPIC-HR trial, the incidence of adverse events was similar for patients who received nirmatrelvir/ritonavir (22.6%) compared with placebo (23.9%).[26] Dysgeusia and diarrhea were more commonly observed in the nirmatrelvir/ritonavir group compared with placebo. Owing to ritonavir's CYP3A4 inhibition, nirmatrelvir/ritonavir's use must account for co-administered medications which interact with the same cytochrome P450 enzyme (eg, phenytoin, cyclosporine, and warfarin).[28] Successful implementation of nirmatrelvir/ritonavir requires systematic approaches to dose monitoring in this subpopulation of patients. There are no clinical data to guide the use of nirmatrelvir/ritonavir in pregnancy, but adverse events after exposure to nirmatrelvir were observed in embryo-fetal developmental studies in mammals.[29,30] The risk of progression to severe COVID-19 should be weighed against potential adverse fetal effects when making a decision on use in pregnancy.

In general, nirmatrelvir/ritonavir is an oral antiviral therapy for preventing disease progression in outpatient persons with COVID-19, and it resulted in an 89% relative risk reduction in hospitalization or all-cause mortality at day 28 in the EPIC-HR trial.[26] Its use requires careful monitoring or discontinuation of co-administered medications that interact with CYP3A4[28]; however, this challenge has been overcome in select patient populations (eg, solid organ transplant recipients[31]). Preliminary reports on "rebound" SARS-CoV-2 infection after nirmatrelvir/ritonavir suggest a mild clinical presentation, but the phenomenon requires further characterization.[32,33] Patients are advised to follow the Centers for Disease Control and Prevention standard COVID-19 isolation protocol in the event of "rebound."[33]

Molnupiravir

Molnupiravir is a ribonucleoside analog of N-hydroxycytidine with antiviral activity against SARS-CoV-2 and related RNA viruses.[34] It becomes activated intracellularly and incorporated into RNA by RNA-dependent RNA polymerase, resulting in mutations and eventual loss of viral replication ability. Similar to nirmatrelvir/ritonavir, it is available under FDA EUA as a 5-day oral treatment course (four 200-mg tablets twice daily).[35] Molnupiravir is intended for outpatients within 5-days of COVID-19 symptoms onset who are at risk for disease progression.[36]

Molnupiravir use is supported by the MOVe-OUT trial, a double-blind RCT comparing molnupiravir ($n = 716$) to placebo ($n = 717$) for nonvaccinated, non-hospitalized adult patients with COVID-19 at risk for disease progression who were within 5 days of symptom onset.[36] For the whole randomized, intention-to-treat population, hospitalization or death at day 29 was lower in the molnupiravir group compared with placebo (6.8% vs 9.7%; 95% CI -5.9 to -0.1). A time-to-event analysis showed a roughly 30% lower rate of hospitalization or death at day 29 for patients who received molnupiravir. Of note, an interim analysis of the same trial showed a 50% decrease in all-cause hospitalization or death at day 29 compared with placebo, suggesting possible computational errors during the trial's data analysis.[37] In contrast to the MOVe-OUT trial,[36] a double-blind RCT evaluating molnupiravir at 3 dose levels (200 mg, 400 mg and 800 mg twice daily) for hospitalized adult patients with COVID-19 within 10 days of symptom onset did not show a meaningful benefit for patients receiving molnupiravir compared with placebo.[38]

In the MOVe-OUT trial, the incidence of adverse events was similar between treatment groups (30.4% in molnupiravir group vs 33% in placebo group).[36] Diarrhea, nausea, and dizziness were the most frequent adverse events deemed to be related to the administered regimen (ie, molnupiravir or placebo). Pregnant persons were excluded from the MOVe-OUT trial,[36] and molnupiravir is not recommended during pregnancy due to evidence of teratogenicity from animal studies.[35] In the absence of alternative therapies, use of molnupiravir in pregnant patients at high risk of progression may be considered beyond 10 weeks of gestation after a documented discussion of risk-benefits between patient and provider.[39] Owing to concerns of mutagenicity, patients of reproductive age are also advised to use reliable forms of contraception during and after administration of molnupiravir (4 days after last dose in women, 3 months after last dose in men).[35]

Similar to nirmatrelvir/ritonavir, molnupiravir is an oral antiviral option for prevention of disease progression in at-risk, outpatient persons with COVID-19. Although molnupiravir increases pill burden (8 pills daily) and did not perform as well as nirmatrelvir/ritonavir in an RCT,[26,36] its administration does not require meticulous monitoring of co-administered medications that interact with CYP3A4. The safety of molnupiravir use in pregnant patients and patients of reproductive age requires further study, and a risk-benefit discussion ought to inform these patients' care.[35] In addition, the effectiveness of oral antiviral agents is less characterized in high-risk, immunocompromised patients due to RCTs' focus on general patient populations, and further data are needed.

MONOCLONAL ANTIBODIES

Monoclonal antibodies are sourced from convalescent patients or humanized mice and can serve as antiviral therapies.[40] For SARS-CoV-2, monoclonal antibody therapies block fusion and entry of virus by binding the receptor-binding domain (RBD) of the Spike protein on the virion particle's surface.[40] Given the natural history of COVID-19,[5] monoclonal antibodies are most effective when administered early after symptom onset, and their use is authorized for outpatient persons with COVID-19. Unvaccinated patients, immunocompromised patients who may not respond to vaccine series, and other at-risk patient populations stand to benefit most from passive immunization with monoclonal therapies.

Studies involving the use of monoclonal antibodies in hospitalized adults have yielded mixed results.[41–44] Nonetheless, it is interesting to note that casirivimab/imdevimab led to a statistically significant ($p = 0.0009$) reduction in 28-day mortality for hospitalized patients without detectable antibodies to SARS-CoV-2 (ie, seronegative patients) in the RECOVERY trial.[41] These data suggest a potential role for monoclonal antibody administration in seronegative hospitalized patients, especially immunocompromised individuals who may not mount a humoral response to vaccines.[45,46]

In addition to serving as antiviral therapy, monoclonal antibodies have been evaluated as preexposure prophylaxis for SARS-CoV-2.[47] Despite previous authorizations, monoclonal antibodies are not currently recommended as postexposure prophylaxis. The following sections summarize monoclonal antibodies with active or prior FDA EUA.

Treatment

Casirivimab/imdevimab

Casirivimab and imdevimab are two monoclonal antibodies identified via high-throughput screening which target the SARS-CoV-2 Spike RBD.[48] The use of casirivimab/imdevimab, administered within 72 hours of a positive viral test and 7 days of symptom onset, was evaluated in an adaptive trial that compared 2 different doses [2400 mg ($n = 1355$) and 1200 mg ($n = 736$)] with placebo [2400 mg placebo ($n = 1341$) and 1200 mg placebo ($n = 748$)] in preventing disease progression in non-hospitalized patients with COVID-19 and ≥ 1 risk for severe disease.[48] At day 29, the primary outcome of COVID-19-related hospitalization or death from any cause had occurred in 1.3% of the 2400 mg group compared with 4.6% in the placebo group (relative risk reduction 71.3%; $p < 0.001$). The 1200 mg group had similar results (relative risk reduction 70.4%; $p = 0.002$). Owing to efficacy concerns related to the Omicron variant, the FDA EUA was withdrawn for casirivimab/imdevimab on January 24, 2022.[49]

Bamlanivimab/etesevimab

Originally isolated from plasma of individuals who recovered from COVID-19, bamlanivimab and etesevimab are recombinant monoclonal antibodies with neutralizing activity against the SARS-CoV-2 Spike protein.[50] In the BLAZE-1 RCT, the combination of bamlanivimab and etesevimab was evaluated as a means to prevent disease progression in at-risk, non-hospitalized patients with COVID-19 within 3 days of laboratory diagnosis.[50] The primary outcome of COVID-19-related hospitalization or all-cause death at day 29 was 4.9 percentage points lower in the bamlanivimab/etesevimab group ($n = 518$) relative to placebo ($n = 517$) (absolute risk difference −4.8%; 95% CI −7.4 to −2.3; $p < 0.001$). Ten deaths occurred in the placebo group versus no deaths in the bamlanivimab/etesevimab group. Owing to concerns of decreased neutralizing activity with the Omicron variant, the EUA for bamlanivimab/etesevimab in the United States was withdrawn on January 24, 2022.[51]

Sotrovimab

Sotrovimab is a monoclonal antibody which targets a conserved epitope of the RBD of the Spike protein on sarbecoviruses, including SARS-CoV-2.[52] Early administration of sotrovimab (within 5 days of symptom onset) was evaluated for prevention of disease progression in non-hospitalized, at-risk adults with COVID-19 in the COMET-ICE trial.[53,54] At the interim analysis, 1% of the patients who received sotrovimab ($n = 291$) experienced the primary outcome of hospitalization or death from any cause at day 29 compared with 7% in the placebo group ($n = 292$) (relative risk reduction 85%; 97.24% CI 44–96; $p = 0.002$). Rates of adverse were similar in the sotrovimab (17%) and placebo (19%) groups, and infusion-related reactions affected 1% of both groups. Despite its initial promise in treating patients with infections due to the Omicron variant, the sustained rise in the Omicron BA.2 sublineage, against which sotrovimab has significantly reduced neutralizing activity,[55] has led to withdrawal of its EUA by the FDA as of April 5, 2022.[56]

Bebtelovimab

Bebtelovimab is a monoclonal antibody which targets the SARS-CoV-2 Spike RBD, with activity against Omicron subvariants[57] and was first authorized for use in the United States on February 11, 2022 under an FDA EUA.[58] Bebtelovimab is indicated for prevention of disease progression in high risk outpatients with mild-to-moderate COVID-19. The clinical evidence supporting bebtelovimab's use stems from the phase 2 BLAZE-4 trial which was notably conducted before the emergence of Omicron.[58,59] The placebo-controlled arm of the study evaluated low-risk, non-hospitalized patients within 3 days of symptom onset and randomized participants in three groups: bebtelovimab ($n = 125$), bebtelovimab/bamlanivimab/etesevimab ($n = 127$), and placebo ($n = 128$). The primary endpoint of persistently elevated viral load (log viral load >5.27) at day 7 occurred in 21% of the placebo group compared with 13% in the combination group and 14% in the bebtelovimab group. Differences between groups were not statistically significant. Further trial data and real-world datasets are needed.

Preexposure Prophylaxis

Tixagevimab/cilgavimab

The monoclonal antibody combination tixagevimab/cilgavimab, which bind to non-overlapping loci of the SARS-CoV-2 Spike protein,[47] received an FDA EUA on December 8, 2021, for the preexposure prophylaxis of COVID-19 for immunocompromised individuals who may not mount an adequate response to available vaccines or individuals with contraindications to current vaccines due to serious adverse events.[60] Its use as preexposure prophylaxis is supported by the PROVENT phase 3 trial which compared tixagevmab/cilgavimab administered as two consecutive injections of 300 mg doses ($n = 3460$) with saline placebo ($n = 1737$).[47] The primary endpoint of symptomatic COVID-19 occurred in 0.2% (8/3441) in the tixagevimab/cilgavimab group versus 1.0% (17/1731) in the placebo group (Relative risk reduction 76.7%; 95% CI 46–90 $p < 0.001$). Unlike other available monoclonal antibodies for SARS-CoV-2, tixagevimab/cilgavimab is not currently authorized for treatment of COVID-19 or postexposure prophylaxis.[60] The combination is expected to have activity against the Omicron BA.2 sublineage, with reduced activity against BA.1 and BA.1.1[60]; however, real-world data are limited. In addition, the PROVENT trial was conducted before the emergence of Omicron, and the dosage of tixagevimab/cilgavimab currently recommended by the FDA (two 600 mg injections) is double the trial's dose.[60] A recent report has highlighted the risk of SARS-CoV-2 infection in the time period following administration and emphasized the need to reinforce masking and social distancing in patients who receive tixagevimab/cilgavimab.[61]

OTHER THERAPIES FOR TREATMENT OF CORONAVIRUS DISEASE-2019

In addition to the direct acting antivirals and monoclonal antibodies discussed above, numerous therapies have been evaluated as treatment options for COVID-19. Some therapies (eg, convalescent plasma)[62,63] have yielded mixed results in clinical trials, whereas others have consistently shown no meaningful benefit. **Supplement Table 1** summarizes data on select therapeutic options not currently recommended as treatment of COVID-19.

MANAGEMENT OF OUTPATIENT CORONAVIRUS DISEASE-2019 AND PREEXPOSURE PROPHYLAXIS

Outpatient management of COVID-19 in at-risk patient populations is essential in preventing hospitalization and progression of disease. **Fig. 3** provides an overview of the Yale New Haven Health System's (YNHHS) clinical pathway for the

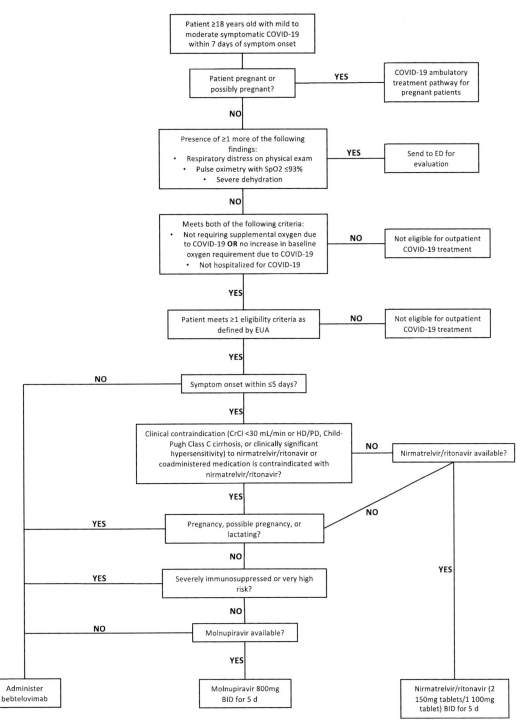

Fig. 3. Clinical pathway for management of outpatient persons with COVID-19. Clinical pathway as of May 16, 2022. Definitions for "severely immunosuppressed" and "very high risk" provided in **Supplement Table 2**. CrCl, creatinine clearance; ED, emergency department; EUA, emergency use authorization; HD, hemodialysis; PD, peritoneal dialysis.

management of mild-to-moderate COVID-19 in the outpatient setting. This pathway is largely consistent with guideline statements published by the NIH[64] and IDSA.[12] When evaluating persons

with COVID-19 in an outpatient setting, providers must first identify and appropriately triage patients who may benefit from hospitalization. To qualify for outpatient therapies, patients must also have symptom lengths within acceptable time frames and have predisposing factors that confer a higher risk for disease progression.

After these initial considerations are addressed, patients' comorbidities and symptom lengths determine which of three treatment options is appropriate. For persons with ≤5 days of symptoms and no contraindications (eg, co-administered medication interacts with CYP3A4), our center prioritizes the use of nirmatrelvir/ritonavir for 5 days. If nirmatrelvir/ritonavir is contraindicated, molnupiravir and bebtelovimab are alternative options. Molnupiravir, administered as a 5-day course, is offered to patients with contraindications to nirmatrelvir/ritonavir who are neither pregnant nor severely immunocompromised. Bebtelovimab is preferred for lactating or pregnant patients, patients who are severely immunocompromised and patients who are beyond 5 days but within 7 days of symptom onset. Our center does not offer remdesivir to outpatient persons with COVID-19 due to logistical constraints; however, remdesivir is a preferred therapy in the NIH guidelines for management of outpatient COVID-19,[64] and its use in outpatient settings is supported by the PINE-TREE trial.[19]

To prevent COVID-19 in immunocompromised patients who may not respond to vaccines and/or patients with severe hypersensitivity reactions to current vaccines, our center offers tixagevimab/cilgavimab as preexposure prophylaxis (**Fig. 4**). In accordance with the FDA's EUA,[60] eligible patients must be ≥ 12 years and weigh ≥40 kilograms with one or more immunocompromising conditions or recent use of immunosuppressive medication(s). Our center's list of qualifying comorbidities includes conditions with functional or numerical deficits in T cells and/or B cells. Patients eligible for tixagevimab/cilgavimab in the YNHHS are required to have received the most recent vaccine dose >2 weeks beforehand.

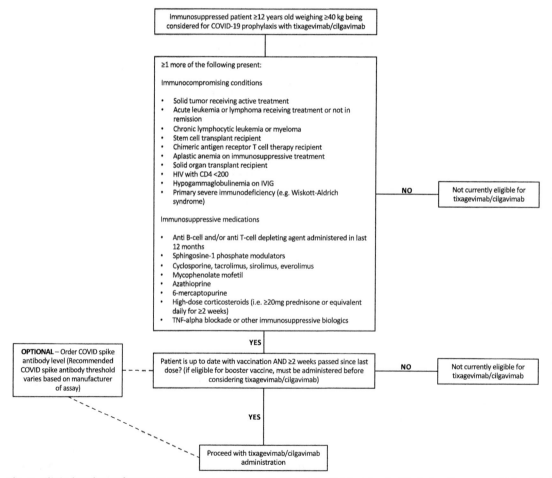

Fig. 4. Clinical pathway for preexposure prophylaxis with tixagevimab/cilgavimab. Clinical pathway as of May 16, 2022. HIV, human immunodeficiency virus; IVIG, intravenous immunoglobulin.

MANAGEMENT OF INPATIENT CORONAVIRUS DISEASE-2019

Management of hospitalized adults with COVID-19 varies based on the severity of COVID-19-related symptoms. **Fig. 5** summarizes the YNHHS clinical pathway for hospitalized adults with known or suspected COVID-19. The pathway is largely consistent with guidelines published by the NIH[13] and IDSA.[12] For asymptomatic infections, no COVID-19-specific treatments are administered, and close monitoring with appropriate isolation is recommended.

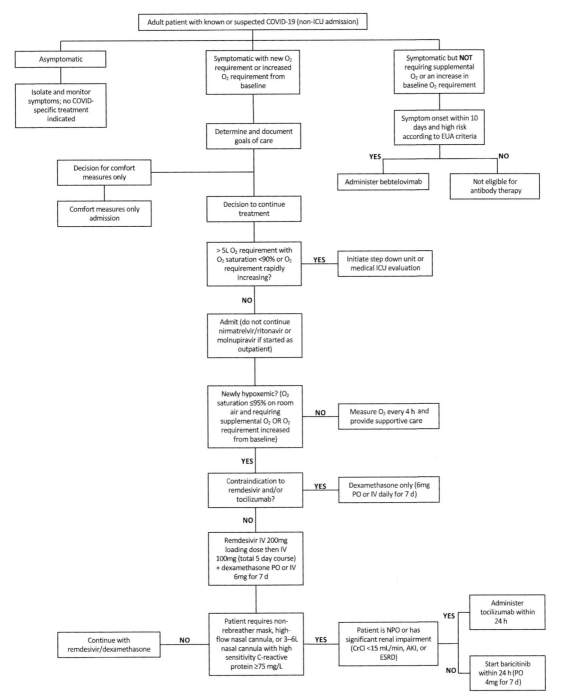

Fig. 5. Clinical pathway for management of inpatient persons with COVID-19. Clinical pathway as of May 16, 2022. AKI, acute kidney injury; CrCl, creatinine clearance; ESRD, end stage renal disease; EUA, emergency use authorization; ICU, intensive care unit; IV, intravenous; NPO, nil per os; PO, per os.

Table 2
Reduction in SARS-CoV-2 lineages' susceptibility to monoclonal antibodies based on pseudotyped virus-like particle neutralization assay

SARS-CoV-2 Lineage	World Health Organization Nomenclature	Casirivimab/Imdevimab[a] Reduction in Susceptibility	Bamlanivimab/Etesevimab[b] Reduction in Susceptibility	Sotrovimab[c] Reduction in Susceptibility	Tixagevimab/Cilgavimab[d] Reduction in Susceptibility	Bebtelovimab[e] Reduction in Susceptibility
B.1.1.7	Alpha	No change	No change	No change	0.5- to 5.2-fold	No change
B.1.351	Beta	No change	431-fold	No change	No change	No change
P.1	Gamma	No change	252-fold	No change	No change	No change
B.1.617.2/AY.3	Delta	No change	No change	No change	No change	No change
AY.1/AY.2 (B.1.617.2 sublineages)	Delta [+K417 N]	Not determined	1235-fold	No change	No change	No change
B.1.427/B.1.429	Epsilon	No change	9-fold	No change	No change	No change
B.1.526	Iota	No change	30-fold	No change	No change	No change
B.1.617.1	Kappa	No change	6-fold	No change	No change	No change
C.37	Lambda	Not determined	No change	No change	No change	No change
B.1.621	Mu	No change	116-fold	No change	7.5-fold	5.3-fold
B.1.1.529/BA.1	Omicron [BA.1]	>1013-fold	>2938-fold	No change	132- to 183-fold	No change
BA.1.1	Omicron [+R346 K]	Not determined	Not determined	No change	424-fold	No change
BA.2	Omicron [BA.2]	Not determined	Not determined	16-fold	No change	No change
BA.2.12.1	Omicron [BA.2 + L452Q]	Not determined	Not determined	Not determined	Not determined	No change
BA.4/BA.5	Omicron [BA.4/BA.5]	Not determined	Not determined	Not determined	No determined	No change

a Casirivimab/imdevimab data from Food & Drug Administration (FDA) fact sheet[49] updated January 24, 2022.
b Bamlanivimab/etesevimab data from FDA fact sheet[51] updated January 24, 2022.
c Sotrovimab data from FDA fact sheet[54] updated March 25, 2022.
d Tixagevimab/cilgavimab data from FDA fact sheet[60] updated May 17, 2022.
e Bebtelovimab data from FDA fact sheet[58] updated June 16, 2022.

For mildly symptomatic patients without a new or increased oxygen requirement, our center recommends bebtelovimab when symptom onset is within 10 days and the patient is considered high risk for disease progression. This subset of patients likely carries COVID-19 as an incidental diagnosis, and the reason for admission is unrelated. Though not a component of published guidelines, our pathway's recommendation of bebtelovimab is designed to prevent further progression of disease in this subset of patients with COVID-19. Our center's decision is in line with bebtelovimab's EUA and motivated by the need to intervene at an earlier timepoint for both immunocompromised persons and patients at higher risk for disease progression.

For symptomatic patients with a new or increased oxygen requirement, management focuses on supportive care (eg, supplemental oxygen) and COVID-19-specific treatments. A 5-day course of remdesivir co-administered with a 7-day course of dexamethasone is recommended for newly hypoxemic patients, and dexamethasone alone is used for patients with contraindications to remdesivir. In addition to these therapies, patients with greater severity of disease and substantial oxygen requirements (eg, high flow nasal cannula) are offered a 7-day course of baricitinib. Owing to tocilizumab shortages, a single dose of tocilizumab is prioritized for patients with significant renal impairment or patients unable to receive orally-administered medications. In each case, it is critical to monitor the illness trajectory of the individual patient, and the level of care must be elevated or deescalated as needed.

IMPACT OF SEVERE ACUTE RESPIRATORY SYNDROME CORONAVIRUS 2 VARIANTS ON TREATMENT

Novel variants of SARS-CoV-2 have emerged at a steady pace since the onset of the pandemic. Detection and characterization of new variants is crucial to determine whether available therapies retain antiviral and neutralizing activity.[65] At this time, the dominant variant remains Omicron and its sublineages.[66] Importantly, the BA.2, BA.2.12.1, BA.4 and BA.5 variants, which are currently dominant in many areas of the world, contain several mutations in the RBD of the Spike protein which render them less susceptible to neutralization with available monoclonal antibodies (**Table 2**).[55] However, bebtelovimab is expected to retain its neutralizing activity against BA.2, BA.2.12.1, BA.4 and BA.5.[57,67] Small molecule antivirals (ie, remdesivir, molnupiravir, and nirmatrelvir) have been shown to retain activity against the BA.2 sublineage.[55] Despite the lower severity of illness observed during the Omicron surge,[68,69] further data on the effectiveness of monoclonal antibodies and small molecule antivirals are still needed, especially in immunocompromised populations.

SUMMARY

Direct acting antivirals and monoclonal antibodies reduce morbidity and mortality associated with SARS-CoV-2 infection. Persons at higher risk for disease progression and hospitalized patients with COVID-19 benefit most from available therapies. Following an emphasis on inpatient treatment of COVID-19 during the early pandemic, several therapeutic options were developed for outpatients with COVID-19. Additional clinical trials and real-world studies are needed to both inform the care of immunocompromised patients and keep pace with the evolving pandemic.

CLINICS CARE POINTS

- Remdesivir and dexamethasone with or without additional immunomodulatory therapy are recommended for hospitalized persons with moderate-to-severe coronavirus disease-2019 (COVID-19)
- Bebtelovimab is the only monoclonal antibody authorized for treatment of SARS-CoV-2 infections caused by circulating Omicron sublineages
- Both molnupiravir and nirmatrelvir/ritonavir are oral antiviral options for outpatient persons with COVID-19; relative and absolute contraindications should be taken into account before prescribing these therapies.

DISCLOSURE

The authors report no potential conflicts of interest or funding sources.

REFERENCES

1. WHO. WHO coronavirus (COVID-19) dashboard. Available at: https://covid19.who.int/. Accessed September 30, 2022.
2. Nguyen KH, Anneser E, Toppo A, et al. Disparities in national and state estimates of COVID-19 vaccination receipt and intent to vaccinate by race/ethnicity, income, and age group among adults ≥ 18 years, United States. Vaccine 2022;40(1):107–13 (In eng).

3. Wagner CE, Saad-Roy CM, Morris SE, et al. Vaccine nationalism and the dynamics and control of SARS-CoV-2. Science 2021;373(6562):eabj7364 (In eng).

4. Gandhi RT, Lynch JB, Del Rio C. Mild or moderate covid-19. N Engl J Med 2020;383(18):1757–66 (In eng).

5. Berlin DA, Gulick RM, Martinez FJ. Severe covid-19. N Engl J Med 2020;383(25):2451–60 (In eng).

6. Wang M, Cao R, Zhang L, et al. Remdesivir and chloroquine effectively inhibit the recently emerged novel coronavirus (2019-nCoV) in vitro. Cell Res 2020;30(3):269–71 (In eng).

7. Warren TK, Jordan R, Lo MK, et al. Therapeutic efficacy of the small molecule GS-5734 against Ebola virus in rhesus monkeys. Nature 2016;531(7594):381–5 (In eng).

8. Jorgensen SCJ, Kebriaei R, Dresser LD. Remdesivir: review of pharmacology, pre-clinical data, and emerging clinical experience for COVID-19. Pharmacotherapy 2020;40(7):659–71 (In eng).

9. Beigel JH, Tomashek KM, Dodd LE, et al. Remdesivir for the treatment of covid-19 - final report. N Engl J Med 2020;383(19):1813–26 (In eng).

10. Goldman JD, Lye DCB, Hui DS, et al. Remdesivir for 5 or 10 Days in patients with severe covid-19. N Engl J Med 2020;383(19):1827–37 (In eng).

11. Mulangu S, Dodd LE, Davey RT, et al. A randomized, controlled trial of Ebola virus disease therapeutics. N Engl J Med 2019;381(24):2293–303 (In eng).

12. IDSA. IDSA Guidelines on the treatment and management of patients with COVID-19. 2022. Available at: https://www.idsociety.org/practice-guideline/covid-19-guideline-treatment-and-management/. Accessed June 4, 2022.

13. Therapeutic NIH. Management of hospitalized adults with COVID-19. 2022. Available at: https://www.covid19treatmentguidelines.nih.gov/management/clinical-management/hospitalized-adults–therapeutic-management/. Accessed June 4, 2022.

14. Kalil AC, Patterson TF, Mehta AK, et al. Baricitinib plus remdesivir for hospitalized adults with covid-19. N Engl J Med 2021;384(9):795–807 (In eng).

15. Wolfe CR, Tomashek KM, Patterson TF, et al. Baricitinib versus dexamethasone for adults hospitalised with COVID-19 (ACTT-4): a randomised, double-blind, double placebo-controlled trial. Lancet Respir Med 2022. https://doi.org/10.1016/S2213-2600(22)00088-1 (In eng).

16. Rosas IO, Diaz G, Gottlieb RL, et al. Tocilizumab and remdesivir in hospitalized patients with severe COVID-19 pneumonia: a randomized clinical trial. Intensive Care Med 2021;47(11):1258–70 (In eng).

17. Salama C, Han J, Yau L, et al. Tocilizumab in patients hospitalized with covid-19 pneumonia. N Engl J Med 2021;384(1):20–30 (In eng).

18. Gordon AC, Mouncey PR, Al-Beidh F, et al. Interleukin-6 receptor antagonists in critically ill patients with covid-19. N Engl J Med 2021;384(16):1491–502 (In eng).

19. Gottlieb RL, Vaca CE, Paredes R, et al. Early remdesivir to prevent progression to severe covid-19 in outpatients. N Engl J Med 2022;386(4):305–15 (In eng).

20. NIH. Remdesivir - LiverTox - NCBI Bookshelf. 2022. Available at: https://www.ncbi.nlm.nih.gov/books/NBK564049/#:~:text=Hepatotoxicity,other%20evidence%20of%20hepatic%20injury. Accessed June 4, 2022.

21. Shah S, Ackley TW, Topal JE. Renal and hepatic toxicity analysis of remdesivir formulations: does what is on the inside really count? Antimicrob Agents Chemother 2021;65(10):e0104521 (In eng).

22. Ackley TW, McManus D, Topal JE, et al. A valid warning or clinical lore: an evaluation of safety outcomes of remdesivir in patients with impaired renal function from a multicenter matched cohort. Antimicrob Agents Chemother 2021;65(2). https://doi.org/10.1128/AAC.02290-20 (In eng).

23. Gandhi S, Klein J, Robertson AJ, et al. De novo emergence of a remdesivir resistance mutation during treatment of persistent SARS-CoV-2 infection in an immunocompromised patient: a case report. Nat Commun 2022;13(1):1547 (In eng).

24. Focosi D, Maggi F, McConnell S, et al. Very low levels of remdesivir resistance in SARS-COV-2 genomes after 18 months of massive usage during the COVID19 pandemic: a GISAID exploratory analysis. Antivir Res 2022;198:105247 (In eng).

25. Owen DR, Allerton CMN, Anderson AS, et al. An oral SARS-CoV-2 M. Science 2021;374(6575):1586–93 (In eng).

26. Hammond J, Leister-Tebbe H, Gardner A, et al. Oral nirmatrelvir for high-risk, nonhospitalized adults with covid-19. N Engl J Med 2022. https://doi.org/10.1056/NEJMoa2118542 (In eng).

27. Pfizer shares top-line results from phase 2/3 EPIC-PEP study of PAXLOVID™ for postexposure prophylactic use. 2022. Available at: https://www.pfizer.com/news/press-release/press-release-detail/pfizer-shares-top-line-results-phase-23-epic-pep-study. Accessed June 4, 2022.

28. Saravolatz LD, Depcinski S, Sharma M. Molnupiravir and nirmatrelvir-ritonavir: oral COVID antiviral drugs. Clin Infect Dis 2022. https://doi.org/10.1093/cid/ciac180 (In eng).

29. Catlin NR, Bowman CJ, Campion SN, et al. Reproductive and developmental safety of nirmatrelvir (PF-07321332), an oral SARS-CoV-2 M. Reprod Toxicol 2022;108:56–61 (In eng).

30. FDA. Fact sheet for healthcare providers: emergency use authorization for Paxlovid™. Available at: https://www.fda.gov/media/155050/download. Accessed June 4, 2022.

31. Salerno DM, Jennings DL, Lange NW, et al. Early clinical experience with nirmatrelvir/ritonavir for treatment of COVID-19 in solid organ transplant recipients. Am J Transpl 2022. https://doi.org/10.1111/ajt.17027 (In eng).

32. Ranganath N, O'Horo JC, Challener DW, et al. Rebound phenomenon after nirmatrelvir/ritonavir treatment of coronavirus disease-2019 in high-risk persons. Clin Infect Dis 2022. https://doi.org/10.1093/cid/ciac481 (In eng).

33. CDC. COVID-19 rebound after paxlovid treatment. 2022. Available at: https://emergency.cdc.gov/han/2022/han00467.asp. Accessed June 4, 2022.

34. Wahl A, Gralinski LE, Johnson CE, et al. SARS-CoV-2 infection is effectively treated and prevented by EIDD-2801. Nature 2021;591(7850):451–7 (In eng).

35. FDA. Fact sheet for healthcare providers: emergency use authorization for Lagevrio™ (molnupiravir) capsules. Available at: https://www.fda.gov/media/155054/download. Accessed June 4, 2022.

36. Jayk Bernal A, Gomes da Silva MM, Musungaie DB, et al. Molnupiravir for oral treatment of covid-19 in nonhospitalized patients. N Engl J Med 2022; 386(6):509–20 (In eng).

37. Thorlund K, Sheldrick K, Mills E. Molnupiravir for covid-19 in nonhospitalized patients. N Engl J Med 2022;386(13):e32 (In eng).

38. Arribas JR, Bhagani S, Lobo SM, et al. Randomized trial of molnupiravir or placebo in patients hospitalized with covid-19. NEJM Evid 2022;1(2). https://doi.org/10.1056/EVIDoa2100044.

39. NIH. Molnupiravir. 2022. Available at: https://www.covid19treatmentguidelines.nih.gov/therapies/antiviral-therapy/molnupiravir/. Accessed June 4, 2022.

40. Taylor PC, Adams AC, Hufford MM, et al. Neutralizing monoclonal antibodies for treatment of COVID-19. Nat Rev Immunol 2021;21(6):382–93 (In eng).

41. Group RC. Casirivimab and imdevimab in patients admitted to hospital with COVID-19 (RECOVERY): a randomised, controlled, open-label, platform trial. Lancet 2022;399(10325):665–76 (In eng).

42. Lundgren JD, Grund B, Barkauskas CE, et al. A neutralizing monoclonal antibody for hospitalized patients with covid-19. N Engl J Med 2021; 384(10):905–14 (In eng).

43. Lundgren JD, Grund B, Barkauskas CE, et al. Responses to a neutralizing monoclonal antibody for hospitalized patients with COVID-19 according to baseline antibody and antigen levels : a randomized controlled trial. Ann Intern Med 2022;175(2):234–43 (In eng).

44. Group A-TflwC-TS. Efficacy and safety of two neutralising monoclonal antibody therapies, sotrovimab and BRII-196 plus BRII-198, for adults hospitalised with COVID-19 (TICO): a randomised controlled trial. Lancet Infect Dis 2022;22(5):622–35 (In eng).

45. Eckerle I, Rosenberger KD, Zwahlen M, et al. Serologic vaccination response after solid organ transplantation: a systematic review. PLoS One 2013; 8(2):e56974 (In eng).

46. Dhodapkar MV, Dhodapkar KM, Ahmed R. Viral immunity and vaccines in hematologic malignancies: implications for COVID-19. Blood Cancer Discov 2021;2(1):9–12 (In eng).

47. Levin MJ, Ustianowski A, De Wit S, et al. Intramuscular AZD7442 (Tixagevimab-Cilgavimab) for prevention of covid-19. N Engl J Med 2022. https://doi.org/10.1056/NEJMoa2116620 (In eng).

48. Weinreich DM, Sivapalasingam S, Norton T, et al. REGEN-COV antibody combination and outcomes in outpatients with covid-19. N Engl J Med 2021; 385(23):e81 (In eng).

49. FDA. Fact sheet for healthcare providers emergency use authorization (EUA) of REGEN-COV (casirivimab and imdevimab). 2022. Available at: https://www.fda.gov/media/145611/download. Accessed June 4, 2022.

50. Dougan M, Nirula A, Azizad M, et al. Bamlanivimab plus etesevimab in mild or moderate covid-19. N Engl J Med 2021;385(15):1382–92 (In eng).

51. FDA. Fact sheet for healthcare providers emergency use authorization (EUA) of bamlanivimab and etesevimab. 2022. Available at: https://www.fda.gov/media/145802/download. Accessed June 4, 2022.

52. Pinto D, Park YJ, Beltramello M, et al. Cross-neutralization of SARS-CoV-2 by a human monoclonal SARS-CoV antibody. Nature 2020;583(7815):290–5 (In eng).

53. Gupta A, Gonzalez-Rojas Y, Juarez E, et al. Early treatment for covid-19 with SARS-CoV-2 neutralizing antibody sotrovimab. N Engl J Med 2021;385(21):1941–50 (In eng).

54. FDA. Fact sheet for healthcare providers emergency use authorization (EUA) of sotrovimab. 2022. Available at: https://www.fda.gov/media/149534/download. Accessed June 20, 2022.

55. Takashita E, Kinoshita N, Yamayoshi S, et al. Efficacy of antiviral agents against the SARS-CoV-2 omicron subvariant BA.2. N Engl J Med 2022;386(15):1475–7 (In eng).

56. FDA. FDA updates Sotrovimab emergency use authorization. 2022. Available at: https://www.fda.gov/drugs/drug-safety-and-availability/fda-updates-sotrovimab-emergency-use-authorization. Accessed June 4, 2022.

57. Iketani S, Liu L, Guo Y, et al. Antibody evasion properties of SARS-CoV-2 Omicron sublineages. Nature 2022. https://doi.org/10.1038/s41586-022-04594-4 (In eng).

58. FDA. Fact sheet for healthcare providers: emergency use authorization for bebtelovimab. 2022. Available at: https://www.fda.gov/media/156152/download. Accessed June 20, 2022.

59. Dougan M, Azizad M, Chen P, et al. Bebtelovimab, alone or together with bamlanivimab and etesevimab, as a broadly neutralizing monoclonal antibody treatment for mild to moderate, ambulatory COVID-19. medRxiv 2022. https://doi.org/10.1101/2022.03.10.22272100.

60. FDA. Fact sheet for healthcare providers: emergency use authorization for Evusheld™ (tixagevimab co-packaged with cilgavimab). 2022. Available at: https://www.fda.gov/media/154701/download. Accessed June 4, 2022.

61. Ordaya EE, Beam E, Yao JD, et al. Characterization of early-onset SARS-CoV-2 infection in immunocompromised patients who received tixagevimab-cilgavimab prophylaxis. Open Forum Infect Dis 2022;ofac283. https://doi.org/10.1093/ofid/ofac283.

62. Simonovich VA, Burgos Pratx LD, Scibona P, et al. A randomized trial of convalescent plasma in covid-19 severe pneumonia. N Engl J Med 2021; 384(7):619–29 (In eng).

63. Libster R, Pérez Marc G, Wappner D, et al. Early high-titer plasma therapy to prevent severe covid-19 in older adults. N Engl J Med 2021;384(7): 610–8 (In eng).

64. NIH. Therapeutic Management of nonhospitalized adults with COVID-19. 2022. Available at: https://www.covid19treatmentguidelines.nih.gov/management/clinical-management/nonhospitalized-adults–therapeutic-management/. Accessed June 4, 2022.

65. Krause PR, Fleming TR, Longini IM, et al. SARS-CoV-2 variants and vaccines. N Engl J Med 2021; 385(2):179–86 (In eng).

66. CDC. CDC COVID data tracker: variant proportions. 2022. Available at: https://covid.cdc.gov/covid-data-tracker/#variant-proportions. Accessed June 5, 2022.

67. Wang Q, Guo Y, Iketani S, et al. SARS-CoV-2 Omicron BA.2.12.1, BA.4, and BA.5 subvariants evolved to extend antibody evasion. bioRxiv 2022. https://doi.org/10.1101/2022.05.26.493517.

68. Maslo C, Friedland R, Toubkin M, et al. Characteristics and outcomes of hospitalized patients in South Africa during the COVID-19 omicron wave compared with previous waves. JAMA 2022; 327(6):583–4 (In eng).

69. Nyberg T, Ferguson NM, Nash SG, et al. Comparative analysis of the risks of hospitalisation and death associated with SARS-CoV-2 omicron (B.1.1.529) and delta (B.1.617.2) variants in England: a cohort study. Lancet 2022;399(10332):1303–12 (In eng).

70. Ison MG, Scheetz MH. Understanding the pharmacokinetics of Favipiravir: implications for treatment of influenza and COVID-19. EBioMedicine 2021;63: 103204 (In eng).

71. Tsuzuki S, Hayakawa K, Doi Y, et al. Effectiveness of favipiravir on nonsevere, early-stage COVID-19 in Japan: a large observational study using the COVID-19 registry Japan. Infect Dis Ther 2022. https://doi.org/10.1007/s40121-022-00617-9 (In eng).

72. Bosaeed M, Alharbi A, Mahmoud E, et al. Efficacy of favipiravir in adults with mild COVID-19: a randomized, double-blind, multicentre, placebo-controlled clinical trial. Clin Microbiol Infect 2022;28(4):602–8 (In eng).

73. Ivashchenko AA, Dmitriev KA, Vostokova NV, et al. AVIFAVIR for treatment of patients with moderate coronavirus disease 2019 (COVID-19): interim results of a phase II/III multicenter randomized clinical trial. Clin Infect Dis 2021;73(3):531–4 (In eng).

74. Chuah CH, Chow TS, Hor CP, et al. Efficacy of early treatment with favipiravir on disease progression among high risk COVID-19 patients: a randomized, open-label clinical trial. Clin Infect Dis 2021. https://doi.org/10.1093/cid/ciab962 (In eng).

75. Udwadia ZF, Singh P, Barkate H, et al. Efficacy and safety of favipiravir, an oral RNA-dependent RNA polymerase inhibitor, in mild-to-moderate COVID-19: a randomized, comparative, open-label, multicenter, phase 3 clinical trial. Int J Infect Dis 2021; 103:62–71 (In eng).

76. Holubar M, Subramanian A, Purington N, et al. Favipiravir for treatment of outpatients with asymptomatic or uncomplicated COVID-19: a double-blind randomized, placebo-controlled, phase 2 trial. Clin Infect Dis 2022. https://doi.org/10.1093/cid/ciac312 (In eng).

77. Cao B, Wang Y, Wen D, et al. A trial of lopinavir-ritonavir in adults hospitalized with severe covid-19. N Engl J Med 2020;382(19):1787–99 (In eng).

78. Pan H, Peto R, Henao-Restrepo AM, et al. Repurposed antiviral drugs for covid-19 - interim WHO solidarity trial results. N Engl J Med 2021;384(6): 497–511 (In eng).

79. van Griensven J, Edwards T, de Lamballerie X, et al. Evaluation of convalescent plasma for Ebola virus disease in Guinea. N Engl J Med 2016;374(1): 33–42 (In eng).

80. Katz LM, Little A. Clarity on convalescent plasma for covid-19. N Engl J Med 2021;384(7):666–8 (In eng).

81. Korley FK, Durkalski-Mauldin V, Yeatts SD, et al. Early convalescent plasma for high-risk outpatients with covid-19. N Engl J Med 2021;385(21):1951–60 (In eng).

82. Sullivan DJ, Gebo KA, Shoham S, et al. Early outpatient treatment for covid-19 with convalescent plasma. N Engl J Med 2022. https://doi.org/10.1056/NEJMoa2119657 (In eng).

83. Lenze EJ, Mattar C, Zorumski CF, et al. Fluvoxamine vs placebo and clinical deterioration in outpatients with symptomatic COVID-19: a randomized clinical trial. JAMA 2020;324(22): 2292–300 (In eng).

84. Reis G, Dos Santos Moreira-Silva EA, Silva DCM, et al. Effect of early treatment with fluvoxamine on risk of emergency care and hospitalisation among patients with COVID-19: the TOGETHER randomised, platform clinical trial. Lancet Glob Health 2022;10(1):e42–51 (In eng).

85. Seftel D, Boulware DR. Prospective cohort of fluvoxamine for early treatment of coronavirus disease 19. Open Forum Infect Dis 2021;8(2):ofab050 (In eng).

86. Sukhatme VP, Reiersen AM, Vayttaden SJ, et al. Fluvoxamine: a review of its mechanism of action and its role in COVID-19. Front Pharmacol 2021;12: 652688 (In eng).

87. Lee TC, Vigod S, Bortolussi-Courval É, et al. Fluvoxamine for outpatient management of COVID-19 to prevent hospitalization: a systematic review and meta-analysis. JAMA Netw Open 2022;5(4): e226269 (In eng).

88. Bhuta S, Khokher W, Kesireddy N, et al. Fluvoxamine in nonhospitalized patients with acute COVID-19 infection and the lack of efficacy in reducing rates of hospitalization, mechanical ventilation, and mortality in placebo-controlled trials: a systematic review and meta-analysis. Am J Ther 2022;29(3): e298–304 (In eng).

89. Markowski MC, Tutrone R, Pieczonka C, et al. A phase 1b/2 study of sabizabulin, a novel oral Cytoskeleton disruptor, in men with metastatic castration-resistant prostate cancer with progression on an androgen receptor targeting agent. Clin Cancer Res 2022. https://doi.org/10.1158/1078-0432.CCR-22-0162 (In eng).

90. Veru's novel COVID-19 drug candidate reduces deaths by 55% in hospitalized patients in interim analysis of phase 3 study; independent data monitoring committee halts study early for overwhelming efficacy. Available at: https://verupharma.com/news/verus-novel-covid-19-drug-candidate-reduces-deaths-by-55-in-hospitalized-patients-in-interim-analysis-of-phase-3-study-independent-data-monitoring-committee-halts-study-early-for-overwhelmin/.

APPENDIX

Supplement Table 1
Numerous therapeutic agents have been investigated as therapies for COVID-19. The above summaries offer brief synopses of the body of evidence surrounding the use of select agents which are not currently recommended as therapies for COVID-19

Therapies not recommended as coronavirus disease-2019 treatment
  Antiviral Agents
    Favipiravir is an orally administered, nucleoside analog that inhibits RNA-dependent RNA polymerase and has antiviral activity against several RNA viruses. [70] Early in the SARS-CoV-2 pandemic, there was enthusiasm around repurposing favipiravir for the treatment of COVID-19, and its use has now been investigated in both outpatient and hospitalized populations in several countries.[71–76] However, several large studies have not reported a significant improvement in clinical outcomes relative to placebo or supportive care. Given its potential for adverse events and complex pharmacokinetic profile, [70] the risk of favipiravir use may outweigh its marginal benefits. Similar to favipiravir, the combination lopinavir/ritonavir was investigated early in the SARS-CoV-2 pandemic, but evidence from multiple trials did not support its use. [77,78]
  Convalescent Plasma
    Based on experience with prior infectious agents such as the Ebola virus, [79] convalescent plasma has been evaluated for the treatment of COVID-19.[80] Plasma from donors who have recovered from COVID-19 generally contains polyclonal antibodies to SARS-CoV-2 thus offering passive immunity if administered to COVID-19 naïve recipients. In practice, the homogeneity of plasma is limited by several factors including the variability of assays used to evaluate the adequacy of antibody titers, time between convalescence and donation, and whether administered plasma is from one or multiple donors.
    Convalescent plasma for COVID-19 has been evaluated in both outpatient and hospitalized patients with mixed results. The PlasmAr trial was a double-blind RCT that evaluated convalescent plasma with a median IgG titer of 1:3200 (n = 228) using the COVIDAR Argentina Consortium enzyme-linked immunosorbent assay (ELISA) compared with placebo (n = 105) for hospitalized adult patients with severe COVID-19. [62] Study participants had a median symptom length of 8 days at time of enrollment, and no significant differences in clinical status at day 30 were observed between the groups. [62] Given the potential benefit of earlier administration, a double-blind RCT compared high-titer (IgG >1:1000 on COVIDAR assay) plasma (n = 80) to placebo (n = 80) in older adult patients with mild COVID-19 within the first 3 days of symptom onset and found a relative risk reduction of 48% for progression to severe respiratory disease in patients who received convalescent plasma. [63]
    In the outpatient setting, convalescent plasma has had variable performance. The SIREN-C3PO trial evaluated high-titer convalescent plasma (defined as 50% inhibitory dilution of 1:250 or more with live-virus, five-dilution plaque reduction neutralization test) (n = 257) compared with placebo (n = 254) for outpatients at risk for disease progression who were within 7 days of symptom onset. [81] The primary outcome of disease progression within 15 days was not significantly different between the groups. [81] A separate, double-blind RCT compared convalescent plasma (n = 592) to control plasma (n = 589) in outpatient, adult persons with COVID-19 within 8 days of symptom onset. [82] Eligible donors had anti-spike IgG titers of 1:320 or greater on one of three ELISAs produced by Euroimmun, Ortho Clinical Diagnostics, or Mount Sinai Laboratory, and plasma transfused after July 2021 had arbitrary units >3.5 at a 1:101 dilution on Euroimmun IgG assay. The primary outcome of COVID-19 related hospitalization within 28 days of transfusion was observed in 2.9% of those receiving convalescent plasma compared with 6.3% in the control group (absolute risk reduction 3.4%; 95% confidence interval 1.0–5.8; p = 0.005).
    Based on available data, convalescent plasma is most likely to be useful when administered early (ideally within 3 days of symptom onset) and in high-titers. Monoclonal antibodies are generally preferred and more widely used due to improved titer standardization, high efficacy and less transfusion reactions, but convalescent plasma is potentially less susceptible to decreased efficacy for emerging viral variants due to polyclonality and matching of circulating strains.
  Fluvoxamine
    Fluvoxamine is a selective serotonin reuptake inhibitor which has been found to have some efficacy in preventing disease progression in patients with COVID-19. [83–85] Its mechanism of action is likely multifactorial with contributions from immune response modulation via the sigma-1 receptor and possible disruption of viral egress. [86] In a small, double-blind RCT (n = 152), fluvoxamine

administered to non-hospitalized adults with mild COVID-19 resulted in a lower proportion of patients with clinical deterioration at day 15 compared with placebo. [83] The larger TOGETHER trial evaluated fluvoxamine ($n = 741$) compared with placebo ($n = 756$) in adult patients with COVID-19 at risk for disease progression. [84] The primary composite outcome was retention in an emergency department for >6 hours or referral for hospitalization due to COVID-19 within 28 days of randomization. Fluvoxamine had a lower proportion of patients meeting the composite outcome (11%) compared with placebo (16%), leading to a relative risk of 0.68 (95% Bayesian credible interval 0.52–0.88); however, this was largely driven by differences in emergency department visits as opposed to hospitalizations. [84] There were no significant differences in COVID-related hospitalization, mechanical ventilation, or death observed between treatment groups.

Two recent meta-analyses used different statistical approaches to evaluate the use of fluvoxamine in outpatient persons with COVID-19, and their results are conflicting. [87,88] The Bayesian meta-analysis on three RCTs (2196 patients) reported a high probability that fluvoxamine was associated with reduced risk of hospitalization [87] whereas the other meta-analysis on 2 RCTs and one prospective cohort study (1762 patients) found no significant reduction in risk of hospitalization, mechanical ventilation, or death. [88] Further data may offer clarity on fluvoxamine's role in the treatment of COVID-19.

Sabizabulin

Sabizabulin (VERU-111) is a small molecule which binds and disrupts microtubules.[89] It was originally investigated as an anti-cancer medication and has now been repurposed as therapy for moderate-to-severe COVID-19 in hospitalized adults (clinicaltrials.gov identifier NCT04842747). Its mechanism of action is thought to stem from both antiviral and anti-inflammatory effects. A phase 3, double-blind RCT comparing standard of care plus a single dose of 9 mg sabizabulin daily for 21 days (or until discharge) versus standard of care plus placebo is ongoing. For the primary endpoint of death within 60 days, the interim analysis reported a 55% relative reduction in mortality for the sabizabulin group ($n = 98$) relative to placebo ($n = 52$).[90] Full trial results are not yet available, but the interim results are promising despite the relatively small sample size and co-administration of standard of care therapies (eg, remdesivir, and IL-6 inhibitors).

Supplement Table 2
The above definitions are used to define select patient populations in the Yale New Haven Health System

Definitions for Yale New Haven Health System pathways

The term "severely immunosuppressed" in **Fig. 3** includes the following conditions: various hematological malignancies (eg, acute myelogenous leukemia or lymphoma on B-cell depleting therapy), allogeneic stem cell transplantation within the last 12 months or active immunosuppressive treatment of graft versus host disease, chimeric antigen receptor-T therapy within the last 12 months, solid organ transplantation within the last 6 months or treatment of rejection within the last 3 months, history of lung transplantation at any time, HIV with CD4 <200, or receipt of select immunosuppressive medications (eg, rituximab, purine analogs, mycophenolate mofetil, and ibrutinib). To be considered "very high risk," patients must meet ≥1 more of the following criteria: complex chronic illness or multiple comorbidities, no receipt of SARS-CoV-2 vaccination.

Immunomodulatory Agents for Coronavirus Disease-2019 Pneumonia

Dayna McManus, PharmD[a],*, Matthew W. Davis, PharmD[a],
Alex Ortiz, MD, MS[b], Clemente Britto-Leon, MD[b],
Charles S. Dela Cruz, MD, PhD[b], Jeffrey E. Topal, MD[a],*

KEYWORDS

- COVID-19 • SARS-CoV-2 • Immunomodulatory treatment • Corticosteroids • JAK inhibitors

KEY POINTS

- Hyperinflammatory response to severe acute respiratory syndrome coronavirus 2 contributes to severe inflammation, acute lung injury, and end-organ damage.
- Many immunomodulatory agents have been tested to attenuate inflammatory responses associated with coronavirus disease-2019 (COVID-19).
- Corticosteroids, specifically dexamethasone, have been shown to reduce mortality in hospitalized patients with COVID-19 who require supplemental oxygen.
- Interleukin-6 antagonists and Janus kinase inhibitors have shown mortality benefits in patients with COVID-19 requiring supplemental oxygen.

INTRODUCTION

The primary cause of morbidity and mortality in coronavirus disease-2019 (COVID-19) pneumonia is acute hypoxemic respiratory failure, an inability to maintain adequate gas exchange caused by severe inflammation and tissue damage in the lungs of individuals infected with severe acute respiratory syndrome coronavirus 2 (SARS-CoV-2).[1–3] The inflammatory response observed in the lungs infected with SARS-CoV-2 is multifactorial and of variable severity, ranging from mild cases that remain largely asymptomatic to cases of severe respiratory failure requiring mechanical ventilation and in some cases, extracorporeal membrane oxygenation (ECMO).[1,4,5] Early on the course of the pandemic, it became clear that these variable clinical presentations reflected individual differences in immune response and inflammation resolution, underscoring the possibility of using immunomodulatory therapies to avoid or mitigate respiratory failure in COVID-19 pneumonia.

The immune response to SARS-CoV-2 infection in the lungs is complex and includes a proinflammatory state characterized by increased innate immune cell activation and an abnormal inflammatory cytokine response that exacerbates local inflammation and immune cell recruitment to the lungs.[4,6–12] In early studies to define circulating and local markers of severe COVID-19 presentations and clinical outcomes, cytokines such as interleukin-1β (IL-1β), IL-6, IL-8, tumor necrosis factor α (TNFα), and other nonspecific markers of inflammation such as C-reactive protein (CRP) and ferritin were frequently dysregulated at different stages, providing an initial focus for the selection and timing of immunomodulatory therapies.[4,6,8,13–15]

Upon entering epithelial cells and interacting with immune cells in the respiratory tract, the double-stranded SARS-CoV-2 RNA activates cytoplasmic pathogen recognition receptors (eg, MDA5, toll-like receptors [TLRs]) to activate an

[a] Department of Pharmacy Services, Yale New Haven Hospital, 20 York Street, New Haven, CT 06510, USA;
[b] Pulmonary, Critical Care & Sleep Medicine, 300 Cedar Street, P.O. Box 208057, New Haven, CT 06520-8057, USA
* Corresponding authors.
E-mail addresses: dayna.mcmanus@ynhh.org (D.M.); Jeffrey.Topal@ynhh.org (J.E.T.)

Clin Chest Med 44 (2023) 299–319
https://doi.org/10.1016/j.ccm.2022.11.009
0272-5231/23/© 2022 Elsevier Inc. All rights reserved.

early but dysfunctional type I and type III interferon (IFN) response.[16–22] Type I and III IFN responses during SARS-CoV-2 induce the expression of numerous antiviral IFN-stimulated genes (ISGs) that promote cytokine secretion, recruitment, and activation of innate immune cells such as mononuclear phagocytes (monocytes and macrophages) and neutrophils, and also the recruitment and activation of adaptive immune cells such as B and T cells that play a critical role in SARS-CoV-2 immunity.[23–26] There is evidence that while early type I and III IFN to SARS-CoV2 may be impaired, delayed IFN responses and their interaction with IL-1β signaling may lead to excessive inflammation through stimulation of IL-6 and TNFα secretion.[14,26–28]

The continued innate immune cell recruitment and activation and a hyperinflammatory response to the virus lead to widespread alveolar epithelial and vascular endothelial damage, associated with capillary extravasation, inflammatory infiltrate, cell death, and microvascular thrombosis.[7,8,29–31] Both alveolar epithelial cell types, AT1 and AT2 are affected in this process, leading not only to impairments in gas exchange through AT2 lesion but the impaired secretion of pulmonary surfactants and host defense proteins through AT1 cell injury.[8,32] In addition to epithelial injury, endothelial damage also contributes to cytokine (IL-6, IL-8, and CCL2) and prothrombotic factor release (eg, PAI1 or SERPINE1), exacerbating inflammatory recruitment, capillary leakage, and microvascular thrombosis.[31,33–35]

In addition to the essential role of epithelial cells in the inflammatory response to SARS-CoV-2, immune cells play a crucial role in COVID-19 pathogenesis.[8,10,32,36] Monocytes and monocyte-derived airway macrophages play a critical role in the development of COVID-19 pathogenesis.[30] Dysfunctional monocyte and macrophage populations were detected in the lungs of those with severe presentations, characterized by impaired antigen presentation, proinflammatory transcriptome profiles, and impaired expression of pro-resolving genes (eg, increased expression of CCL2 CCL3, CXCL1, CXCL3, CXCL8, CXCL10, IL-1β, and TNFα).[8,10,11,22,37,38] In addition to recruited cells, alveolar macrophages expressed high levels of CCL7, CCL8, and CCL13, which may further exacerbate adaptive and innate immune cell recruitment to affected areas.[11] Although neutrophils are not the predominant cell type encountered in the airways of patients with COVID-19, they play an essential role as effectors of these pro-inflammatory changes and likely drivers of tissue injury in COVID-19.[8,39,40] The excessive release of neutrophil extracellular traps (NETs) and tissue proteases by neutrophils and abnormal cell survival programs expressed by these cells exacerbate the alveolar and epithelial injury and promote further lung inflammation through cell death and poor clearance of inflammatory debris.[37,41,42]

On the basis of these findings, a large number of studies were published in the past three years targeting specific cell populations or inflammatory cytokines, aiming to minimize the proinflammatory features of COVID-19 to minimize its clinical impact or enhance the protective effects of early IFN response.[15,43–45] For example, depletion of mononuclear phagocyte populations in animal models infected with SARS-CoV2 improved survival from infection, mediated through decreased CCL2, TNFα, and IL-6 signaling.[22] Consistently, CCR2-deficient mice, with impaired ability to recruit monocytes had increased cytokines responses and viremia, suggesting that monocytes and their products are essential to COVID-19 pathogenesis.[46] Concurrently, immune modulation studies in human subjects diverged into a broad immunosuppressive approach using corticosteroids or targeted approaches aimed at minimizing the effects of excessive cytokine responses as was the case with targeted IL-6 and IFN signaling modulation.[15,43,45,47]

Corticosteroids

Corticosteroids are broad immunosuppressing agents that can reduce systemic inflammatory responses and therefore decrease the severity of illness in several infectious syndromes.[44,48,49] Corticosteroids were commonly used for this reason during the 2002 to 2004 severe acute respiratory syndrome (SARS) and were shown to improve oxygenation, decrease fever, and overall hospital length of stay and mortality.[49] Therefore, corticosteroids were thought to be potentially beneficial during the COVID-19 pandemic.[44,48,49] Table 1 summarizes the key studies that sought to evaluate the role of corticosteroids in the treatment of COVID-19.

The Randomized Evaluation of COVID-19 Therapy (RECOVERY) trial demonstrated that the use of corticosteroids decreased mortality in patients who are hospitalized for COVID-19.[44] This decreased mortality, however, has only been demonstrated in patients with severe COVID, that is, those who are hospitalized and require supplemental oxygen. Benefit has not been demonstrated in non-severe COVID-19, that is, nonhospitalized patients or those who are hospitalized but are not requiring oxygen.[50,51] Furthermore, studies have revealed hospitalized patients

Table 1
Systemic corticosteroids

Clinical Trial Name	Study Type	Study Population	Interventions	Outcomes	Limitations	Conclusion
RECOVERY[44]	Open-label RCT	Hospitalized patients with COVID-19	2:1 random assignment of usual standard of care (SOC) alone ($n = 4321$) or standard of care plus oral of IV dexamethasone ($n = 2104$) 6 mg daily for up to 10 days (or hospital discharge whichever was sooner)	All-cause mortality at 28 days: All patients: 23% in dexamethasone arm versus 26% in SOC arm (RR 0.83; 95% CI, 0.75–0.93; $P < 0.001$) Receipt of mechanical ventilation (MV) or ECMO at randomization: 29% in dexamethasone vs 41% in SOC (RR 0.64, 95% CI 0.51–0.81) Receipt of supplemental oxygen but not MV at randomization: 23% dexamethasone versus 26% in SOC (RR 0.82; 95% CI,0.72–0.94) Patients not requiring supplemental oxygen at randomization: 18% dex versus 14% SOC (RR 1.19, 95% CI, 0.92–1.55)	Open-label Did not evaluate cause-specific mortality, adverse events and subgroups to look at comorbidities Patients on supplemental oxygen had varying degrees of severity	Dexamethasone reduced 28-day mortality in hospitalized patients who required supplemental oxygen with the greatest benefit being demonstrated in patient requiring MV.

(continued on next page)

Table 1
(continued)

Clinical Trial Name	Study Type	Study Population	Interventions	Outcomes	Limitations	Conclusion
CoDEX[52]	Open-label RCT	Hospitalized COVID-19 patients with MV within 48 h of meeting criteria for moderate-to-severe ARDs (PaO2/FiO2 ≤ 200 mm HG)	Random 1:1 assignment of dexamethasone 20 mg IV daily for 5 days then 10 mg daily for 5 days or until ICU discharge (n = 151) or SOC (n = 148)	Mean number of days alive and free from MV by Day 28: 7 in dexamethasone arm vs 4 in SOC arm (P = 0.04) No differences between arms in all-cause mortality (56% vs 62%), number of ICU-free days, duration of MV, or score on 6-point OS Mean SOFA score at Day 7: 6.1 in DEX arm vs 7.5 in SOC arm (P = 0.004) Post hoc analysis of probability of death or MV by Day 15: 68% in dexamethasone arm vs 80% in SOC arm (OR 0.46)	Open-label Underpowered Patient discharged before 28 days were not followed for re-hospitalization or death Approximately 25% of patients who were randomized to SOC alone received corticosteroids	Dexamethasone increased the number of days alive and MV free in 28 days in moderate-to-severe ARDS patients with COVID-19.

REMAP-CAP[53]	Randomized Open-label adaptive trial	Hospitalized COVID-19 patients with severe COVID-19 requiring ICU admission for respiratory or cardiovascular support	1:1:1 randomization of hydrocortisone 50 mg IV every 6 h for 7 days (n = 137), shock-dependent hydrocortisone 50 mg IV every 6 h for up to 28 days (n = 146), or no hydrocortisone (n = 101)	No difference between in median number of organ support-free days at Day 21 (0 in each arm) No difference between arms in in-hospital mortality (30% in fixed-dose hydrocortisone arm vs 26% in shock-dependent hydrocortisone arm vs 33% in no hydrocortisone arm)	Open-label Terminated early therefore underpowered	Hydrocortisone did not increase median number of support-free days
Crothers et al.[51]	Observational cohort study	27,168 patients admitted to a VA hospital for COVID-19 within 14 days after testing positive	Corticosteroids (95% of patients received dexamethasone) administered within 48 h of admission (n = 7507) Compared with no corticosteroids administered (n = 7433)	Risk of all-cause mortality at 90 days was higher in those who received dexamethasone: For combination of those not on supplemental oxygen and those on low-flow nasal cannula oxygen: HR 1.59; 95% CI, 1.39–1.81 For those not on supplemental oxygen: HR 1.76; 95% CI, 1.47–2.12 For those on low-flow nasal cannula oxygen: HR 1.08; 95% CI, 0.86–1.36	Retrospective observational study Variation in other therapies patients received	Dexamethasone in hospitalized COVID-19 patients who were receiving low-flow nasal cannula during the first 48 h of admission did not show a mortality benefit. There was an increase in mortality seen in patients who received dexamethasone who were not on supplemental oxygen within the first 48 h after admission.

not requiring supplemental oxygen may have worse outcomes when corticosteroids are used, as suggested by a large observational cohort study done in veterans administration (VA) patients.[51] Corticosteroids are not without their side effects, which include hyperglycemia, secondary infection, and psychiatric effects. Therefore, use in mild COVID-19 is not recommended at this time due to the lack of adequate positive data and potential for side effects.[44,50,51]

The COVID-19 Dexamethasone study (CoDEX) and *Randomised, Embedded, Multi-factorial, Adaptive Platform Trial for Community-Acquired Pneumonia* (REMAP-CAP) are the two largest studies done to date looking specifically at the role of corticosteroids for COVID-19 in the hospital setting.[52,53] CoDEX, which was a randomized open-label trial, demonstrated that dexamethasone increased the number of days alive and mechanical ventilation-free days in patients with moderate-to-severe acute respiratory distress syndrome (ARDS) COVID-19 patients. However, this study was terminated early and therefore was underpowered. In addition, many of the patients in the standard-of-care arm also received corticosteroids, which makes interpreting the results of the trial challenge.[52] REMAP-CAP compared outcomes using a fixed dose, shock-dependent dosing of hydrocortisone versus the standard of care with no hydrocortisone. There was no difference in the number of days alive and mechanical ventilation-free days in patients with severe COVID-19 requiring respiratory or cardiovascular support.[53]

The differences in the clinical outcomes in these studies suggest that the timing of corticosteroids in the treatment of COVID-19 is important. Using corticosteroids early in treatment may result in worsening outcomes given the effect of corticosteroids on the immune system's ability to fight off the virus earlier on in the infection. As the disease progresses and the cytokine storm begins corticosteroids become beneficial in preventing additional damage and subsequently poor outcomes. However, once there is progression to a severe disease requiring respiratory or cardiovascular support, the benefit may be diminished due to the extensive damage that likely has already been done.[48,49,52,53]

The systemic corticosteroid that has been most studied is dexamethasone. However, the current National Institute of Health (NIH) guidelines recommend that if dexamethasone cannot be used that other equivalent dose of a systemic corticosteroid is substituted. A few studies have evaluated the effects of different doses of dexamethasone but given the mixed results of those studies 6 mg daily is the recommended dose at this time. Therefore,

equivalent doses for dexamethasone 6 mg would be prednisone 40 mg, methylprednisolone 32 mg, or hydrocortisone 160 mg. As dexamethasone has a longer half-life, it is given daily whereas prednisone and methylprednisolone are recommended to be given once or twice daily and hydrocortisone is recommended to be given two to four times daily.[53,54] The guidelines only recommend this therapy for hospitalized patients who require supplemental oxygen. It is important to note that this therapy is recommended for 10 days or until hospital discharge; it is not recommended to discharge patients on this therapy. The guidelines recommend against the use of dexamethasone or other systemic corticosteroids specifically for the non-hospitalized patient given the lack of data for this population. If patients are on a corticosteroid for another indication the guidelines recommend continuing it.[54]

In addition to systemic corticosteroids, inhaled corticosteroids, given their direct anti-inflammatory effects on the lungs, have also been studied for the treatment of COVID-19.[55–58] **Table 2** summarizes the four main randomized controlled trials that sought to evaluate the effects of this therapy on the treatment of COVID-19. PRINCIPLE and SOTIC used budesonide comparison to standard of care and CONTAIN and a study by Clemency and colleagues used ciclesonide compared with placebo.[55–58] CONTAIN used ciclesonide both as an inhalation as well as an intranasal preparation.[58] All of these studies evaluated non-hospitalized patients with COVID-19. PRINCIPLE evaluated high-risk patients, whereas the other studies were conducted in any patients who were not hospitalized. PRINCIPLE found a reduction in the time to patient's self-reported recovery, whereas the study by Clemency and colleagues and CONTAIN did not. PRINCIPLE did not find a reduction in COVID-19-reported hospitalization or death, whereas STOIC and the study by Clemency and colleagues found a decrease in need for urgent care/emergency department assessment and hospitalization. However, these trials had small sample sizes making conclusions from them difficult to interpret.[55–58] Given the mixed outcomes, the use of inhaled corticosteroids for the treatment of COVID-19 is not recommended at this time.[50]

Interleukin-6 Inhibitors

Early data from patients with COVID-19 suggested a correlation of elevated IL-6 levels with a hyperinflammatory response and severe ARDS. The elevated IL-6 was also linked to increased mortality.[13,48,59] This led to the idea that the use of IL-6

Table 2
Inhaled corticosteroids

Clinical Trial Name	Study Type	Study Population	Interventions	Outcomes	Limitations	Conclusion
PRINCIPLE[55]	Open-label RCT	Nonhospitalized COVID-19 patients with ≤ 14 days of symptoms and age ≥ 65 or ≥ 50 with comorbidities	1:1 random assignment of usual standard of care (SOC) alone (n = 787) or standard of care plus budesonide 800 mcg inhaled twice daily for 14 days (n = 1069)	Patients who were hospitalized or died due to COVID-19 within 28 days: 6.8% in budesonide arm vs 8.8% in usual care arm (OR 0.75; 95% CrI, 0.55–1.03) Median time to reported recovery: 11.8 days in budesonide arm vs 14.7 days in usual care arm (HR 1.21; 95% CrI, 1.08–1.36)	Open-label Relied on patient's self-report for time to recovery	Inhaled budesonide reduced time to patient's self-reported recovery, but not COVID-19-reported hospitalization or death.
STOIC[56]	Open-label phase 2 RCT	Nonhospitalized COVID-19 patients with ≤ 7 days of symptoms and age ≥ 18	1:1 random assignment of usual standard of care (SOC) alone (n = 73) or standard of care plus budesonide 800 mcg inhaled twice daily until symptom resolution (n = 73)	Median duration of budesonide use: 7 days Percentage of patients with COVID-19-related urgent care visit or hospitalization: 1% in budesonide arm versus 14% in usual care arm (relative risk reduction 91%).	Open-label Small sample size	Inhaled budesonide may reduce the need for urgent care or ED assessment and/or hospitalization in adult outpatients with mild COVID-19.

(continued on next page)

Table 2
(continued)

Clinical Trial Name	Study Type	Study Population	Interventions	Outcomes	Limitations	Conclusion
Clemency et al.[57]	Double-blind randomized controlled trial	Nonhospitalized COVID-19 patients with a positive test in the last 72 h age ≥ 12 with ≥ 1 symptom of fever, cough, or dyspnea	1:1 random assignment of placebo meter dose inhaler (MDI) (n = 203) or ciclesonide MDI 160 μg/actuation, 2 actuations twice a day for 30 days (n = 197)	Median time to alleviation of all COVID-19-related symptoms: 19 days in ciclesonide arm vs 19 days in placebo arm (HR 1.08; 95% CI, 0.84–1.38) By Day 30: Alleviation of COVID-19-related symptoms: 70.6% in ciclesonide arm vs 63.5% in placebo arm Subsequent ED visit or hospital admission for COVID-19: 1% in ciclesonide arm vs 5.4% in placebo arm (OR 0.18; 95% CI, 0.04–0.85) Hospital admission or death: 1.5% in ciclesonide arm vs 3.4% in placebo arm (OR 0.45; 95% CI, 0.11–1.84) No deaths seen at 30 days in either group	Relied on patient's self-report for alleviation of all symptoms Small sample size particularly for ED/hospitalization outcome	Inhaled ciclesonide did not reduce time to reported recovery; however, there was decrease in ED visits and hospitalization in the small sample size of events.

| Contain[58] | Double-blind randomized controlled trial | Nonhospitalized COVID-19 patients age ≥ 18 with ≥ 1 symptom of fever, cough, or dyspnea and symptoms for ≤ 6 days | 1:1 random assignment of saline placebo MDI and intranasal saline twice daily for 14 days (n = 98) or ciclesonide MDI 600 μg/actuation and intranasal ciclesonide 100 μg twice a day for 14 days (n = 105) | Percentage of patients with resolution of fever and all respiratory symptoms at Day 7: 40% in ciclesonide arm vs 35% in the placebo arm (adjusted risk difference 5.5%; 95% CI, −7.8% to 18.8%)

Percentage of patients with resolution of fever and all respiratory symptoms at Day 14: 66% in ciclesonide arm vs 58% in placebo arm (adjusted risk difference 7.5%; 95% CI, −5.9% to 20.8%)

Percentage of patients who were admitted to the hospital by Day 14: 6% in ciclesonide arm vs 3% in placebo arm (adjusted risk difference 2.3%; 95% CI, −3.0% to 7.6%) | Small sample size | Inhaled plus intranasal ciclesonide did not improve resolution of fever and respiratory symptoms in young healthy nonhospitalized patients with COVID-19 |

inhibitors could help mitigate the inflammatory response and reduce pathological damage from COVID-19 infection.[60]

This idea was not novel, as IL-6 inhibitors have been previously studied in the treatment of cytokine release syndrome. Tocilizumab, siltuximab, and sarulimab have been found to be effective in cytokine storm diseases such as hemophagocytic lymphohistiocytosis (HLH), idiopathic multicentric Castleman's disease and chimeric antigen receptor (CAR) T-cell-induced cytokine storm.[60–66]

The potential benefits of IL-6 inhibitors have been well studied, specifically with tocilizumab. Several randomized controlled trials demonstrated a benefit for tocilizumab in the treatment of COVID-19 (**Table 3**). The RECOVERY trial was a large open-label randomized controlled trial that studied the addition of tocilizumab in patients with hypoxemia and CRP $\geq$ 75. Tocilizumab resulted in a reduction in 28-day mortality/mechanical ventilation and increased hospital discharge; notably, 16% of participants in the tocilizumab arm did not actually receive the drug.[67] REMAP-CAP showed a reduction in mortality and an increase in organ-free support days when tocilizumab was administered within 24 h of ICU admission after starting organ support, which included the need for noninvasive or invasive mechanical ventilation, vasopressors, or inotropes. Sarilumab had a similar outcome in this trial, but the sample size for these patient groups was very low.[68] EMPACTA found a reduction in the need for mechanical ventilation but no difference in mortality in hospitalized patients not requiring mechanical ventilation; the treatment arm ended up including a portion of patients who did not require any oxygen at all.[69]

Randomized controlled clinical trials of tocilizumab that demonstrated unfavorable outcomes have potential flaws in study design involving timing of administration. REMDACTA was a well-designed study that showed no benefit of tocilizumab when administered to patients requiring > 6L of oxygen. This could potentially be too late in the hyperinflammatory phase as some patients may have lower oxygen requirements but increasing inflammatory markers necessitating earlier administration of the drug.[70]

CONVACTA was another well-designed study showing no benefit of tocilizumab, but receipt of corticosteroids was allowed which likely confounded the effect of tocilizumab. There were also a significant number of patients who were mechanically ventilated or on ECMO, which represents a disease stage too late to benefit from tocilizumab as end-organ damage may have already occurred.[71] The BACC Bay study showed no difference for the prevention of intubation or death but included a portion of patients with COVID-19 who were not requiring any oxygen and had a small sample size.[72] The CORIMUNO-19 study targeted patients requiring at least 3L of oxygen and showed a numerical benefit of tocilizumab but was not statistically significant likely due to the lack of an adequate sample size.[73] In addition, the primary endpoint was set at 14 days, which is likely not long enough to appreciate significant differences given the protracted course of the disease. Lescure and colleagues was the only randomized controlled trial evaluating the use of sarilumab alone and showed no benefit in time to clinical improvement compared with placebo but was limited in their sample size.[74,75]

Collectively, these randomized controlled trials demonstrate the importance of tocilizumab as a treatment of COVID-19 for a high-risk patient at the optimal time during the course of disease before significant end-organ damage. This includes patients with escalating oxygen requirements and elevated inflammatory markers, such as CRP while receiving remdesivir and dexamethasone. Patients who are not showing these signs of a hyperinflammatory syndrome may not benefit from this drug. In addition, timing of administration is important as patients who have reached mechanical ventilation or ECMO may already have irreversible end organ damage from viral infection that may not be reversed by additional immunomodulating therapies. As of this writing, the other IL-6 inhibitors have not been well studied enough to recommend use.

Janus Kinase Inhibitors

As immune modulators, Janus kinase (JAK) inhibitors are potent molecules that inhibit the JAK/STAT pathway which results in reduced production of IL-1 and IL-6. Baricitinib reversibly inhibits JAK1/JAK2 which prevents the production of inflammatory cytokines.[76] In addition, baricitinib exerts an antiviral effect by inhibiting the clathrin-associated viral entry by suppressing 2 host kinases, AP2-associated protein kinase 1 (AAK1) and cyclin G-associated kinase (GAK) which are responsible for clathrin-mediated endocytosis and viral endocytosis, respectively.[77] The immunomodulatory effects of baricitinib in SARS-CoV-2 infection were first noted in an in-vitro study of blood samples of patients with COVID-19 infection in which following the administration of 1000 nM of baricitinib, levels of interferon-gamma, IL-1β, IL-6, TNF-α, and other inflammatory cytokines were reduced.[78] Another study using the rhesus macaque model of COVID-19 infection reported

Table 3
Overview of randomized controlled trials for interleukin 6 inhibitors with the benefit

	Study Type	Study Population	Interventions	Outcomes	Limitations	Conclusion
RECOVERY[56]	Open-label RCT	Hospitalized COVID-19 patients with hypoxia and a CRP ≥75 mg/L	1:1 random assignment of tocilizumab 400–800 mg (n = 621) or placebo (n = 729) in addition to standard care	28-day mortality: 31% vs 35% (RR 0.85, 95%CI, 0.76–0.94; P = 0.003) Hospital discharge within 28 days: 57% vs 50% (RR 1.22, 95% CI, 1.12–1.33;P < 0.0001) Receipt of mechanical ventilation or death: 35% vs 42% (RR0.84, 95% CI0.77–0.92;P < 0.0001)	Open-label 16% of patients in tocilizumab actually did not receive treatment Random CRP cutoff	Tocilizumab reduced the probability of progression to mechanical ventilation and/or death and increased the probability of hospital discharge within 28 days.
REMAP-CAP[57]	Open-label adaptive platform RCT	Hospitalized patients with COVID-19 admitted in the ICU within 24 h after starting organ support	Random assignment of tocilizumab 8 mg/kg (n = 353), sarilumab 400 mg (n = 48), or standard care (n = 402)	*Tocilizumab vs control* Median organ support free-days (IQR): 10 (−1 to 16) vs 0 (−1 to 15) In-hospital survival: 28% vs 36% (aOR 1.64; 95% credible interval 1.14–2.35) *Sarilumab vs control* Median organ support free-days (IQR): 11 (0 to 16) vs 0 (−1 to 15) In-hospital survival: 22% vs 36% (aOR 2.01; 95% credible interval 1.18–4.71)	Open-label Control arm closed early	Tocilizumab and sarilumab increased the amount of organ-free support days and reduced in-hospital mortality.

(continued on next page)

Table 3
(continued)

	Study Type	Study Population	Interventions	Outcomes	Limitations	Conclusion
EMPACTA[58]	Double-blind placebo-controlled RCT	Hospitalized patients with COVID-19 not receiving mechanical ventilation	2:1 random assignment of tocilizumab 8 mg/kg (n = 249) or placebo (n = 128) in addition to standard care	Mechanical ventilation or death at day 28: 12% vs 19.3% (HR 0.56, 95% CI 0.33–0.97; $P = 0.04$) Death at day 28: 10.4% vs 8.6% (weighted difference 2 95% CI, −5.2 to 7.8)	Sample size somewhat small especially in placebo group 9% of patients did not require oxygen at baseline, this population may not benefit from this therapy	Tocilizumab reduced the need for mechanical ventilation but did not have an effect on mortality.

baricitinib reducing inflammation and lung pathology.[79] Several studies using JAK inhibitors have shown positive results (**Table 4**).

The first randomized, placebo-controlled clinical trial which assessed baricitinib for the treatment of COVID-19 was the Adaptive Covid-19 Treatment Trial 2 (ACTT-2). In this trial, patients were randomized to receive remdesivir plus baricitinib versus remdesivir plus placebo. The primary clinical endpoint was time to recovery and the main secondary outcome was clinical status at day 15 using an ordinal scale. In both groups, the majority of patients were receiving supplemental oxygen (86%) with 20.9% and 10.7% of patients receiving oxygen through high-flow devices/noninvasive ventilation and invasive mechanical ventilation/ECMO, respectively.[80] The patients who received combination therapy with remdesivir and baricitinib recovered a median 1 day faster than the control group who received remdesivir and placebo (median 7 days versus 8 days, respectively), with a hazard ratio 1.15. The effect of baricitinib was most pronounced for the group receiving high-flow oxygen/noninvasive ventilation where the median time to recovery was 10 days in the combination group and 18 days in the control group with a rate ratio [RR] for recovery of 1.51. For the key secondary outcome of odds of clinical improvement at day 15, the overall odds ratio (OR) of improvement was greater in the combination group than the control group (OR 1.3). As with the primary outcome, the OR of clinical improvement was greatest in the group receiving high-flow oxygen/noninvasive ventilation at 2.2. Finally, 28-day mortality was 5.1% in the combination therapy group compared with 7.6% in the control group with a hazard ratio (HR) for death to be 0.65. The greatest difference in mortality between the two groups was noted in the group receiving supplemental oxygen, 1.9% versus 4.7% (HR 0.40) and in the group receiving high flow oxygen/noninvasive ventilation 7.5% versus 12.9% (HR 0.55).[80]

A major limitation of the ACTT-2 trial was the low usage of concomitant glucocorticoids as part of the treatment regimen for COVID-19. The study was conducted before the results of the RECOVERY trial which revealed a mortality benefit for patients in COVID-19 in the dexamethasone treatment group. Of the whole cohort in the ACTT-2 trial, only 223 patients (21.5%) received glucocorticoids. An analysis of this group of patients revealed a ratio for recovery of 1.06 and a lack of an effect on the overall results for the ACTT-2 trial. However, even with this caveat, the ACTT-2 trial demonstrated that immune modulation with baricitinib benefited patients requiring oxygenation, especially those who required high-flow/noninvasive ventilation. The lack of benefit in patients receiving mechanical ventilation or ECMO suggested that the end organ damage due to COVID-19 inflammatory effects was not responsive to the immunomodulatory effects of baricitinib.[80]

The COV-BARRIER study evaluated baricitinib in hospitalized patients, who were randomized to receive baricitinib, 4 mg daily, versus matched placebo for up to 14 days. The composite primary endpoint was the proportion of patients who progressed to high-flow oxygen, noninvasive ventilation, invasive mechanical ventilation, or death by day 28.[45] 88% of the patient enrolled required supplemental oxygen. Of the 1518 patients in the trial, 1204 received systemic corticosteroids, a key therapy that reduced mortality in this patient population. Only a minority of patients (18.9%) received remdesivir.[45] Of the baricitinib group, 27.8% compared with 30.5% receiving placebo progressed to meet the composite the primary endpoint (OR 0.85, $P = 0.180$). However, there was a significant mortality benefit for hospitalized patients with COVID-19. The endpoint of 28-day all-cause mortality was 8% in the baricitinib group compared with 13% in the placebo group (HR 0.57, $P = 0.0018$). This was a 38.2% relative reduction in mortality with an estimated 1 additional death prevented per every 20 patients treated with baricitinib.[45]

The RECOVERY trial was the largest study to evaluate baricitinib in hospitalized patients with COVID-19. Patients were randomly allocated to usual care plus baricitinib 4 mg daily for 10 days or until discharge (if sooner) versus usual care. A total of 8156 patients were randomly allocated to receive baricitinib plus usual care in addition to usual care alone. In this patient population, 95% of the patients received corticosteroids and 32% received tocilizumab either at the time of randomization or within 24 h of randomization. Overall, 514 (12%) of 4148 patients in the baricitinib group versus 546 (14%) of 4008 patients allocated to usual care died within 28 days (age-adjusted rate ratio 0·87; $P = 0·028$), for a reduction in mortality of 13%. was smaller than seen in smaller studies.[81]

Other JAK inhibitors which have been studied in the treatment of COVID-19 include ruxolitinib and tofacitinib. Although the initial ruxolitinib studies had favorable outcomes data, the sample sizes were small and the study designs were either retrospective, or non-randomized prospective studies.[82–85] However, in the largest international randomized, double-blind placebo-controlled studies with ruxolitinib, favorable results were not seen. RUXCOVID was a phase III study that evaluated the efficacy and safety of ruxolitinib versus

Table 4
Overview of negative clinical studies of immunotherapeutic targets and respective trials

Drug	Target/ Mechanism of Action	Trial Name	Study Type	Study Population	Inflammatory Requirements for Enrollment	Respiratory Requirements for Enrollment	Primary Endpoint	n in Intervention Arm; n in Placebo Arm	Conclusion
Adalimumab[90]	TNF inhibitor	N/A	Double-Blind RCT	Hospitalized patients with severe COVID-19 Pneumonia receiving remdesivir and dexamethasone	N/A	SpO2 <93% on room air or mechanical ventilation or ARDS	Mechanical ventilation, ICU admission, and rate of mortality	34; 34	No benefit to using adalimumab in combination with remdesivir and dexamethasone
Canakinumab[86]	IL-1β antagonist	CAN-COVID	Double-Blind RCT	Hospitalized patients with Severe COVID-19 Pneumonia	CRP >20 mg/L or ferritin >600 mg/L	Hypoxemic but not mechanically ventilated	Survival without the need for invasive mechanical ventilations from Days 3 through 29	227; 227	No statistical difference between intervention and placebo arms in proportion of patients who survived without mechanical ventilation
Mavrilimumab[91]	GM-CSF Inhibitor	MASH-COVID	Double-Blind RCT	Hospitalized Patients with Severe COVID-19 pneumonia and systemic hyperinflammation	CRP >5 mg/dL	SpO2 <92% on room air or required supplemental oxygen, patients on MV excluded	Alive and off supplemental oxygen at day 14	21; 19	No evidence of improved supplemental oxygen-free survival by Day 14

Otilimab[92]	GM-CSF inhibitor	OSCAR	Double-Blind RCT	Hospitalized patients with Severe COVID-19 pneumonia	CRP or ferritin > ULN	HFNC Oxygen, NIV, or MV < 48 h before dosing	Alive and free of respiratory failure at Day 28	395; 398	No evidence of reduced probability of respiratory failure of death
Ruxolitinib[89]	JAK-1 and JAK-2 inhibitor	RUXCOVID	Double-Blind RCT	Hospitalized patients with confirmed COVID-19 who were not mechanically ventilated or in the ICU	N/A	Respiratory rate greater than 30 breaths per minute, requiring supplementary oxygen, oxygen saturation of 94% or less on room air, P/F ratio of less than 300 mm Hg	Composite of death, respiratory failure (requiring invasive mechanical ventilation), or ICU care, by day 29	284; 144	No statistical difference in composite endpoint nor in secondary individual outcomes
Vilobelimab[93]	C5a inhibitor	PANAMO	Double-Blind RCT	Hospitalized patients with severe PCR- and radio-graphically confirmed COVID-19	N/A	Mechanically ventilated patients	28-day all-cause mortality	185; 184	No statistical difference in mortality[a]

[a] Prespecified subanalysis of patients showed a statistically significant reduction in mortality.

placebo in hospitalized patients with severe COVID-19 requiring oxygen support. However, patients who were intubated or in the ICU at the time of randomization were excluded from the evaluation of the primary outcome. A total of 432 patients were randomized in a 2:1 fashion to receive ruxolitinib 5 mg every 12 h versus placebo. An equal number of patients received corticosteroids and remdesivir in each arm. There were no differences in the composite primary endpoint of death and respiratory failure requiring mechanical ventilation between the two groups. Secondary outcomes of mortality and ICU care by day 29, and duration of hospitalization were also similar in both groups. The RUXCOVID trial did not demonstrate the efficacy of ruxolitinib compared with a placebo in the treatment of severe COVID-19.[86]

Tofacinitib was evaluated in the STOP-COVID trial where 289 patients with severe COVID-19 were randomized to receive tofacitinib 10 mg versus placebo every 12 h up to 14 days (or until day of discharge, which was sooner). Patients who were receiving noninvasive or invasive mechanical ventilation as well as ECMO were excluded. Baseline characteristics were similar in both groups where 63.2% of the tofacitinib group received supplemental oxygen and 13.2% received high-flow oxygen compared with 62.1% and 12.4% in the placebo group, respectively. Approximately 80% of patients in each arm received corticosteroids. The antiviral oseltamivir was administered in 13.9% of the tofacitinib group compared with 12.4% in the placebo group.[87] The primary outcome of death or respiratory failure through day 28 occurred in 18.1% of the patients who received tofacitinib compared with 29.0% who received placebo (risk ratio 0.63; 95% CI, 0.41 to 0.97, $P = 0.04$).[87]

Which immune modulator is best for the treatment of severe COVID-19 remains an unresolved question. Aside from corticosteroids, tociluzimab and baricitinib have been the most extensively studied. Baricitinib is an oral agent and can also be administered via an enteral feeding tube in critically ill patients. However, it cannot be administered to patients with severely impaired renal function (ie, eGFR < 15 mL/min).[88] Tocilizumab is usually administered intravenously in hospitalized patients which may be useful in patients who are cannot take anything enterally. On the contrary, tocilizumab can be administered safely in patients with an (eGFR<15 mL/min).[89] However, there is no prospective, randomized controlled trial comparing the two agents in the treatment of COVID-19. A retrospective, multicenter cohort compared baricitinib to tocilizumab, of the 382 patients, 194 (50.8%) received tocilizumab, and 188 (49.2%) received baricitinib and found no significant difference in the outcomes of hospital discharge within 60 days alive and freedom from mechanical ventilation.[90]

Baricitinib reduces mortality in hospitalized patients with COVID-19 who require supplemental oxygen in addition to standard care which included corticosteroid therapy. The cumulative efficacy data led the US Food and Drug Administration to grant approval to baricitanib for the treatment of severe COVID.[91] Further research is needed to assess whether baricitinib and tocilizumab are equivalent therapies for severe COVID-19 in hospitalized patients.

Additional immunomodulatory agents that have not demonstrated benefit

Although some therapeutics targeting immunomodulation have been found to be efficacious in clinical trials, many more, even within the same drug class, have not. Much emphasis has been placed on the IL-6 and IL-1 axis as the data for these targets have been the most promising to date. However, the trial results have not all been congruent with clinical improvement. Canakinumab, an IL-1β antagonist, has shown no improvement in survival without mechanical ventilation in a randomized control trial of 454 patients with COVID-19 pneumonia.[92] On the contrary, anakinra, another IL-1 antagonist, was shown to have some potential clinical benefit.[93,94] However, differences in the designs of these trials may have directly affected the results. In the canakinumab trial, CRP and ferritin were used as indicators of acute inflammation, whereas in the anakinra trial soluble urokinase plasminogen activator receptor (suPAR) was used. Chronic inflammatory conditions such as obesity and smoking are known to lead to increased suPAR levels whereas CRP is generally unaffected by these levels. By using suPAR in lieu of CRP, the anakinra trial may have selected for a group of patients who were demonstrating acute on chronic inflammation as opposed to the acute inflammation required for enrollment in the canakinumab trial. This may indicate that canakinumab, and other IL-1β antagonists may prove to have increased benefit when used earlier in the disease process.

In a similar scenario, ruxolitinib, a JAK inhibitor, did not show any improvement in death, worsening respiratory failure, or ICU admission at 28 days.[89] This is compared with other kinase inhibitors such as baricitinib and tofacitinib which have demonstrated at least partial benefit in patients hospitalized with severe COVID-19 pneumonia.[68] One of the key differences between these trials, however, were the respiratory requirements to enroll patients. In REMAP-CAP, patients were eligible for enrollment if they were receiving either invasive or noninvasive ventilation, whereas in RUXCOVID the patients were required to not be mechanically ventilated. This may indicate that additional studies into ruxolitinib, and other JAK inhibitors, would be best designed for patients with higher degrees of respiratory support.

Other potential immunomodulatory therapeutic targets that have not yet panned out clinically include TNF-inhibitors such as adalimumab; granulocyte-macrophage colony-stimulating factor inhibitors such as mavrilimumab and otilimab; and C5a inhibitors such as vilobelimab.[95–98] Some of these trials have failed to reach statistical significance due to being underpowered, whereas others have found benefit only in subgroups. For example, vilobelimab was able to reach statistical significance in 28-day all-cause mortality in a pre-specified sub-analysis of patients from Western European countries but not when all the patients were included.[93] There remain several promising therapies that target the hyperactivation of the immune system against COVID-19, but whether they will join the growing list of beneficial agents remains to be determined.

SUMMARY

Early in the COVID-19 pandemic, it became evident that the immune response to SARS-CoV-2 infection could lead to a hyperinflammatory state resulting in severe end-organ damage such as ARDS. To attenuate the immune response, studies of immunomodulatory agents were rapidly initiated to determine which potential agents and in which patient populations such agents would be of benefit. Consequently, we now know that patients with severe COVID-19 who require supplemental oxygen but do not require mechanical ventilation or ECMO may derive the greatest benefit from immunomodulatory therapy. Of the agents studied to date, the corticosteroid, dexamethasone, has the most robust state supporting its in reducing mortality in the patient who require supplemental oxygenation. Other agents, such as tocilizumab and the JAK inhibitors, baricitinib, and tofacitinib, have been also shown to reduce mortality in patients requiring high levels of supplemental oxygen despite the use of corticosteroids and/or remdesivir. Although much has been learned during the pandemic regarding attenuating the pathologic hyperinflammatory state associated with COVID-19, more research is still needed to determine if the IL-6 antagonism of tocilizumab or the JAK inhibitors are equivalent in their salutary effects in treating severe COVID-19 or if combining such agents would lead to a greater improvement in mortality.

CLINICS CARE POINTS

- Dexamethasone use should be limited to those who are hospitalized are require supplemental oxygen.
- Duration of treatment with dexamethasone for COVID-19 should be a maximum of 10 days or until hospital discharge whichever is first.
- If a patient requires additional immunomodulatory therapy in addition to dexamethasone interleukin-6 antagonist, tocilizimab, or Janus kinase inhibitor, baracitinib, should be considered as adjunctive therapy.

DISCLOSURE

The authors declare they have no conflict of interests.

REFERENCES

1. Wang D, Hu B, Hu C, et al. Clinical characteristics of 138 hospitalized patients with 2019 novel coronavirus–infected pneumonia in Wuhan, China. JAMA 2020;323(11):1061–9.
2. Zhou F, Yu T, Du R, et al. Clinical course and risk factors for mortality of adult inpatients with COVID-19 in Wuhan, China: a retrospective cohort study. Lancet 2020;395(10229):1054–62.
3. Berlin DA, Gulick RM, Martinez FJ. Severe covid-19. N Engl J Med 2020;383(25):2451–60.
4. Del Valle DM, Kim-Schulze S, Huang HH, et al. An inflammatory cytokine signature predicts COVID-19 severity and survival. Nat Med 2020;26(10):1636–43.
5. Bradley BT, Maioli H, Johnston R, et al. Histopathology and ultrastructural findings of fatal COVID-19 infections in Washington State: a case series. Lancet 2020;396(10247):320–32.
6. Herold T, Jurinovic V, Arnreich C, et al. Elevated levels of IL-6 and CRP predict the need for mechanical ventilation in COVID-19. J Allergy Clin Immunol 2020;146(1):128–36.e4.
7. Carsana L, Sonzogni A, Nasr A, et al. Pulmonary post-mortem findings in a series of COVID-19 cases from northern Italy: a two-centre descriptive study. Lancet Infect Dis 2020;20(10):1135–40.
8. Melms JC, Biermann J, Huang H, et al. A molecular single-cell lung atlas of lethal COVID-19. Nature 2021;595(7865):114–9.

9. Maucourant C, Filipovic I, Ponzetta A, et al. Natural killer cell immunotypes related to COVID-19 disease severity. Sci Immunol 2020;5(50). https://doi.org/10.1126/sciimmunol.abd6832.

10. Liao M, Liu Y, Yuan J, et al. Single-cell landscape of bronchoalveolar immune cells in patients with COVID-19. Nat Med 2020;26(6):842–4.

11. Grant RA, Morales-Nebreda L, Markov NS, et al. Circuits between infected macrophages and T cells in SARS-CoV-2 pneumonia. Nature 2021;590(7847):635–41.

12. Lowery SA, Sariol A, Perlman S. Innate immune and inflammatory responses to SARS-CoV-2: implications for COVID-19. Cell Host Microbe 2021;29(7):1052–62.

13. Chen N, Zhou M, Dong X, et al. Epidemiological and clinical characteristics of 99 cases of 2019 novel coronavirus pneumonia in Wuhan, China: a descriptive study. Lancet 2020;395(10223):507–13.

14. Karki R, Sharma BR, Tuladhar S, et al. Synergism of TNF-α and IFN-γ triggers inflammatory cell death, tissue damage, and mortality in SARS-CoV-2 infection and cytokine shock syndromes. Cell 2021;184(1):149–68.e17.

15. Price CC, Altice FL, Shyr Y, et al. Tocilizumab treatment for cytokine release syndrome in hospitalized patients with coronavirus disease 2019: survival and clinical outcomes. Chest 2020;158(4):1397–408.

16. Yin X, Riva L, Pu Y, et al. MDA5 governs the innate immune response to SARS-CoV-2 in lung epithelial cells. SSRN Electron J 2020. https://doi.org/10.2139/ssrn.3682826.

17. Sampaio NG, Chauveau L, Hertzog J, et al. The RNA sensor MDA5 detects SARS-CoV-2 infection. Sci Rep 2021;11(1):13638.

18. Han L, Zhuang MW, Deng J, et al. SARS-CoV-2 ORF9b antagonizes type I and III interferons by targeting multiple components of the RIG-I/MDA-5-MAVS, TLR3-TRIF, and cGAS-STING signaling pathways. J Med Virol 2021;93(9):5376–89.

19. Khanmohammadi S, Rezaei N. Role of Toll-like receptors in the pathogenesis of COVID-19. J Med Virol 2021;93(5):2735–9.

20. Kayesh MEH, Kohara M, Tsukiyama-Kohara K. An overview of recent insights into the response of TLR to SARS-CoV-2 infection and the potential of TLR agonists as SARS-CoV-2 vaccine adjuvants. Viruses 2021;13(11). https://doi.org/10.3390/v13112302.

21. Venet M, Sa Ribeiro M, Décembre E, et al. Severe COVID-19 patients have impaired plasmacytoid dendritic cell-mediated control of SARS-CoV-2-infected cells. bioRxiv 2021. https://doi.org/10.1101/2021.09.01.21262969.

22. Channappanavar R, Fehr AR, Vijay R, et al. Dysregulated type I interferon and inflammatory monocyte-macrophage responses cause lethal pneumonia in SARS-CoV-infected mice. Cell Host Microbe 2016;19(2):181–93.

23. Chiale C, Greene TT, Zuniga EI. Interferon induction, evasion, and paradoxical roles during SARS-CoV-2 infection. Immunol Rev 2022. https://doi.org/10.1111/imr.13113.

24. Znaidia M, Demeret C, van der Werf S, et al. Characterization of SARS-CoV-2 evasion: interferon pathway and therapeutic options. Viruses 2022;14(6). https://doi.org/10.3390/v14061247.

25. Eskandarian Boroujeni M, Sekrecka A, Antonczyk A, et al. Dysregulated interferon response and immune hyperactivation in severe COVID-19: targeting STATs as a novel therapeutic strategy. Front Immunol 2022;13:888897.

26. Walker FC, Sridhar PR, Baldridge MT. Differential roles of interferons in innate responses to mucosal viral infections. Trends Immunol 2021;42(11):1009–23.

27. Greene TT, Zuniga EI. Type I interferon induction and exhaustion during viral infection: plasmacytoid dendritic cells and emerging COVID-19 findings. Viruses 2021;13(9). https://doi.org/10.3390/v13091839.

28. Kim YM, Shin EC. Type I and III interferon responses in SARS-CoV-2 infection. Exp Mol Med 2021;53(5):750–60.

29. Menter T, Haslbauer JD, Nienhold R, et al. Postmortem examination of COVID-19 patients reveals diffuse alveolar damage with severe capillary congestion and variegated findings in lungs and other organs suggesting vascular dysfunction. Histopathology 2020;77(2):198–209. https://doi.org/10.1111/his.14134.

30. Bonaventura A, Vecchié A, Dagna L, et al. Endothelial dysfunction and immunothrombosis as key pathogenic mechanisms in COVID-19. Nat Rev Immunol 2021;21(5):319–29.

31. Varga Z, Flammer AJ, Steiger P, et al. Endothelial cell infection and endotheliitis in COVID-19. Lancet 2020;395(10234):1417–8.

32. Delorey TM, Ziegler CGK, Heimberg G, et al. COVID-19 tissue atlases reveal SARS-CoV-2 pathology and cellular targets. Nature 2021;595(7865):107–13.

33. Georg P, Astaburuaga-García R, Bonaguro L, et al. Complement activation induces excessive T cell cytotoxicity in severe COVID-19. Cell. 2022;185(3):493–512.e25.

34. Zuo Y, Warnock M, Harbaugh A, et al. Plasma tissue plasminogen activator and plasminogen activator inhibitor-1 in hospitalized COVID-19 patients. Sci Rep 2021;11(1):1580.

35. Mackman N, Antoniak S, Wolberg AS, et al. Coagulation abnormalities and thrombosis in patients infected with SARS-CoV-2 and other pandemic viruses. Arterioscler Thromb Vasc Biol 2020;40(9):2033–44.

36. Lamers MM, Haagmans BL. SARS-CoV-2 pathogenesis. Nat Rev Microbiol 2022;20(5):270–84.

37. Schulte-Schrepping J, Reusch N, Paclik D, et al. Severe COVID-19 is marked by a dysregulated myeloid cell compartment. Cell. 2020;182(6):1419–40.e23.
38. Wendisch D, Dietrich O, Mari T, et al. SARS-CoV-2 infection triggers profibrotic macrophage responses and lung fibrosis. Cell. 2021;184(26):6243–61.e27.
39. Rendeiro AF, Ravichandran H, Bram Y, et al. The spatial landscape of lung pathology during COVID-19 progression. Nature 2021;593(7860):564–9.
40. Wu P, Chen D, Ding W, et al. The trans-omics landscape of COVID-19. Nat Commun 2021;12(1):4543.
41. Wilk AJ, Rustagi A, Zhao NQ, et al. A single-cell atlas of the peripheral immune response in patients with severe COVID-19. Nat Med 2020;26(7):1070–6.
42. Skendros P, Mitsios A, Chrysanthopoulou A, et al. Complement and tissue factor–enriched neutrophil extracellular traps are key drivers in COVID-19 immunothrombosis. J Clin Invest 2020;130(11):6151–7.
43. WHO Rapid Evidence Appraisal for COVID-19 Therapies (REACT) Working Group, Sterne JAC, Murthy S, et al. Association between administration of systemic corticosteroids and mortality among critically ill patients with COVID-19: a meta-analysis. JAMA 2020;324(13):1330–41.
44. RECOVERY Collaborative Group, Horby P, Lim WS, et al. Dexamethasone in hospitalized patients with COVID-19. N Engl J Med 2021;384(8):693–704. Available at: https://www.ncbi.nlm.nih.gov/pubmed/32678530.
45. Marconi VC, Ramanan AV, de Bono S, et al. Efficacy and safety of baricitinib for the treatment of hospitalised adults with COVID-19 (COV-BARRIER): a randomised, double-blind, parallel-group, placebo-controlled phase 3 trial. Lancet Respir Med 2021;9(12):1407–18.
46. Vanderheiden A, Thomas J, Soung AL, et al. CR2 signaling restricts SARS-CoV-2 infection. MBio 2021;12(6):e0274921.
47. Salvarani C, Dolci G, Massari M, et al. Effect of tocilizumab vs standard care on clinical worsening in patients hospitalized with COVID-19 pneumonia: a randomized clinical trial. JAMA Intern Med 2021;181(1):24–31.
48. Fajgenbaum DC, June CH. Cytokine storm. N Engl J Med 2020;383(23):2255–73. https://doi.org/10.1056/NEJMra2026131.
49. Cordeiro LP, Linhares EONN, Nogueira FGO, et al. Perspectives on glucocorticoid treatment for COVID-19: a systematic review. Pharmacol Rep 2021;73(3):728–35.
50. Crothers K, DeFaccio R, Tate J, et al. Dexamethasone in hospitalised coronavirus-19 patients not on intensive respiratory support. Eur Respir J 2022;60(1):2102532.
51. Tomazini BM, Maia IS, Cavalcanti AB, et al. Effect of dexamethasone on days alive and ventilator-free in patients with moderate or severe acute respiratory distress syndrome and COVID-19: the CoDEX randomized clinical trial. JAMA 2020;324(13):1307–16.
52. Angus DC, Derde L, Al-Beidh F, et al. Effect of hydrocortisone on mortality and organ support in patients with severe COVID-19: the REMAP-CAP COVID-19 corticosteroid domain randomized clinical trial. JAMA 2020;324(13):1317–29. Available at: https://www.ncbi.nlm.nih.gov/pubmed/32876697.
53. Czock D, Keller F, Rasche FM, et al. Pharmacokinetics and pharmacodynamics of systemically administered glucocorticoids. Clin Pharmacokinet 2005;44(1):61–98.
54. Coronavirus disease 2019 (COVID-19) treatment guidelines. National Institutes of Health. Available at: https://www.covid19treatmentguidelines.nih.gov/. Accessed August 1, 2022.
55. Yu LM, Bafadhel M, Dorward J, et al. Inhaled budesonide for COVID-19 in people at high risk of complications in the community in the UK (PRINCIPLE): a randomised, controlled, open-label, adaptive platform trial. Lancet 2021;398(10303):843–55. Available at: https://www.ncbi.nlm.nih.gov/pubmed/34388395.
56. Ramakrishnan S, Nicolau DV Jr, Langford B, et al. Inhaled budesonide in the treatment of early COVID-19 (STOIC): a Phase 2, open-label, randomised controlled trial. Lancet Respir Med 2021;9(7):763–72. Available at: https://www.ncbi.nlm.nih.gov/pubmed/33844996.
57. Clemency BM, Varughese R, Gonzalez-Rojas Y, et al. Efficacy of inhaled ciclesonide for outpatient treatment of adolescents and adults with symptomatic COVID-19: a randomized clinical trial. JAMA Intern Med 2022;182(1):42–9.
58. Ezer N, Belga S, Daneman N, et al. Inhaled and intranasal ciclesonide for the treatment of COVID-19 in adult outpatients: CONTAIN Phase II randomised controlled trial. BMJ 2021;375:e068060. Available at: https://www.ncbi.nlm.nih.gov/pubmed/34728476.
59. Clinical characteristics of 113 deceased patients with coronavirus disease 2019: retrospective study. BMJ 2020;368:m1295.
60. Huang C, Wang Y, Li X, et al. Clinical features of patients infected with 2019 novel coronavirus in Wuhan, China. Lancet 2020;395:497–506.
61. Sarosiek S, Shah R, Munshi NC. Review of siltuximab in the treatment of multicentric Castleman's disease. Ther Adv Hematol 2016;7(6):360–6.
62. Yip RML, Yim CW. Role of interleukin 6 inhibitors in the management of rheumatoid arthritis. J Clin Rheumatol 2021;27(8):e516–24.

63. Kotch C, Barrett D, Teachey DT. Tocilizumab for the treatment of chimeric antigen receptor T cell-induced cytokine release syndrome. Expert Rev Clin Immunol 2019;15(8):813–22.

64. Anonymous. Acetemra® (tocilizumab) prescribing information, Available at: https://www.accessdata.fda.gov/drugsatfda_docs/label/2021/125276s131lbl.pdf, 2022. Accessed July 7, 2022.

65. Anonymous. Kevzara® (sarilumab) prescribing information, Available at: https://www.accessdata.fda.gov/drugsatfda_docs/label/2017/761037s000lbl.pdf, 2017. Accessed July 7, 2022.

66. Anonymous. Sylvant® (siltuximab) prescribing information, Available at: https://www.accessdata.fda.gov/drugsatfda_docs/label/2018/125496s013lbl.pdf, 2018. Accessed July 7, 2022.

67. RECOVERY Collaborative Group. Tocilizumab in patients admitted to hospital with COVID-19 (RECOVERY): a randomised, controlled, open-label, platform trial. Lancet 2021;397(10285):1637–45.

68. REMAP-CAP Investigators, Gordon AC, Mouncey PR, et al. Interleukin-6 receptor antagonists in critically ill patients with covid-19. N Engl J Med 2021;384(16):1491–502.

69. Salama C, Han J, Yau L, et al. Tocilizumab in patients hospitalized with covid-19 pneumonia. N Engl J Med 2021;384(1):20–30.

70. Tatham KC, Shankar-Hari M, Arabi YM. The REMDACTA trial: do interleukin receptor antagonists provide additional benefit in COVID-19? Intensive Care Med 2021;47(11):1315–8.

71. Rosas IO, Bräu N, Waters M, et al. Tocilizumab in hospitalized patients with severe covid-19 pneumonia. N Engl J Med 2021;384(16):1503–16.

72. Stone JH, Frigault MJ, Serling-Boyd NJ, et al. Efficacy of tocilizumab in patients hospitalized with covid-19. N Engl J Med 2020;383(24):2333–44.

73. Hermine O, Mariette X, Tharaux PL, et al. Effect of tocilizumab vs usual care in adults hospitalized with COVID-19 and moderate or severe pneumonia: a randomized clinical trial. JAMA Intern Med 2021;181(1):32–40. published correction appears in JAMA Intern Med. 2021 Jan 1;181(1):144] [published correction appears in JAMA Intern Med. 2021 Jul 1;181(7):1021.

74. Lescure FX, Honda H, Fowler RA, et al. Sarilumab in patients admitted to hospital with severe or critical COVID-19: a randomised, double-blind, placebo-controlled, phase 3 trial. Lancet Respir Med 2021;9(5):522–32.

75. Stebbing J, Phelan A, Griffen I, et al. COVID-19: combining antiviral and anti-inflammatory treatment. Lancet Infect Dis 2020;20:400–2.

76. Richardson P, Griffin I, Tucker C, et al. Baricitinib as potential treatment for 2019-nCoV acute respiratory disease. Lancet 2020;395:e30–1.

77. Kaksonen M, Roux A. Mechanisms of clathrin-mediated endocytosis. Nat Rev Mol Cell Biol 2018;19(5):313–26.

78. Petrone L, Petruccioli E, Alonzi T, et al. In-vitro evaluation of the immunomodulatory effects of baricitinib: implication for COVID-19 therapy. J Infect 2021;82:58–66.

79. Hoang TN, Pino M, Boddapati AK, et al. Baricitinib treatment resolves lower-airway macrophage inflammation and neutrophil recruitment in SARS-CoV-2-infected rhesus macaques. Cell 2021;184:460–75.e21.

80. Kalil AC, Patterson TF, Mehta AK, et al. Baricitinib plus remdesivir for hospitalized adults with COVID-19. N Engl J Med 2021;384:795–807.

81. Recovery Collaborative Group. Baricitinib in patients admitted to hospital with COVID-19 (RECOVERY): a randomised, controlled, open-label, platform trial and updated meta-analysis. Lancet 2022;400(10349):359–68.

82. Vannucchi AM, Sordi B, Morettini A, et al. Compassionate use of JAK1/2 inhibitor ruxolitinib for severe COVID-19: a prospective observational study. Leukemia 2021;35:1121–33.

83. La Rosée F, Bremer HC, Gehrke I, et al. The Janus kinase 1/2 inhibitor ruxolitinib in COVID-19 with severe systemic hyperinflammation. Leukemia 2020;34:1805–15.

84. D'Alessio A, Del Poggio P, Bracchi F, et al. Low-Dose ruxolitinib plus steroid in severe SARS-CoV-2 pneumonia. Leukemia 2021;35:635–8.

85. Cao Y, Wei J, Zou L, et al. Ruxolitinib in treatment of severe coronavirus disease 2019 (COVID-19): a multicenter, singleblind, randomized controlled trial. J Allergy Clin Immunol 2020;146:137–46.

86. Han MK, Antila M, Ficker JH, et al. Ruxolitinib in addition to standard of care for the treatment of patients admitted to hospital with COVID-19 (RUXCOVID): a randomised, double-blind, placebo-controlled, phase 3 trial. Lancet Rheumatol 2022;4(5):e351–61.

87. Guimaraes PO, Quirk D, Furtado RH, et al. Tofacitinib in patients hospitalized with covid-19 pneumonia. N Engl J Med 2021;385(5):406–15.

88. Anonymous. Olumiant® (baricitinib) prescribing information, Available at: https://www.accessdata.fda.gov/drugsatfda_docs/label/2022/207924s006lbl.pdf, 2022. Accessed July 10, 2022.

89. Anonymous. Fact sheet of healthcare providers: emergency use authorization for Actemra® (tocilizumab), Available at: https://www.fda.gov/media/150321/download, 2021. Accessed July 10, 2022.

90. Roddy J, Wells D, Schenk K, et al. Tocilizumab versus baricitinib in patients hospitalized with COVID-19 pneumonia and hypoxemia: a multicenter retrospective cohort study. Crit Care Explor 2022;4(5):e0702.

91. US Food and Drug Administration, Supplement to NDA 207924 for baricitinib for the treatment of COVID-19 in hospitalized adults requiring supplemental oxygen, non-invasive or invasive mechanical ventilation, or ECMO, Available at: https://www.fda.gov/media/143822/download. Accessed July 10, 2022.

92. Caricchio R, Abbate A, Gordeev I, et al. Effect of canakinumab vs placebo on survival without invasive mechanical ventilation in patients hospitalized with severe COVID-19. JAMA 2021;326(3):230.

93. Kyriazopoulou E, Panagopoulos P, Metallidis S, et al. An open label trial of anakinra to prevent respiratory failure in COVID-19. eLife 2021;10:e66125.

94. Kyriazopoulou E, Poulakou G, Milionis H, et al. Early treatment of COVID-19 with anakinra guided by soluble urokinase plasminogen receptor plasma levels: a double-blind, randomized controlled phase 3 trial. Nat Med 2021;27(10):1752–60.

95. Fakharian A, Barati S, Mirenayat M, et al. Evaluation of adalimumab effects in managing severe cases of COVID-19: a randomized controlled trial. Int Immunopharmacol 2021;99:107961.

96. Cremer PC, Abbate A, Hudock K, et al. Mavrilimumab in patients with severe COVID-19 pneumonia and systemic hyperinflammation (MASH-COVID): an investigator initiated, multicentre, double-blind, randomised, placebo-controlled trial. Lancet Rheumatol 2021;3(6):e410–8.

97. Patel J, Beishuizen A, Ruiz XB, et al. A randomized trial of otilimab in severe COVID-19 pneumonia (OSCAR). Eur Respir J 2022;2101870.

98. Vlaar APJ, De Bruin S, Busch M, et al. Anti-C5a antibody IFX-1 (vilobelimab) treatment versus best supportive care for patients with severe COVID-19 (PANAMO): an exploratory, open-label, phase 2 randomised controlled trial. Lancet Rheumatol 2020;2(12):e764–73.

Lessons Learned in Mechanical Ventilation/ Oxygen Support in Coronavirus Disease 2019

Laura Dragoi, MD, MHSc[a],*, Matthew T. Siuba, DO, MS[b,c], Eddy Fan, MD, PhD[d,e]

KEYWORDS

- COVID-19 • SARS-CoV-2 • ARDS • Mechanical ventilation

KEY POINTS

- Evidence-based treatment principles for patients with non-COVID ARDS apply to patients with COVID-19 ARDS as well.
- A trial of HFNC or NIPPV can be offered.
- Once intubated, provide lung protective ventilation. Prone positioning should be considered in patients with persistent hypoxemia or when lung protective ventilation targets cannot be achieved.
- Rescue therapies such as recruitment maneuvers, inhaled pulmonary vasodilators and ECMO should be considered on a case-by-case basis.

BACKGROUND

After its first description in Wuhan, China, in December 2019, the coronavirus disease 2019 (COVID-19) caused by the severe acute respiratory syndrome coronavirus-2 (SARS-CoV-2) spread worldwide at a rapid pace, causing the WHO to declare a pandemic on March 11, 2020.[1] Two years later, there have been more than 480 million confirmed cases and more than 6 million confirmed deaths.[2] The spectrum of the disease ranges from asymptomatic infection or mild respiratory symptoms to pneumonia, with severe cases leading to the acute respiratory distress syndrome (ARDS) with multiorgan involvement. Data from the first months of the pandemic reported that approximately 14% of infected individuals required hospitalization and 5% intensive care unit (ICU) admission.[3]

Faced with a global health crisis caused by a previously unknown disease entity, the medical and scientific community felt the imperative to disseminate even preliminary observations and data. Information emerged in real time and clinical management was adjusted as more evidence became available, thus creating certain trends that changed over the course of the pandemic.

This article will review how the ventilatory management of patients with COVID-19 evolved during the course of the pandemic and review the data that are currently available. We will conclude with current evidence-based recommendations.

[a] Interdepartmental Division of Critical Care, University of Toronto, Toronto General Hospital – MaRS Centre, Room 9026, 585 University Avenue, Toronto, Ontario M5G 2N2, Canada; [b] Department of Critical Care Medicine, Respiratory Institute, Cleveland Clinic, Cleveland Clinic Main Campus, 9500 Euclid Avenue, Cleveland, OH 44195, USA; [c] Cleveland Clinic Lerner College of Medicine of Case Western Reserve University; [d] Interdepartmental Division of Critical Care, University of Toronto, Toronto General Hospital – MaRS Centre, Room 9013, 585 University Avenue, Toronto, Ontario M5G 2N2, Canada; [e] Institute of Health Policy, Management and Evaluation, University of Toronto
* Corresponding author.
E-mail address: laura.dragoi@mail.utoronto.ca

Clin Chest Med 44 (2023) 321–333
https://doi.org/10.1016/j.ccm.2022.11.010
0272-5231/23/© 2022 Elsevier Inc. All rights reserved.

chestmed.theclinics.com

SEARCH STRATEGY

To inform our review, we searched MEDLINE/PubMed from inception to February 24, 2022, using a combination of the terms COVID-19, SARS-CoV-2, ARDS, acute respiratory distress syndrome, critical care, mechanical ventilation, and oxygen supplementation. We reviewed relevant references cited in selected articles and added relevant publications.

DISCUSSION
COVID-19 Phenotypes

It became evident early on during the pandemic that respiratory failure is one of the main features of severe COVID-19 disease, with a large number of patients with COVID-19 requiring oxygen supplementation and mechanical ventilation. Although clinical features of this new entity typically met the Berlin definition criteria for ARDS,[4] there was initial concern that lung involvement in COVID-19 might represent a specific disease with distinctive phenotypes, potentially requiring a unique approach to ventilatory support. In a small case series, Gattinoni and colleagues[5] described profound hypoxemia associated with near normal compliance of the respiratory system (Crs), which is rarely seen in cases of ARDS. The authors made a distinction between this non-ARDS, type 1 presentation as opposed to "typical" ARDS, which they called type 2 presentation.[6] These 2 subtypes were soon renamed to Phenotype L—characterized by low elastance, low VA/Q ratio, low lung weight, and low recruitability—and Phenotype H characterized by high elastance, high right-to-left shunt, high lung weight, and high recruitability.[7] Although recognized as being time-dependent manifestations on the same disease spectrum, postulating different phenotypes raised the question of a tailored, different therapeutic approach. Recommendations were made to favor noninvasive approaches or—once intubated—lower positive end-expiratory pressure (PEEP) and more liberal tidal volumes (8–9 mL/kg predicted body weight [PBW]) in type L.[7] Once transitioned to type H, the patient would be treated as a "typical" ARDS patient with low tidal volumes and prone positioning.[7,8]

ARDS is a heterogenous syndrome, and efforts are continuously made to identify subtypes based on biological, clinical, or radiological characteristics—both in non-COVID[9–12] and COVID patients with ARDS.[13,14] Different phenotypic patterns based on the compliance of the respiratory system (Crs) as observed by Gattinoni and colleagues[5] seem to be present in non-COVID-19 ARDS[15] as well, and represent most likely progression of the disease entity. The postulation of the distinct phenotypes L and H requiring different approaches to ventilation has led to discussions in the published literature[16–19]; however, with little additional data to support a dichotomous phenotypic distribution, or the need for a tailored approach to ventilation as suggested by these phenotypes, this concept has been largely deemphasized in the later phases of the pandemic.

Use of Noninvasive Respiratory Support

The COVID-19 pandemic saw a renewed interest in noninvasive forms of respiratory support—including high-flow nasal cannula (HFNC) and noninvasive ventilation (NIV) for the treatment of COVID-19-associated respiratory failure. This was due in part to the initial reports of high mortality in patients on invasive mechanical ventilation[20] and in part to the limited availability of ventilators in some jurisdictions. The early observation of preserved lung compliance and increased shunt fraction in patients with COVID-19[5] also seemed to favor maintaining spontaneous breathing. Using a helmet interface for NIV, rather than more typical mask interfaces, was suggested to reduce risk of airborne transmission[21,22] because NIV and HFNC were initially considered aerosolizing procedures. Evidence that their use did not produce additional viral contamination emerged in later phases of the pandemic.[23] Early observational studies with considerable limitations reported safe usage of HFNC[24] and NIV,[25] both in the ICU and outside the ICU setting, and variable rates of escalation to intubation.[26–28] The Helmet Noninvasive Ventilation vs High-Flow Nasal Oxygen on Days Free of Respiratory Support in Patients with COVID-19 and Moderate to Severe Hypoxemic Respiratory Failure (HENIVOT) randomized clinical trial[29] compared helmet NIV followed by HFNC versus HFNC alone in 109 patients with COVID-19 induced moderate-to-severe respiratory failure (PaO2/FiO2 < 200 mm Hg and PaCO2 $\leq$ 45). This trial failed to show a difference in respiratory support-free days at 28 days (mean difference, 2 days [95% CI, −2 to 6]); however, the incidence of intubation was significantly lower in the helmet NIV group compared with the HFNC group (30% vs 51%; difference −21% [95% CI -38% to −3%], p = 0.03).

The use of noninvasive respiratory support continued through the course of the pandemic, with both HFNC and NIV being used. A recent parallel group, adaptative, randomized clinical trial of 1273 hospitalized patients with COVID-19-associated hypoxemic respiratory failure (RECOVERY-RS) compared the use of either continuous positive airway pressure (CPAP), HFNC, or conventional oxygen therapy with the primary composite outcome of tracheal intubation or mortality within 30 days.[30] The trial was discontinued early due to declining numbers of patients with COVID-19 and termination of the funded recruitment period. The primary outcome was significantly lower in the group randomized to CPAP as compared with conventional oxygen therapy (36.3% vs 44.4%, absolute difference, −8% [95% CI, −15% to −1%]). This was mainly driven by the reduction in the need for intubation (33.4% vs 41.3%). There was no statistically significant difference in the primary outcome between the HFNC group versus the conventional oxygen therapy group (44.3% vs 45.1%, absolute difference, −1% [95% CI, −8% to 6%]). Safety events were more common in the CPAP arm (130/380–34.2%) compared with the HFNC arm (86/418–20.6%) and the conventional oxygen therapy arm (66/475 or 13.9%). In a post hoc analysis, CPAP was compared with HFNC in 570 participants randomized across all 3 groups, with the primary outcome occurring in 34.6% (91/263) of participants in the CPAP group and in 44.3% (136/307) of participants in the HFNO group (absolute difference 10% [95%CI, −18% to −2%]). This is the largest study of NIV in COVID-19-induced respiratory failure to date. The main limitation of the trial consists in its early termination, which could lead to an overestimation of the results. Additionally, patients, clinicians, and outcome assessors were unblinded and the clinical criteria for intubation were left to provider discretion.

In the HiFLo-Covid trial,[31] 199 patients with suspected or confirmed infection with SARS-CoV-2, acute hypoxemic respiratory failure with a PaO2/FIO2 less than 200 and clinical signs of respiratory distress were randomized to either HFNC or conventional oxygen therapy. Intubation occurred in 34 (34.3%) patients randomized to the high-flow oxygen therapy and in 51 (51%) patients randomized to receive conventional oxygen therapy. In addition, patients treated with HFNC had a median time to recovery of 11 days (IQR, 9–14) vs 14 (IQR 11–19) days in the conventional oxygen therapy group.

Given the lack of evidence demonstrating a mortality benefit in the usage of one noninvasive modality over the other, both HFNC and NIV are acceptable initial therapeutic modalities for patients with COVID-19 with hypoxemic respiratory failure. Further research is needed to confirm the advantage of CPAP over HFNC, as demonstrated in the post hoc analysis of 570 participants of the RECOVERY-RS trial.

Timing of Intubation

Determining the optimal timing for intubation remains challenging and should be done on a case-by-case basis. Intubation is considered a high-risk, aerosol-generating procedure but the magnitude of the infection risk for health-care personnel is difficult to quantify.[32,33] During the beginning of the pandemic, there was a controversy regarding whether "early" intubation is necessary to prevent patient self-inflicted lung injury[8,34] or not.[35,36] This in keeping with data from patients with non-COVID-19 induced moderate-to-severe ARDS and a PO2/FiO2 ratio of less than 150, in which the use of NIV instead of early intubation was associated with higher mortality.[37] In addition, early intubation was thought to minimize the risks of aerosol transmission and infection of health-care workers by avoiding the exposure of NIV and HFNC, which are considered aerosolizing generating medical procedures. However, what exactly constitutes an "early" timing was never defined. In addition, there were concerns around high mortality in intubated patients,[38,39] which led to some practitioners tolerating high oxygen requirements and low saturations and basing the decision of intubation on the patient's subjective work of breathing.

The literature published during the pandemic around timing of intubation in COVID-19 consists mainly of retrospective observational studies and does not show a significant association between timing of intubation and mortality.[27,40–44] Thus, given the lack of evidence to the contrary, the decision to intubate a patient in respiratory failure due to COVID-19 should be individualized and follow the same decision-making algorithm as the decision to intubate any patient in respiratory failure.

Lung Protective Ventilation

Pressure-limited, low-tidal volume ventilation improves outcomes in patients with ARDS[45] and without ARDS[46]. In the first months of the pandemic, there was a recommendation to consider liberalizing tidal volumes in patients with the L-phenotype who had difficult to control hypercapnia.[7] This increases the potential risk of ventilator-induced lung injury (VILI) through tidal volumes higher than 6 mL/kg PBW, especially considering the possibility that type L and type H phenotypes represent the temporal evolution of the course in severe pneumonia/ARDS. A scoping review published by Grasselli and colleagues[47] showed that settings for mechanical ventilation used in COVID-19 ARDS generally followed recommendations for lung protective ventilation. A cohort study of 1503 patients with ARDS secondary to COVID-19[48] reported that the use of lung protective settings of mechanical ventilation (defined as a tidal volume less than 8 mL/kg PBW and a plateau pressure less than 30 cm H2O in the first 24 hours after admission to the ICU) was associated with an increased survival at 28 days (HR 0.763, 95%CI 0.605–0.963), and remained associated with increased survival after adjusting for PEEP, compliance, PaO2/FiO2 (P/F) ratio and pH (aHR 0.73, 95% CI 0.57–0.94). The median plateau pressure and driving pressure were higher in nonsurvivors than in survivors (23 vs 22 cmH2O and 13 vs 12 cmH2O). The distribution of static compliance did not suggest the identification of dichotomous phenotypes.

The evidence available to date supports providing mechanical ventilation for patients with COVID-19 ARDS in the same way as for non-COVID-19 ARDS, aiming for a pressure-limited low tidal volume ventilation—as is reflected in current guideline recommendations.[49–52] Similar to non-COVID-19 ARDS, the optimal level of PEEP remains elusive in the COVID-19 ARDS population, with observational studies showing a variable range applied in clinical practice.[47,53]

Prone Positioning

Proning, the positioning of a patient face-down for a period of time in a 24-hour cycle, is standard of care in the therapy for intubated patients with moderate-to-severe ARDS, and high-quality evidence has shown that proning has a mortality benefit in these patients.[54–56] During prone positioning, oxygenation improves by decrease of the shunt fraction as a result of more homogenous lung aeration and strain distribution with perfusion patterns remaining relatively constant.[57] The improvement in gas exchange however does not seem to be the sole driver of the survival benefit.[58] In addition, prone positioning is thought to attenuate VILI by recruiting lung parenchyma in dependent regions and reducing hyperinflation in nondependent regions.[57]

Small, observational studies published early in the pandemic[59–62] showed improved oxygenation through prone positioning, and further observational data described reduced mortality in those patients on mechanical ventilation who were proned.[63–65] Proning protocols were developed, and some centers created specific proning teams to provide relief for the core intensive care team.[66–68] Intermittent prone positioning became standard of care for intubated patients with ARDS secondary to COVID-19, mainly based on literature showing reduction in mortality in non-COVID ARDS.[54–56]

Proning had been shown to provide improvement in oxygenation in awake, nonintubated patients even before the COVID-19 pandemic,[69,70] and its use in COVID-19 awake patients has been shown to be feasible and effective in terms of an oxygenation benefit.[71] Ehrmann and colleagues[72] demonstrated additionally that prone positioning in awake patients reduces the incidence of treatment failure and the need for intubation, without increasing adverse events. In the recently published COVID-PRONE trial—prone positioning of patients with moderate hypoxemia due to COVID-19 multicenter pragmatic randomized trial—257 patients were randomized to prone positioning or standard of care.[73] The rate of the primary outcome—a composite of in-hospital death, mechanical ventilation of worsening respiratory failure defined as needing at least 60% FiO2 for more than 24 hours—was similar in both groups. The investigators also report a low adherence to the prone position, with "discomfort" being anecdotally cited as the main reason. The trial was discontinued early for futility.

In a recent systematic review and meta-analysis on awake prone positioning in COVID-19-related acute hypoxemic respiratory failure, aggregate data of 10 RCTs showed that awake prone positioning significantly reduced the need for intubation in patients who received advanced respiratory support (HFNC or NIV) and those in intensive care setting.[74]

Although robust data showing that self-proning in awake patients reduces mortality is still lacking, it is now part of standard of care in many centers for the COVID-19 patient with increased oxygen requirements.

Timing of Tracheostomy

The optimal timing for tracheostomy is a matter of debate even in prolonged mechanical ventilation outside the context of COVID-19. In the early days of the pandemic, tracheostomies were often deferred until the patients were confirmed to be no longer infectious (ie, using polymerase chain reaction), given that tracheostomy was generally considered a high-risk procedure. Emerging data showed that both recommendations and practice vary from institution to institution and transition to tracheostomy is performed anywhere between 3 and 21 days after intubation,[75] similar to the non-COVID-19 population. Some have suggested support for earlier timing due to emerging data on reduction of sedation and analgesia in patients undergoing tracheostomy.[76] Current guidelines recommend performing a tracheostomy in intubated patients with COVID-19 who are anticipated to require prolonged mechanical ventilation, with no specific recommendation on the timing of the procedure. In order to mitigate the infectious risk for health-care workers, the use of enhanced protective equipment (airborne precautions) is advised.

POTENTIAL RESCUE THERAPIES AND OTHER CONSIDERATIONS
Recruitment Maneuvers

Previous experience from non-COVID-19 ARDS has shown that the effect of recruitment maneuvers varies from patient to patient, often improving oxygenation but with conflicting results on mortality. Recruitment maneuvers are most likely to be beneficial in patients who have a high potential for recruitment.[77] The assessment of recruitability at the bedside can be determined with the recruitment to inflation (R/I) ratio—the ratio between the compliance of the recruited lung and ventilated lung at low PEEP,[78] which can be calculated using an online calculator (https://crec.coemv.ca/).[79] The R/I ratio has only been evaluated in small studies in the COVID-19 population, although with promising results.[59,80,81] Should a recruitment maneuver be performed, most guidelines are currently recommending against the use of a staircase (incremental PEEP increase) maneuver.[50,82]

Airway Pressure Release Ventilation

Airway pressure release ventilation (APRV) has the theoretical physiologic benefit of optimizing alveolar recruitment and allowing for spontaneous breathing at the same time. However, studies failed to show a consistent benefit in non-COVID-19 hypoxemic respiratory failure and ARDS. In a recent RCT, Ibarra-Estrada and colleagues[83] randomized 90 patients with COVID-19 ARDS to receive either low tidal volume ventilation or APRV. There was no difference in ventilator-free days, sedation or analgesia requirements, or barotrauma between the 2 groups. Further evidence is needed before APRV can have an established role in the treatment of COVID-19 ARDS.

Pulmonary Vasodilators

The role of pulmonary vasodilators as a rescue therapy has been established in the non-COVID-19 ARDS population, with improvement in physiologic parameters but no mortality benefit.[84] The current evidence regarding the use of inhaled pulmonary vasodilators as a rescue therapy in refractory hypoxic respiratory failure secondary to COVID-19 ARDS is limited[85–88] and does not allow for definitive conclusions. Current guidelines recommend against the routine use of inhaled nitric oxide and for the use of a trial of inhaled pulmonary vasodilators as a rescue therapy.[50,82]

Extracorporeal Membrane Oxygenation

The indication to use extracorporeal membrane oxygenation (ECMO) as a rescue therapy for refractory hypoxemic respiratory failure secondary to COVID-19 ARDS follows traditional selection criteria while considering availability of resources, as discussed in detail in a separate article of this series.

Resource Shortages Affecting Approach to Respiratory Support

Shortage and need can often lead to bold, new solutions. In August 1952, the Blegdam Hospital in Copenhagen faced a polio epidemic, and there was only one iron lung to treat a large number of patients who required negative pressure ventilation. It was in this context that the anesthesiologist Bjorn Ibsen brought forward and implemented the idea of ventilation with positive pressure through a tracheostomy. It soon became the lifesaving treatment during the polio epidemic, thanks to the coordinated efforts of the University of Copenhagen's medical and dental students, who provided ventilation by hand—around the clock.[89]

The COVID-19 pandemic underscored a fear of lack of sufficient resources to provide ventilatory support. The anticipated shortage of ventilators in the beginning of the pandemic led to a discussion around the use of shared ventilation, with one ventilator supporting 2 patients. A review published by Branson and Rodriguez in 2021 summarizes the proposed technical solution, the limited evidence in human trials as well as neglected ethical aspects, concluding that shared ventilation should be seen as a last resort procedure.[90] Shared ventilation appeared to be safe in a small case series and for a limited time (48 hours) but generalizability is yet untested.[91] Another proposed approach was the use of anaesthesia ventilators for prolonged mechanical ventilation.[92]

These technical aspects of increasing the number of available ventilators can only be one part of a complex response to increased demand for acute and critical care services. During the course of the pandemic, most countries and/or administrative divisions developed protocols to give legal and ethical guidance under a crisis standard of care, with the aim to direct resource allocation for the individual institutions aiming at maximizing resources, discussing how to efficiently redeploy health-care professionals to areas of need and

Table 1
Overview of recommendations made by different societies regarding mechanical ventilation in coronavirus disease 2019 acute respiratory distress syndrome

	Surviving Sepsis Campaign	NIH COVID-19 Treatment Guideline	WHO: Clinical Management of Patients with COVID-19: Living Guideline	Australian Guidelines for the Clinical Care of People with Covid-19 v62.
Supplemental oxygen	Suggestion to start supplemental oxygen if SpO2 <92% Recommendation to start supplemental oxygen if SpO2 <90%	Target an SpO2 of 92% to 96%	Target SpO2 >90%	Target SpO2 of 92%–96% in most patients Target SpO2 of 88%–92% in patients at risk of hypercapnia
HFNC, NIPPV	HFNC over conventional oxygen therapy HFNC over NIPPV	HFNC oxygen over NIV (NIPPV)	HFNC over standard oxygen therapy HFNC, CPAP, or NIV—no recommendation to chose one device over another	Consider using CPAP. If CPAP is not available or not tolerated, consider HFNC as an alternative to conventional oxygen delivery
Awake proning	No recommendation	Trial of awake proning recommended Awake proning should not be used as a rescue therapy	Awake proning suggested in severely ill hospitalized patients	Consider awake prone positioning
Mechanical Ventilation				
Tidal volumes	Low Vt ventilation (4-8 mL/ kg PBW) over higher tidal volumes (>8 mL/kg PBW)	Low Vt ventilation (4-8 mL/ kg PBW) over higher tidal volumes (>8 mL/kg PBW)	Lower tidal volumes (4-8 mL/kg PBW)	
Plateau pressure	Target plateau pressure <30 cm H2O	Target plateau pressure <30 cm H2O	Target plateau pressure <30 cm H2O	
PEEP	Higher PEEP strategy over lower PEEP strategy	Higher PEEP strategy over lower PEEP strategy	Trial of higher PEEP instead of lower PEEP is suggested	Higher PEEP strategy over lower PEEP strategy

Rescue therapies

| Recruitment maneuvers | If using recruitment maneuvers, strong recommendation against staircase (incremental PEEP) maneuvers | If using recruitment maneuvers, recommends against using staircase (incremental PEEP) maneuvers | If recruitment maneuvers are used, recommendation to not use staircase (incremental PEEP) recruitment |
| Inhaled pulmonary vasodilators | Recommendation against the routine use of inhaled nitric oxide Suggestion for a trial of inhaled pulmonary vasodilators as a rescue therapy | Reasonable to attempt an inhaled pulmonary vasodilator as a rescue therapy | |

Table 2
Overview of recommendations for ventilation in coronavirus disease 2019 acute respiratory distress syndrome

	Recommendation	Available Evidence
Oxygen supplementation and noninvasive ventilation	Trial of HFNC or noninvasive positive pressure ventilation The use of CPAP possibly reduces the need for intubation	No evidence demonstrating a mortality benefit in usage of one noninvasive modality over the other RECOVERY-RS[30]: CPAP seems to reduce the need for intubation when compared with the use of conventional oxygen therapy Strength of the trial: • Large, multicenter RCT of NIV in respiratory failure secondary to COVID-19 • Allocation concealment Limitations of the trial: • Stopped early—results might be overestimated • No criteria for when to intubate patients • Unblinded
Timing of intubation	No recommendation, individualized decision requiring clinical judgment	No high-quality evidence available
Lung protective ventilation	Tidal volumes limited to 4–6 cc/kg Plateau pressures limited to <30 cmH2O Driving pressures <15 cmH2O	Evidence for pressure limited low tidal volumes as well as limitation of driving pressures in non-COVID ARDS[45] No high-quality evidence available in the COVID-19 population
Prone positioning	In nonintubated patients: trial of awake self proning In intubate patients with moderate to severe ARDS: proning recommended	Awake self proning reduces the incidence of treatment failure and need for intubation in patients with COVID-19 induced hypoxic respiratory failure[72] Evidence showing that proning improves mortality in intubated patients with non-COVID-19 ARDS[54] No high-quality evidence for the benefit of proning in the COVID-19 ARDS population
Timing of tracheostomy	Tracheostomy recommended in patients anticipated to require prolonged mechanical ventilation No recommendation on timing of tracheostomy	Possible benefit from reduction of analgesia and sedation with early tracheostomy in the COVID-19 ARDS population[76]

providing guidance if triage were to become necessary.

Overview of Recommendation from Current Guidelines

The Surviving Sepsis Campaign Guidelines[50] provided an update on their recommendations on the management of adults with COVID-19 in the ICU in March 2021. There continues to be a strong recommendation for oxygen supplementation to keep SpO2 between 92% and 96%, lung protective ventilation with low tidal volumes and limited plateau pressure, a higher PEEP strategy over a lower PEEP strategy, and a strong recommendation against the use of staircase recruitment maneuvers. As a weak recommendation, HFNC is suggested over NIV. No recommendation was made regarding the use of helmet NIPPV compared with mask NIV. As an addition to the previous guideline, there was no recommendation regarding the use of awake prone positioning due to insufficient evidence. Of note, the update to the Surviving Sepsis Campaign Guidelines was released before evidence becoming available showing that awake self-proning reduced the need for intubation without a signal for harm.[72–74]

The NIH COVID-19 Treatment Guidelines,[82] last updated in December 2021, provide similar recommendations, stating that there is no evidence that ventilator management of patients with ARDS secondary to COVID-19 should differ from ventilator management of patients with ARDS secondary to other causes. The guideline does recommend a trial of awake prone positioning for patients with persistent hypoxia requiring HFNC oxygen and adds a recommendation against using awake proning as a rescue therapy to avoid intubation.

The WHO Living guidance for clinical management of COVID-19[49] does suggest awake prone positioning in severely ill patients with COVID-19 who require supplemental oxygen (including HFNC) or NIV. Their recommendations for mechanical ventilation do not differ from recommendations for ventilation in non-COVID-19 ARDS, emphasizing pressure limited low-tidal volume ventilation.

The Australian National COVID-19 Clinical Evidence Taskforce's continuously updated Living Guideline[51] on Caring for people with COVID-19 provides similar recommendations.

Table 1 provides an overview of these societies' recommendations.

SUMMARY

Nearly 3 years since the beginning of the pandemic, it is clear that COVID-19 ARDS does not differ substantially from non-COVID-19 ARDS and that treatment principles of ARDS based on high-quality prepandemic evidence are applicable to COVID-19 as well.

Patients with increased oxygen requirements should be supported with either HFNC or NIPPV. The generally recommended target of SpO2 is between 92% and 96%. Awake self-proning is recommended for patients awake and still hypoxemic despite oxygen supplementation. The timing of intubation remains a challenging decision that should be individualized, with the aim to avoid delaying a necessary intubation. Once intubated, the mainstay of supportive therapy consists in lung protection with pressure-limited and volume-limited mechanical ventilation. Prone positioning should be considered in patients with persistent low PaO_2/FiO_2 ratios or when parameters of lung protective ventilation cannot be achieved. Rescue therapies such as recruitment maneuvers, inhaled pulmonary vasodilators, and ECMO should be considered on a case-by-case basis. As in non-COVID-19-associated ARDS, tracheostomy should be performed when prolonged mechanical ventilation is anticipated.

Table 2 summarizes these recommendations for ventilation in COVID-19 ARDS.

CLINICS CARE POINTS

- Evidence-based treatment principles for patients with non-COVID ARDS apply to patients with COVID-19 ARDS as well.
- A trial of HFNC or NIPPV can be offered.
- Once intubated, provide lung protective ventilation. Prone positioning should be considered in patients with persistent hypoxemia or when lung protective ventilation targets cannot be achieved.
- Rescue therapies such as recruitment maneuvers, inhaled pulmonary vasodilators and ECMO should be considered on a case-by-case basis.

DISCLOSURE

Dr E. Fan reports personal fees from ALung Technologies, Aerogen, Baxter, GE Healthcare, Inspira, and Vasomune outside the submitted work. All other authors declare that they have no conflict of interest.

REFERENCES

1. World Health Organization. WHO Director-General's opening remarks at the media briefing on COVID-19 - 11 March 2020. Available at: https://www.who.int/director-general/speeches/detail/who-director-general-s-opening-remarks-at-the-media-briefing-on-covid-19—11-march-2020. Accessed 30 March, 2022.
2. Our World in Data. Cumulative confirmed COVID-19 cases and deaths, world. Available at: https://ourworldindata.org/grapher/cumulative-deaths-and-cases-covid-19. Accessed 30 March, 2022.
3. Wu Z, McGoogan JM. Characteristics of and important lessons from the coronavirus disease 2019 (COVID-19) outbreak in China: summary of a report of 72314 cases from the Chinese center for disease control and prevention. JAMA 2020;323(13):1239–42.
4. Force ADT, Ranieri VM, Rubenfeld GD, et al. Acute respiratory distress syndrome: the Berlin Definition. JAMA 2012;307(23):2526–33.
5. Gattinoni L, Coppola S, Cressoni M, et al. COVID-19 does not lead to a "typical" acute respiratory distress syndrome. Am J Respir Crit Care Med 2020;201(10):1299–300.
6. Gattinoni L, Chiumello D, Rossi S. COVID-19 pneumonia: ARDS or not? Crit Care (London, England) 2020;24(1):154.
7. Gattinoni L, Chiumello D, Caironi P, et al. COVID-19 pneumonia: different respiratory treatments for different phenotypes? Intensive Care Med 2020;46(6):1099–102.
8. Marini JJ, Gattinoni L. Management of COVID-19 respiratory distress. JAMA 2020;323(22):2329–30.
9. Sinha P, Delucchi KL, McAuley DF, et al. Development and validation of parsimonious algorithms to classify acute respiratory distress syndrome phenotypes: a secondary analysis of randomised controlled trials. Lancet Respir Med 2020;8(3):247–57.
10. Calfee CS, Delucchi K, Parsons PE, et al. Subphenotypes in acute respiratory distress syndrome: latent class analysis of data from two randomised controlled trials. Lancet Respir Med 2014;2(8):611–20.
11. Wilson JG, Calfee CS. ARDS subphenotypes: understanding a heterogeneous syndrome. Crit Care 2020;24(1):102.
12. Duggal A, Kast R, Van Ark E, et al. Identification of acute respiratory distress syndrome subphenotypes de novo using routine clinical data: a retrospective analysis of ARDS clinical trials. BMJ Open 2022;12(1):e053297.
13. Bos LDJ, Sjoding M, Sinha P, et al. Longitudinal respiratory subphenotypes in patients with COVID-19-related acute respiratory distress syndrome: results from three observational cohorts. Lancet Respir Med 2021;9(12):1377–86.
14. Ranjeva S, Pinciroli R, Hodell E, et al. Identifying clinical and biochemical phenotypes in acute respiratory distress syndrome secondary to coronavirus disease-2019. EClinicalMedicine 2021;34:100829.
15. Panwar R, Madotto F, Laffey JG, van Haren FMP. Compliance phenotypes in early acute respiratory distress syndrome before the COVID-19 pandemic. Am J Respir Crit Care Med 2020;202(9):1244–52.
16. Bos LDJ, Sinha P, Dickson RP. The perils of premature phenotyping in COVID-19: a call for caution. Eur Respir J 2020;56:2001768. https://doi.org/10.1183/13993003.01768-2020.
17. Gattinoni L, Camporota L, Marini JJ. COVID-19 phenotypes: leading or misleading?Eur Respir J 2020;56:2002195. https://doi.org/10.1183/13993003.02195-2020.
18. Rajendram R. Building the house of CARDS by phenotyping on the fly Eur Respir J 2020;56:2002429. https://doi.org/10.1183/13993003.02429-2020.
19. Zhao Z, Kung WH, Chang HT, et al. COVID-19 pneumonia: phenotype assessment requires bedside tools. Crit Care 2020;24(1):272.
20. Richardson S, Hirsch JS, Narasimhan M, et al. Presenting characteristics, comorbidities, and outcomes among 5700 patients hospitalized with COVID-19 in the New York city area. JAMA 2020;323(20):2052–9.
21. Amirfarzan H, Cereda M, Gaulton TG, et al. Use of Helmet CPAP in COVID-19 - a practical review. Pulmonology 2021;27(5):413–22.
22. Cabrini L, Landoni G, Zangrillo A. Minimise nosocomial spread of 2019-nCoV when treating acute respiratory failure. Lancet 2020;395(10225):685.
23. Winslow RL, Zhou J, Windle EF, et al. SARS-CoV-2 environmental contamination from hospitalised patients with COVID-19 receiving aerosol-generating procedures. Thorax 2022;77(3):259–67.
24. Delbove A, Foubert A, Mateos F, et al. High flow nasal cannula oxygenation in COVID-19 related acute respiratory distress syndrome: a safe way to avoid endotracheal intubation? Ther Adv Respir Dis 2021;15. 17534666211019555.
25. Coppadoro A, Benini A, Fruscio R, et al. Helmet CPAP to treat hypoxic pneumonia outside the ICU: an observational study during the COVID-19 outbreak. Crit Care 2021;25(1):80.
26. Menzella F, Barbieri C, Fontana M, et al. Effectiveness of noninvasive ventilation in COVID-19 related-acute respiratory distress syndrome. Clin Respir J 2021;15(7):779–87.
27. Covid-Icu group ftRnC-ICUi. Benefits and risks of noninvasive oxygenation strategy in COVID-19: a multicenter, prospective cohort study (COVID-ICU) in 137 hospitals. Crit Care (London, England) 2021;25(1):421.
28. Menga LS, Cese LD, Bongiovanni F, et al. High failure rate of noninvasive oxygenation strategies in

critically ill subjects with acute hypoxemic respiratory failure due to COVID-19. Respir Care 2021; 66(5):705–14.

29. Grieco DL, Menga LS, Cesarano M, et al. Effect of helmet noninvasive ventilation vs high-flow nasal oxygen on days free of respiratory support in patients with COVID-19 and moderate to severe hypoxemic respiratory failure: the HENIVOT randomized clinical trial. JAMA 2021;325(17):1731–43.

30. Perkins GD, Ji C, Connolly BA, et al. Effect of noninvasive respiratory strategies on intubation or mortality among patients with acute hypoxemic respiratory failure and COVID-19: the RECOVERY-RS randomized clinical trial. JAMA 2022;327(6): 546–58.

31. Ospina-Tascon GA, Calderon-Tapia LE, Garcia AF, et al. Effect of high-flow oxygen therapy vs conventional oxygen therapy on invasive mechanical ventilation and clinical recovery in patients with severe COVID-19: a randomized clinical trial. JAMA 2021; 326(21):2161–71.

32. El-Boghdadly K, Wong DJN, Owen R, et al. Risks to healthcare workers following tracheal intubation of patients with COVID-19: a prospective international multicentre cohort study. Anaesthesia 2020;75(11): 1437–47.

33. Parotto M, Cavallin F, Bryson GL, et al. Risks to healthcare workers following tracheal intubation of patients with known or suspected COVID-19 in Canada: data from the intubateCOVID registry. Can J Anaesth 2021;68(3):425–7.

34. Weaver L, Das A, Saffaran S, et al. High risk of patient self-inflicted lung injury in COVID-19 with frequently encountered spontaneous breathing patterns: a computational modelling study. Ann Intensive Care 2021;11(1):109.

35. Tobin MJ, Laghi F, Jubran A. Caution about early intubation and mechanical ventilation in COVID-19. Ann Intensive Care 2020;10(1):78.

36. Tobin MJ, Laghi F, Jubran A. P-SILI is not justification for intubation of COVID-19 patients. Ann Intensive Care 2020;10(1):105.

37. Bellani G, Grasselli G, Cecconi M, et al. Noninvasive ventilatory support of patients with COVID-19 outside the intensive care units (WARd-COVID). Ann Am Thorac Soc 2021;18(6):1020–6.

38. Cummings MJ, Baldwin MR, Abrams D, et al. Epidemiology, clinical course, and outcomes of critically ill adults with COVID-19 in New York City: a prospective cohort study. Lancet 2020;395(10239):1763–70.

39. Yang X, Yu Y, Xu J, et al. Clinical course and outcomes of critically ill patients with SARS-CoV-2 pneumonia in Wuhan, China: a single-centered, retrospective, observational study. Lancet Respir Med 2020;8(5):475–81.

40. Hernandez-Romieu AC, Adelman MW, Hockstein MA, et al. Timing of intubation and mortality among

critically ill coronavirus disease 2019 patients: a single-center cohort study. Crit Care Med 2020; 48(11):e1045–53.

41. Lee YH, Choi K-J, Choi SH, et al. Clinical significance of timing of intubation in critically ill patients with COVID-19: a multi-center retrospective study. J Clin Med 2020;9(9):2847. https://doi.org/10.3390/jcm9092847.

42. Matta A, Chaudhary S, Bryan Lo K, et al. Timing of intubation and its implications on outcomes in critically ill patients with coronavirus disease 2019 infection. Crit Care Explor 2020;2(10):e0262.

43. Papoutsi E, Giannakoulis VG, Xourgia E, et al. Effect of timing of intubation on clinical outcomes of critically ill patients with COVID-19: a systematic review and meta-analysis of non-randomized cohort studies. Crit Care 2021;25(1):121.

44. Fayed M, Patel N, Yeldo N, et al. Effect of intubation timing on the outcome of patients with severe respiratory distress secondary to COVID-19 pneumonia. Cureus 2021;13(11):e19620.

45. Acute Respiratory Distress Syndrome N, Brower RG, Matthay MA, et al. Ventilation with lower tidal volumes as compared with traditional tidal volumes for acute lung injury and the acute respiratory distress syndrome. N Engl J Med 2000;342(18): 1301–8.

46. Serpa Neto A, Cardoso SO, Manetta JA, et al. Association between use of lung-protective ventilation with lower tidal volumes and clinical outcomes among patients without acute respiratory distress syndrome: a meta-analysis. JAMA 2012;308(16): 1651–9.

47. Grasselli G, Cattaneo E, Florio G, et al. Mechanical ventilation parameters in critically ill COVID-19 patients: a scoping review. Crit Care 2021;25(1):115.

48. Ferreira JC, Ho YL, Besen B, et al. Protective ventilation and outcomes of critically ill patients with COVID-19: a cohort study. Ann Intensive Care 2021;11(1):92.

49. World Health Organization (WHO). Clinical management of COVID-19 patients: living guideline, 23 November 2021. Available at: https://app.magicapp.org/#/guideline/j1WBYn. Accessed 23 Apr, 2022.

50. Alhazzani W, Evans L, Alshamsi F, et al. Surviving Sepsis Campaign guidelines on the management of adults with coronavirus disease 2019 (COVID-19) in the ICU: first update. Crit Care Med 2021; 49(3):e219–34.

51. National COVID-19 clinical evidence Taskforce. Caring for people with COVID-19. Available at: https://covid19evidence.net.au/#living-guidelines. Accessed 28 03, 2022.

52. Griffiths M, Meade S, Summers C, et al. RAND appropriateness panel to determine the applicability of UK guidelines on the management of acute

respiratory distress syndrome (ARDS) and other strategies in the context of the COVID-19 pandemic. Thorax 2022;77(2):129–35.

53. Botta M, Tsonas AM, Pillay J, et al. Ventilation management and clinical outcomes in invasively ventilated patients with COVID-19 (PRoVENT-COVID): a national, multicentre, observational cohort study. Lancet Respir Med 2021;9(2):139–48.

54. Guerin C, Reignier J, Richard JC, et al. Prone positioning in severe acute respiratory distress syndrome. N Engl J Med 2013;368(23):2159–68.

55. Munshi L, Del Sorbo L, Adhikari NKJ, et al. Prone Position for acute respiratory distress syndrome. A systematic review and meta-analysis. Ann Am Thorac Soc 2017;14(Supplement_4):S280–8.

56. Park SY, Kim HJ, Yoo KH, et al. The efficacy and safety of prone positioning in adults patients with acute respiratory distress syndrome: a meta-analysis of randomized controlled trials. J Thorac Dis 2015;7(3):356–67.

57. Scholten EL, Beitler JR, Prisk GK, et al. Treatment of ARDS with prone positioning. Chest 2017;151(1):215–24.

58. Albert RK, Keniston A, Baboi L, et al. Prone position-induced improvement in gas exchange does not predict improved survival in the acute respiratory distress syndrome. Am J Respir Crit Care Med 2014;189(4):494–6.

59. Pan C, Chen L, Lu C, et al. Lung recruitability in COVID-19-associated acute respiratory distress syndrome: a single-center observational study. Am J Respir Crit Care Med 2020;201(10):1294–7.

60. Weiss TT, Cerda F, Scott JB, et al. Prone positioning for patients intubated for severe acute respiratory distress syndrome (ARDS) secondary to COVID-19: a retrospective observational cohort study. Br J Anaesth 2021;126(1):48–55.

61. Langer T, Brioni M, Guzzardella A, et al. Prone position in intubated, mechanically ventilated patients with COVID-19: a multi-centric study of more than 1000 patients. Crit Care 2021;25(1):128.

62. Ziehr DR, Alladina J, Wolf ME, et al. Respiratory Physiology of Prone Positioning With and Without Inhaled Nitric Oxide Across the Coronavirus Disease 2019 Acute Respiratory Distress Syndrome Severity Spectrum. Crit Care Explor 2021;3(6):e0471.

63. Mathews KS, Soh H, Shaefi S, et al. Prone Positioning and Survival in Mechanically Ventilated Patients With Coronavirus Disease 2019-Related Respiratory Failure. Crit Care Med 2021;49(7):1026–37.

64. Shelhamer MC, Wesson PD, Solari IL, et al. Prone positioning in moderate to severe acute respiratory distress syndrome due to COVID-19: a cohort study and analysis of physiology. J Intensive Care Med 2021;36(2):241–52.

65. Behesht Aeen F, Pakzad R, Goudarzi Rad M, et al. Effect of prone position on respiratory parameters, intubation and death rate in COVID-19 patients: systematic review and meta-analysis. Sci Rep 2021;11(1):14407.

66. Kimmoun A, Levy B, Chenuel B, et al. Usefulness and safety of a dedicated team to prone patients with severe ARDS due to COVID-19. Crit Care 2020;24(1):509.

67. Miguel K, Snydeman C, Capasso V, et al. Development of a prone team and exploration of staff perceptions during COVID-19. AACN Adv Crit Care 2021;32(2):159–68.

68. O'Donoghue SC, Church M, Russell K, et al. Development, implementation, and impact of a proning team during the COVID-19 intensive care unit surge. Dimens Crit Care Nurs 2021;40(6):321–7.

69. Ding L, Wang L, Ma W, et al. Efficacy and safety of early prone positioning combined with HFNC or NIV in moderate to severe ARDS: a multi-center prospective cohort study. Crit Care 2020;24(1):28.

70. Li J, Luo J, Pavlov I, et al. Awake prone positioning for non-intubated patients with COVID-19-related acute hypoxaemic respiratory failure: a systematic review and meta-analysis. Lancet Respir Med 2022;10(6):573–83.

71. Coppo A, Bellani G, Winterton D, et al. Feasibility and physiological effects of prone positioning in non-intubated patients with acute respiratory failure due to COVID-19 (PRON-COVID): a prospective cohort study. Lancet Respir Med 2020;8(8):765–74.

72. Ehrmann S, Li J, Ibarra-Estrada M, et al. Awake prone positioning for COVID-19 acute hypoxaemic respiratory failure: a randomised, controlled, multinational, open-label meta-trial. Lancet Respir Med 2021;9(12):1387–95.

73. Fralick M, Colacci M, Munshi L, et al. Prone positioning of patients with moderate hypoxaemia due to covid-19: multicentre pragmatic randomised trial (COVID-PRONE). BMJ 2022;376:e068585.

74. Li J, Luo J, Pavlov I, et al. Awake prone positioning for non-intubated patients with COVID-19-related acute hypoxaemic respiratory failure: a systematic review and meta-analysis. Lancet Respir Med 2022.

75. Bier-Laning C, Cramer JD, Roy S, et al. Tracheostomy during the COVID-19 pandemic: comparison of international perioperative care protocols and practices in 26 countries. Otolaryngol Head Neck Surg 2021;164(6):1136–47.

76. Kapp CM, Latifi A, Feller-Kopman D, et al. Sedation and analgesia in patients undergoing tracheostomy in COVID-19, a multi-center registry. J Intensive Care Med 2022;37(2):240–7.

77. Gattinoni L, Caironi P, Cressoni M, et al. Lung recruitment in patients with the acute respiratory distress syndrome. N Engl J Med 2006;354(17):1775–86.

78. Chen L, Del Sorbo L, Grieco DL, et al. Potential for lung recruitment estimated by the recruitment-to-inflation ratio in acute respiratory distress syndrome. A clinical trial. Am J Respir Crit Care Med 2020; 201(2):178–87.

79. Published recruitement to inflation ratio. Available at: https://crec.coemv.ca/. Accessed August 28, 2022.

80. Mauri T, Spinelli E, Scotti E, et al. Potential for lung recruitment and ventilation-perfusion mismatch in patients with the acute respiratory distress syndrome from coronavirus disease 2019. Crit Care Med 2020;48(8):1129–34.

81. Zerbib Y, Lambour A, Maizel J, et al. Respiratory effects of lung recruitment maneuvers depend on the recruitment-to-inflation ratio in patients with COVID-19-related acute respiratory distress syndrome.

82. COVID-19 treatment guidelines panel. Coronavirus disease 2019 (COVID-19) treatment guidelines. National institute of health. Available at: https://www.covid19treatmentguidelines.nih.gov/. Accessed 28 03, 2022.

83. Ibarra-Estrada MA, Garcia-Salas Y, Mireles-Cabodevila E, et al. Use of airway pressure release ventilation in patients with acute respiratory failure due to COVID-19: results of a single-center randomized controlled trial. Crit Care Med 2022;50(4): 586–94.

84. Adhikari NK, Dellinger RP, Lundin S, et al. Inhaled nitric oxide does not reduce mortality in patients with acute respiratory distress syndrome regardless of severity: systematic review and meta-analysis. Crit Care Med 2014;42(2):404–12.

85. Bonizzoli M, Lazzeri C, Cianchi G, et al. Effects of rescue inhaled nitric oxide on right ventricle and pulmonary circulation in severe COVID-related acute respiratory distress syndrome. J Crit Care 2022;153987.

86. Chiles JW 3rd, Vijaykumar K, Darby A, et al. Use of inhaled epoprostenol with high flow nasal oxygen in non-intubated patients with severe COVID-19. J Crit Care 2022;69:153989.

87. Lubinsky AS, Brosnahan SB, Lehr A, et al. Inhaled pulmonary vasodilators are not associated with improved gas exchange in mechanically ventilated patients with COVID-19: a retrospective cohort study. J Crit Care 2022;69:153990.

88. Sonti R, Pike CW, Cobb N. Responsiveness of inhaled epoprostenol in respiratory failure due to COVID-19. J Intensive Care Med 2021;36(3): 327–33.

89. Wunsch H. The outbreak that invented intensive care, Nature, 2020. Available at: https://www.nature.com/articles/d41586-020-01019-y. Accessed April 03, 2020.

90. Branson RD, Rodriquez D Jr. 2020 Year in review: shared ventilation for COVID-19. Respir Care 2021; 66(7):1173–83.

91. Beitler JR, Mittel AM, Kallet R, et al. Ventilator sharing during an acute shortage caused by the COVID-19 pandemic. Am J Respir Crit Care Med 2020;202(4):600–4.

92. Gouel-Cheron A, Couffignal C, Elmaleh Y, et al. Preliminary observations of anaesthesia ventilators use for prolonged mechanical ventilation in intensive care unit patients during the COVID-19 pandemic. Anaesth Crit Care Pain Med 2020;39(3):371–2.

The Use of Extracorporeal Membrane Oxygenation for COVID-19: Lessons Learned

Madhavi Parekh, MD[a],*, Darryl Abrams, MD[a], Cara Agerstrand, MD[a],
Jenelle Badulak, MD[b], Amy Dzierba, PharmD[c], Peta M.A. Alexander, MBBS[d,e],
Susanna Price, MBBS[f,g], Eddy Fan, MD, PhD[h], Dana Mullin, MS, CCP, LP[i],
Rodrigo Diaz, MD[j], Carol Hodgson, PhD[k,l,1], Daniel Brodie, MD[a,1]

KEYWORDS

- ECMO • Acute respiratory distress syndrome • ARDS • COVID-19 • Respiratory failure

KEY POINTS

- The coronavirus disease 2019 (COVID-19) pandemic has posed challenges on multiple levels in the implementation of extracorporeal membrane oxygenation (ECMO) support for patients with severe acute respiratory distress syndrome around the world.
- Real-time data gathering and new approaches to research have helped evaluate the utility of ECMO during an ongoing pandemic.
- Regional, national, and international coordination has been crucial in knowledge sharing, research collaboration, and development of guidelines.

INTRODUCTION

The use of extracorporeal membrane oxygenation (ECMO) in the management of severe acute respiratory distress syndrome (ARDS) has been well established in recent years[1–4] but the ongoing coronavirus disease 2019 (COVID-19) pandemic has presented new limitations in knowledge and has complicated the implementation of ECMO. Severe COVID-19 frequently presents with acute respiratory failure in the form of ARDS, and the pandemic has been characterized by surges in the volume of critically ill patients with ARDS worldwide.

Episodic surges in patients with COVID-19-related ARDS have been accompanied by strain both on health-care resources (eg, beds, staffing, medical supplies) and in the ability to provide

[a] Division of Pulmonary, Allergy, and Critical Care Medicine, Department of Medicine, Columbia University Vagelos College of Physicians and Surgeons, 622 West 168th Street, PH8-101, New York, NY 10023, USA; [b] Department of Emergency Medicine, Division of Pulmonary, Critical Care and Sleep Medicine, University of Washington, 4408 S Holly Street, Seattle, WA 98118, USA; [c] Department of Pharmacy, NewYork-Presbyterian Hospital, 622 West 168th Street, VC Basement (pharmacy), New York, NY 10032, USA; [d] Department of Cardiology, Boston Children's Hospital, 300 Longwood Avenue, Boston, MA 02115, USA; [e] Department of Pediatrics, Harvard Medical School, Boston, MA, USA; [f] Royal Brompton & Harefield Hospitals, Guys and St Thomas's NHS Foundation Trust, Sydney Street, London, SW3 6NP, UK; [g] National Heart and Lung Institute, Imperial College, London, UK; [h] Interdepartmental Division of Critical Care Medicine, University of Toronto, Toronto General Hospital, 585 University Avenue, 9-MaRS-9013, Toronto, Ontario, M5G 2N2, Canada; [i] Department of Clinical Perfusion and Anesthesia Support Services, NewYork-Presbyterian Hospital, New York, NY, USA; [j] Clinica Las Condes, Clinica Red Salud Santiago CCHC, Camino El Cajon 18274, casa 5, Lo Barnechea, Santiago, 7710260, Chile; [k] Department of Epidemiology and Preventive Medicine, Australian and New Zealand Intensive Care-Research Centre, Monash University, 3/553 Street Kilda Road, Melbourne 3004, Australia; [l] Department of Intensive Care, Alfred Health, Melbourne, Australia
[1] Cosenior authors.
* Corresponding author. 622 West 168th Street, PH8-101, New York, NY 10023.
E-mail address: mp2654@cumc.columbia.edu

Clin Chest Med 44 (2023) 335–346
https://doi.org/10.1016/j.ccm.2022.11.016

equitable access to care, all of which is further exaggerated when considering the application of ECMO, a highly resource-intensive and specialized technology.

As the pandemic has evolved, the medical community has learned not only about the role of ECMO for COVID-19 from a clinical standpoint but also about how to gather knowledge in real-time about the use of ECMO for a novel disease, the limitations in our ability to equitably deliver health-care resources across the globe, and how to devise best strategies for care in light of substantial resource constraints. The use of ECMO for cardiac or circulatory failure, including for extracorporeal cardiopulmonary resuscitation, has been relatively limited in the setting of COVID-19; we will focus on the use of ECMO for respiratory failure.

Early Experience

Registry data and large cohort studies from early in the pandemic suggested patients managed with ECMO for COVID-19-related ARDS had a mortality rate comparable to similar patients with ARDS before COVID-19 (**Table 1**); mortality rates of 31% at 60 days in a large single-center experience from Paris, France,[5] 33.2% at 60 days in a cohort study across 60 hospitals in the United States,[6] and an estimated 37.4% in-hospital mortality at 90 days from the Extracorporeal Life Support Organization (ELSO) Registry, including 213 hospitals across 36 countries.[7] A meta-analysis of studies spanning December 1, 2019, through January 10, 2021, tallying 1896 patients, reported an in-hospital mortality rate of 37.1%[8]; these analyses were heavily weighted by the aforementioned large cohort studies.

Evolving Mortality Over Time

Despite encouraging data early on, additional data gathered as the pandemic continued suggested increasing mortality and duration of ECMO over time. An analysis of a survey from the European chapter of ELSO found a mortality of 56% for patients with COVID-19 managed with ECMO between September 15, 2020, and March 8, 2021, as compared with 47% before that time period.[9] Similarly, data from 24 centers in Spain and Portugal suggested a higher in-hospital mortality after June 30, 2020 (60.1%) than before that date (41.1%).[10] The Paris-Sorbonne University Hospital Network found a 90-day mortality of 48% in patients after July 1, 2020, as compared with 36% before July (HR 2.27, 95% CI 1.02–5.07).[11] Further analysis of the ELSO registry database, encompassing 4812 patients, also noted a higher 90-day in-hospital mortality for patients after May 1, 2020, as compared with earlier (51.9% vs 36.9%, RR 0.82, 95% CI 0.7–0.96), with a longer duration of ECMO support in the latter cohort (20 vs 14 days).[12] Data published from Germany demonstrated a high in-hospital mortality (68%) for all patients supported with ECMO (n = 3,397) for COVID-19-related ARDS from the start of the pandemic through May 31, 2021, despite a lack of resource constraints.[13] An updated meta-analysis of 52 studies (18,211 patients) reporting data between December 1, 2019, to January 26, 2022, revealed a pooled mortality rate of 48.8% (95% CI 44.8–52.9%) among patients with COVID-19 receiving ECMO, with increasing mortality in the second half of 2020 (46.4%) compared with the first half (41.2%), and an even higher mortality (62%) in the first half of 2021. Predictors of increased mortality included age, later time of

Table 1
Early experience of extracorporeal membrane oxygenation for coronavirus disease 2019–related acute respiratory distress syndrome

Data Source	Timeframe	Number of Patients	Mortality
Single-center observational experience from Paris, France[5]	Patients admitted between March 8 and May 2, 2020	83	31% at 60 d
Cohort study across 60 hospitals in the United States[6]	Patients admitted between March 1 and July 1, 2020	190	33.2% at 60-d
ELSO registry, including 213 hospitals across 36 countries[7]	Patients in whom ECMO was initiated between Jan 16 and May 1, 2020	1035	37.4% in-hospital mortality at 90-d
Meta-analysis of 22 studies[8]	December 1, 2019, through January 10, 2021	1896	37.1% in-hospital mortality

enrollment, higher proportion of patients receiving corticosteroids, and reduced duration of ECMO run.[14]

Several potential reasons for increasing mortality over time have been speculated, including greater selection over time for treatment-refractory disease (those who did not respond to COVID-19-directed therapies that were increasingly used during the course of the pandemic, eg, corticosteroid therapy),[9–12] increased use of noninvasive ventilatory support before intubation, and ECMO (which may contribute to preendotracheal intubation self-inflicted lung injury),[10–12] an increase in superimposed bacterial pneumonia in the setting of immunosuppressive treatments for COVID-19,[10,15,16] emergence of SARS-CoV-2 variants with differential effects on prognosis, increased use of ECMO by less experienced centers,[10,12] and variations in patient selection criteria for ECMO.[10]

Although the mortality of patients managed with ECMO may have increased during the course of the pandemic, ECMO may still benefit selected patients with severe COVID-19-related ARDS.[17–19] A multicenter international emulation trial, which applies principles of randomized controlled trials (RCTs) to the analysis of observational data, including 7345 patients between January 3, 2020, and August 29, 2021, found a reduction in 60-day in-hospital mortality with a risk ratio of 0.78 (95% CI 0.75–0.82). Adherence adjusted mortality, which accounts for adherence to the treatment assignment, was 26% for patients managed with ECMO as compared with conventional treatment (33.2%). Secondary analyses suggested ECMO was most effective in patients aged younger than 65 years, those with a Pao_2 to Fio_2 ratio of less than 80 mm Hg, a driving pressure greater than 15 cmH_2O, or during the first 10 days of mechanical ventilation. Although this was not a traditional RCT, the emulation design allowed for a more rigorous analysis of real-world effectiveness of ECMO than a traditional observational study.[17] Additionally, a study conducted in the United Kingdom demonstrated an absolute mortality reduction of 18.2% (44% vs 25.8%; OR 0.44; 95% CI 0.29–0.68, $P < .001$) for those receiving ECMO compared with matched controls.[18] These data should be interpreted cautiously, as residual confounding may have accounted for some of the benefit, especially as those receiving ECMO were managed at highly specialized centers, whereas those not offered ECMO remained in their original facilities for ongoing care.

The true efficacy of ECMO for severe COVID-19-related ARDS remains uncertain in the absence of high-quality RCTs. The fact that RCTs could not be implemented despite thousands of ECMO cases highlights the challenges faced in conducting research, especially RCTs, during a constantly changing pandemic with substantial limitations in infrastructure and resources, including staffing and time.[20] Ongoing evaluation of emerging data will be necessary to help determine optimal patient selection and management strategies; until then, use of conventional inclusion and exclusion criteria based on pre-COVID-19 ECMO data,[1,21] modified by factors identified in large registry analyses to be predictive of outcomes, seems to be a reasonable approach.[1,22]

CLINICAL CARE
Patient Selection

Criteria for ECMO initiation in patients with COVID-19-related ARDS remain the same as those recommended before the pandemic,[21–25] and fall within the standard approach to ARDS algorithm (**Fig. 1**), because there is no good evidence to support deviation from these preestablished guidelines when resources are available. Outcomes with delayed initiation may in fact be worse and can lead to longer duration of ECMO support, which may in turn offset the benefit of an attempt of conservation of resources. However, resource constraints during the pandemic have overwhelmed the ability to provide ECMO at varying times in different regions of the world. As such, selection criteria may need to be more flexible and potentially stringent at any given time, depending on available resources and coordination locally. Criteria may need to evolve as well, as increasing knowledge arises regarding prognostic factors.[26]

Cannulation and Transport

Conventional cannulation strategies are generally recommended for patients undergoing ECMO initiation for severe COVID-19-related ARDS because there is a paucity of data to support alternative strategies.[22] These include two-site or single-site, dual-lumen venovenous (V-V) cannulation, with additional arterial support depending on whether there is concomitant cardiogenic shock.[23] Some centers have used a veno-pulmonary artery configuration through a single dual-lumen catheter inserted through the internal jugular or subclavian vein in an attempt to provide right ventricular protection[27] because some reports suggest a higher incidence of right ventricular dysfunction in patients with COVID-19-related ARDS[28] but more data is needed to support this strategy either with a dual-lumen cannula or with dual-site cannulation with 2 separate cannulae. Mobile ECMO or

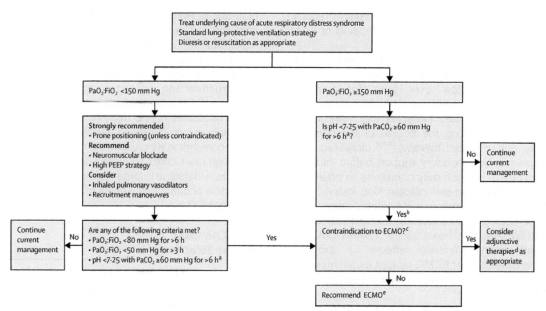

Fig. 1. Algorithm flowsheet for the management of ARDS including indications for ECMO. PEEP, positive end-expiratory pressure. Pao$_2$:Fio$_2$, ratio of partial pressure of oxygen in arterial blood to the fractional concentration of oxygen in inspired air. ECMO = extracorporeal membrane oxygenation. Paco$_2$, partial pressure of carbon dioxide in arterial blood. [a]With respiratory rate increased to 35 breaths per minute and mechanical ventilation settings adjusted to keep a plateau airway pressure of 32 cm or less of water. [b]Consider neuromuscular blockade. [c]There are no absolute contraindications that are agreed on except end-stage respiratory failure when lung transplantation will not be considered; exclusion criteria used in the extracorporeal membrane oxygenation for severe acute respiratory distress syndrome (EOLIA)EOLIA trial[1] can be taken as a conservative approach to contraindications to ECMO. [d]For example, neuromuscular blockade, high PEEP strategy, inhaled pulmonary vasodilators, recruitment maneuvers, high-frequency oscillatory ventilation. [e]Recommend early ECMO as per EOLIA trial criteria; salvage ECMO, which involves deferral of ECMO initiation until further decompensation (as in the crossovers to ECMO in the EOLIA control group), is not supported by the evidence but might be preferable to not initiating ECMO at all in such patients. (*Reprinted* with permission from Elsevier. The Lancet, February 2019, 7 (2), 108-110.)

ECMO transport with cannulation at the originating hospital and transfer to another institution seems to be safe from a health-care exposure standpoint when accompanied by protocols incorporating adequate protective measures.[29,30] However, it is important to note that the coordination and feasibility of ECMO transport varies across regions and, consequently, rates of transport do as well. This may be due in part to differences in practice, training, certification, and regulation.

Ongoing care while receiving extracorporeal membrane oxygenation

Management strategies of patients requiring ECMO support for COVID-19-related ARDS remain similar to those recommended before the pandemic (see **Fig. 1**) but specific factors should be considered (**Fig. 2**).[23,31] From a safety and feasibility standpoint, several procedures and techniques have been successfully performed during the course of the pandemic. Endotracheal extubation while awake during ECMO has been

performed, although data are very limited[27]; in contrast, awake ECMO without intubation in highly selected patients has been associated with potentially worse outcomes in one small cohort.[32] Prone

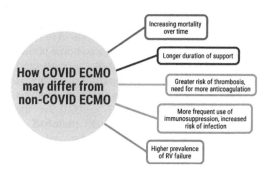

Fig. 2. Specific considerations for ECMO for COVID-19-related ARDS that may differ from ECMO for non-COVID-19 ARDS. RV, right ventricular. (*From* Brodie D, Abrams D, MacLaren G, et al. Extracorporeal Membrane Oxygenation during Respiratory Pandemics: Past, Present, and Future. Am J Respir Crit Care Med. 2022;205(12):1382-1390.)

positioning[5,33,34] and early mobilization[27] seem feasible in patients with COVID-19 requiring ECMO support; however, data remain too limited to support specific recommendations. Percutaneous tracheostomy seems to be safe in patients with COVID-19.[35] From an infection control standpoint, there is no evidence to suggest virions can be expelled through an ECMO circuit.[36] Cytokine removal devices, which use an absorber to remove excess cytokines from whole blood, have been proposed as adjunctive therapies in patients receiving ECMO for COVID-19-related ARDS. However, clinicians should proceed cautiously and consider only using cytokine-removal devices in such patients in the setting of research, given that recent evidence suggests possible harm.[37]

COVID-19 has been associated with coagulopathy, including an increase in risk of both significant thrombosis and bleeding.[38,39] Hematological complications—including circuit clotting,[40,41] pulmonary embolism,[5] and intracranial hemorrhage[42–45]—have been reported as occurring more frequently in patients with COVID-19 supported with ECMO than in non-COVID ECMO cases but when normalized to ECMO run duration, such complication rates seem similar to historical data.[12] In the setting of observational data, the similar normalized rates must be interpreted with caution. Multiple centers have adjusted their anticoagulation thresholds but there are insufficient data to support anticoagulation strategies and monitoring other than usual practices.[46] Additionally, there is no evidence to suggest different blood transfusion thresholds for patients with COVID-19 during ECMO support.[47]

Extracorporeal Membrane Oxygenation as a Bridge to Lung Transplantation

COVID-19-related ARDS has often demonstrated a more prolonged recovery process than what is typically seen for ARDS of other causes, and the duration of ECMO support for patients with severe disease has increased as the pandemic has evolved.[12] Lung transplantation may be considered in select patients who have persistent severe respiratory failure—assuming otherwise appropriate candidacy with preserved extrapulmonary organ function—and may be particularly relevant for those who are unable to wean from ECMO, with initial reports demonstrating posttransplant outcomes comparable to those with non-COVID end-stage lung disease.[48,49] However, determination of the potential for recovery of native lung function and optimal timing of transplantation remain areas of uncertainty that warrant further investigation.[50,51]

SURGE CAPACITY AND EXTRACORPOREAL MEMBRANE OXYGENATION
Crisis Standards of Care

During the pandemic, surges in case volume often led to the implementation of contingency or crisis standards of care, requiring triage of critical care resources, including intensive care unit beds, medical supplies, and staffing. At the same time, there was an increased demand for ECMO—a highly resource-intensive intervention with potential for prolonged use of critical care services[52]—due to the high incidence of severe, refractory ARDS among patients with COVID-19. Many institutions, in an effort to provide medical care to the greatest number of patients, became more stringent with patient selection for ECMO—or abandoned the use of ECMO altogether.[53–56] For those centers that continued to perform ECMO despite resource constraints, nontraditional staffing models were helpful in maintaining operations.[57] In settings of reduced ECMO capacity, it may be necessary to apply more stringent exclusion criteria based on patient characteristics associated with increased mortality and longer ECMO run duration (**Fig. 3**).[22] Predesigned triage systems may be useful in standardizing which patients should receive ECMO at varying levels of capacity and may also help achieve equitable access to ECMO by establishing allocation policies that avoid discrimination based on age, race, ethnicity, disability, or socioeconomic status.[55]

Regional and National Coordination

During the course of the pandemic, the coordination of ECMO programs at regional and national levels was leveraged to more effectively standardize ECMO candidacy and allocate resources. In Paris, a regional network coordinated care of 17 hospitals to pool resources, systematize ECMO candidacy evaluations, and expanded mobile ECMO capacity in an effort to improve resource utilization, streamline workflow for clinicians, optimize management of patients before ECMO initiation, and facilitate data collection.[58,59] Chile used a National Advisory Commission to help coordinate ECMO referrals, provide consistent patient selection, optimize capacity, and distribute educational materials.[60] The United Kingdom modified a preexisting national system to balance ECMO cases among centers in order to help manage capacity.[61] The creation or utilization of existing regional or national ECMO networks has been encouraged by the ELSO, which has an "ECMO Availability Map" to help guide such coordination efforts.[22,62] The purported effectiveness of these examples also

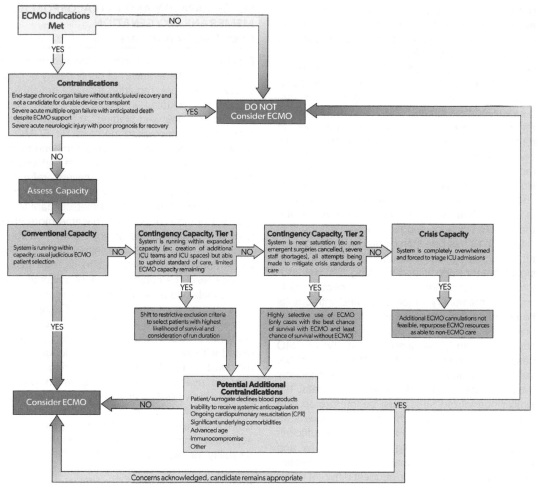

Fig. 3. Patient selection and contingency flowsheet for ECMO during a pandemic. Contraindications algorithm for V-A and V-V ECMO use (COVID-19 and non-COVID-19) during a pandemic based on system capacity. [a]The impact of duration on high-flow nasal cannula and/or noninvasive mechanical ventilation in addition to invasive mechanical ventilation is unknown. COVID-19, coronavirus disease 2019; CPR, cardiopulmonary resuscitation; ECMO, extracorporeal membrane oxygenation; ICU, intensive care unit; Paco$_2$, partial pressure of carbon dioxide in arterial blood; Pao$_2$:Fio$_2$, ratio of partial pressure of oxygen in arterial blood to the fractional concentration of oxygen in inspired air; PEEP, positive end-expiratory pressure; V-A, venoarterial; V-V, venovenous. (*From* Badulak J, Antonini MV, Stead CM, et al. Extracorporeal Membrane Oxygenation for COVID-19: Updated 2021 Guidelines from the Extracorporeal Life Support Organization. ASAIO J. 2021;67(5):485-495.)

provides a rationale for establishing new networks where none currently exists. However, the ability to coordinate ECMO across a region will depend, in large part, on the established health-care systems in that area.

DEVELOPMENT OF NEW EXTRACORPOREAL MEMBRANE OXYGENATION CENTERS

Initial guidance early in the pandemic recommended against the development of new ECMO centers,[24,63] given the concerns during the implementation of a resource-heavy intervention in inexperienced centers that may be dealing with simultaneous surge capacity issues. Retrospective

data from new ECMO centers developed in the Middle East and India—under the guidance of established centers—did report acceptable survival in these new programs overall compared with established ECMO centers (55% vs 45%, OR 1.65; 95% CI 0.75–3.67), although, as the authors note, patient selection likely differed between the centers with selection bias favoring the new centers. In light of this relative success, and recognizing the potential need for ECMO in regions that otherwise would not have access to ECMO, ELSO has updated its guidance to recommend that establishment of new ECMO centers may be considered in select cases where regional resources exist to support these programs, there is sufficiently high demand, and there is close collaboration with experienced centers to optimize outcomes.[22]

EVALUATING EFFECTIVENESS OF EXTRACORPOREAL MEMBRANE OXYGENATION IN AN ONGOING PANDEMIC
Surveillance and Study Design Approaches

Early data during a pandemic of a novel disease must be interpreted with caution given the potential for misleading data due to study designs and population characteristics. Determining the effectiveness of ECMO during an evolving pandemic requires ongoing surveillance as well as design and implementation of studies that have the ability to assess both short-term and long-term outcomes, and especially patient-centered outcomes.[64] National and international registries are useful in centralizing data and may serve as platforms for analysis and dissemination of information.[31] As the course of a pandemic takes shape and data begins to accumulate, especially results from clinical trials, the community must learn to pivot toward practices that are more evidence-based.

Although traditional RCTs are considered the "gold standard" for providing credible, unbiased evidence for the efficacy of an intervention, they can be difficult to organize and perform in real-time during a rapidly evolving pandemic, especially with a resource-intensive therapy such as ECMO, substantial limitations in staffing and funding to conduct such trials, and a perceived lack of clinical equipoise for randomization. Several different study designs have been used during the COVID-19 pandemic in an effort to approximate an RCT using observational data (**Table 2**), including emulation trials,[6,17] registry RCTs, and matched-pair analyses.[18] Adaptive platform trials and weighted lottery systems can also provide a more rapid assessment of ECMO efficacy, the latter of which can provide potentially large sample sizes and a more equitable approach to resource allocation.[65] Given that temporal changes during the pandemic—including emergence of viral variants and evolution of management strategies—are likely to impact ECMO efficacy and effectiveness, more adaptive and flexible study designs are likely to have the greatest success in providing high-quality evidence in a timely fashion.[20]

Communication and Collaboration

Through the course of the pandemic, regional, national, and international coordination has been crucial in knowledge sharing, research collaboration, and development of guidelines. Remote learning and communication became a key component of health-care provider education

---

Table 2
Study designs in a pandemic, pros and cons

Study Design	Pros	Cons
RCT	• Gold standard design • Minimizes bias and confounding • Best at determining efficacy	• Time consuming and expensive making it difficult to perform in real time during a pandemic • Would need clinical equipoise
Emulation of target trial or RCT	• Can simulate RCT with preexisting observational data • Less time consuming and expensive • No ethical concerns	• May still have residual bias and confounding
Registry RCT	• RCT that is less time consuming and expensive • No ethical concerns	• Registries may lack necessary clinical information
Matched-pair analyses	• Allows for evaluation of treatment effect in an observational design	• May still have residual bias and confounding
Adaptive platform trial	• Allows evaluation of multiple interventions that can be added or dropped during the study • Is useful when mechanism of disease is not well understood • Requires fewer patients	• Requires multiple points of interim analysis

throughout the pandemic. Educational webinars and conferences by ELSO and other ECMO networks have been used to disseminate new data to both experienced and new ECMO centers and practitioners.[22]

Pediatric Access to Extracorporeal Membrane Oxygenation During the Pandemic

Children were generally less susceptible to severe illness associated with COVID-19 infection, although a new postviral pathologic process, multisystem inflammatory syndrome in children, was identified during the pandemic.[66–68] Access to ECMO for children with non-COVID-19 critical illness, congenital anomalies and emergent perioperative indications, in addition to the infrequent pediatric patients who were critically ill with COVID-19, was preserved in many regions and recommended in guidelines.[22,69–73] In addition, many established pediatric ECMO centers expanded their admission criteria to facilitate the care of adult patients with COVID-19 who required ECMO and offload regional centers at capacity.[69,70,74] Although there are many examples of successful shared resource allocation protocols, particular care was required to address the unique challenges of assessing mortality risk in the neonatal and pediatric populations. The COVID-19 pandemic highlighted that at times of critical care shortages, protocols that ensure equity across the life span should be used.[72,75]

Health-Care Providers and Extracorporeal Membrane Oxygenation

The COVID-19 pandemic has affected health-care workers in a multitude of ways, notably through occupational stress and provider burnout.[76,77] Surge situations and crisis standards of care have only amplified the pressure placed on health-care providers through unfavorable changes in staffing models and increases in provider responsibilities, ethical dilemmas, and patient mortality, among others. Contingency and crisis standards for ECMO implementation during the COVID-19 pandemic have added to provider stress through a potentially heavy ethical burden of rationing care, potentially resulting in an inability, during surge conditions, to provide ECMO to those who meet standard criteria for initiation and would otherwise have received ECMO under less strained conditions. Prolonged ECMO run times and longer than usual time-to-recovery for these patients with ARDS[12] can also contribute to health-care provider burnout. Triage committees have been proposed to relieve bedside providers of these burdens by objectively and independently setting standards and developing guidelines for rationing decisions. However, operationalizing a triage committee amid a crisis is a complex and fraught undertaking that requires direct input from community leaders in order to address ethical and legal issues, along with the need for equity. The major function of an oversight committee under crisis conditions may simply be to offload the overburdened clinicians on the front lines.[54]

SUMMARY

The COVID-19 pandemic has led to a marked increase in cases of ARDS globally, leading to a concomitant increase in demand for ECMO support. The utilization of ECMO during the pandemic has been complicated by numerous factors, including limited knowledge of ECMO-related outcomes, challenges in performing real-time, high-quality research in an ongoing evolving pandemic, difficulties in patient selection during episodic severe capacity restraints, the ethical dilemmas of rationing care, and excess strain not only on health-care systems but on providers as well. As the pandemic eventually recedes and resources become more readily and consistently available to provide ECMO, both coordinated research and tailoring of guidelines will be necessary to understand the role of ECMO, provide the best care possible to patients with severe COVID-19-related ARDS, and to anticipate needs for future potential pandemics.

CLINICS CARE POINTS

- The COVID-19 pandemic has led to an increase in severe ARDS cases globally, increasing the demand for ECMO.
- Outcomes of patients with COVID-19 managed with ECMO have evolved during the pandemic, with early data suggesting mortality rates similar to those with non-COVID-19 causes of ARDS but later data suggesting increasing mortality and longer ECMO duration of support over time.
- Eligibility criteria, cannulation, and management strategies for patients with severe ARDS requiring ECMO thus far remain largely the same for patients with COVID-19.
- Episodic surge capacity requirements have often led to crisis standards of care, which may include the rationing or tailoring of eligibility criteria of ECMO, particularly with respect to more stringent exclusion criteria.
- Regional, national, and international collaboration will continue to help inform ECMO

- providers, disseminate new information and aid in resource allocation.
- Ongoing surveillance data and new research techniques will continue to inform the role of ECMO in the management of COVID-19-related ARDS.

DISCLOSURE

D. Brodie receives research support from and consults for LivaNova. He has been on the medical advisory boards for Abiomed, Xenios, Medtronic, Inspira, and Cellenkos. He is the President-elect of the ELSO and the Chair of the Executive Committee of the International ECMO Network. P.M.A. Alexander reported receiving grant funding from the National Institute of Child Health and Human Development, National Institutes of Health, Pediatric ECMO Anticoagulation Collaborative, outside the submitted work and serving on the Board of the Extracorporeal Life Support Organization as Treasurer.

REFERENCES

1. Combes A, Hajage D, Capellier G, et al. Extracorporeal membrane oxygenation for severe acute respiratory distress syndrome. N Engl J Med 2018; 378(21):1965–75.
2. Goligher EC, Tomlinson G, Hajage D, et al. Extracorporeal membrane oxygenation for severe acute respiratory distress syndrome and posterior probability of mortality benefit in a post hoc bayesian analysis of a randomized clinical trial. JAMA 2018;320(21): 2251–9.
3. Munshi L, Walkey A, Goligher E, et al. Venovenous extracorporeal membrane oxygenation for acute respiratory distress syndrome: a systematic review and meta-analysis. Lancet Respir Med 2019;7(2): 163–72.
4. Combes A, Peek GJ, Hajage D, et al. ECMO for severe ARDS: systematic review and individual patient data meta-analysis. Intensive Care Med 2020; 46(11):2048–57.
5. Schmidt M, Hajage D, Lebreton G, et al. Extracorporeal membrane oxygenation for severe acute respiratory distress syndrome associated with COVID-19: a retrospective cohort study. Lancet Respir Med 2020;8(11):1121–31.
6. Shaefi S, Brenner SK, Gupta S, et al. Extracorporeal membrane oxygenation in patients with severe respiratory failure from COVID-19. Intensive Care Med 2021;47(2):208–21.
7. Barbaro RP, MacLaren G, Boonstra PS, et al. Extracorporeal membrane oxygenation support in COVID-19: an international cohort study of the Extracorporeal Life Support Organization registry. Lancet 2020;396(10257):1071–8.
8. Ramanathan K, Shekar K, Ling RR, et al. Extracorporeal membrane oxygenation for COVID-19: a systematic review and meta-analysis. Crit Care 2021; 25(1):211.
9. Broman LM, Eksborg S, Lo Coco V, et al. Extracorporeal membrane oxygenation for COVID-19 during first and second waves. Lancet Respir Med 2021; 9(8):e80–1.
10. Riera J, Roncon-Albuquerque R Jr, Fuset MP, et al. Increased mortality in patients with COVID-19 receiving extracorporeal respiratory support during the second wave of the pandemic. Intensive Care Med 2021;47(12):1490–3.
11. Schmidt M, Langouet E, Hajage D, et al. Evolving outcomes of extracorporeal membrane oxygenation support for severe COVID-19 ARDS in Sorbonne hospitals, Paris. Crit Care 2021;25(1): 355.
12. Barbaro RP, MacLaren G, Boonstra PS, et al. Extracorporeal membrane oxygenation for COVID-19: evolving outcomes from the international extracorporeal life support organization registry. Lancet 2021;398(10307):1230–8.
13. Karagiannidis C, Slutsky AS, Bein T, et al. Complete countrywide mortality in COVID patients receiving ECMO in Germany throughout the first three waves of the pandemic. Crit Care 2021;25(1):413.
14. Ling R, Ramanathan K, et al. Evolving outcomes of extracorporeal membrane oxygenation during the first 2 years of the COVID-19 pandemic: a systematic review and meta-analysis. Crit Care 2022;26:147.
15. Abrams D, Grasselli G, Schmidt M, et al. ECLS-associated infections in adults: what we know and what we don't yet know. Intensive Care Med 2020; 46(2):182–91.
16. Carbonell R, Urgelés S, Rodríguez A, et al. Mortality comparison between the first and second/third waves among 3,795 critical COVID-19 patients with pneumonia admitted to the ICU: a multicentre retrospective cohort study. Lancet Reg Health Eur 2021;11:100243.
17. Urner M, Barnett AG, Bassi GL, et al. Venovenous extracorporeal membrane oxygenation in patients with acute covid-19 associated respiratory failure: comparative effectiveness study. Bmj 2022;377: e068723.
18. Whebell S, Zhang J, Lewis R, et al. Survival benefit of extracorporeal membrane oxygenation in severe COVID-19: a multi-centre-matched cohort study. Intensive Care Med 2022;48(4):467–78.
19. Gannon WD, Stokes JW, Francois SA, et al. Association between availability of ECMO and mortality in COVID-19 patients eligible for ECMO: a natural experiment. Am J Respir Crit Care Med 2022; 205(11):1354–7.

20. Granholm A, Alhazzani W, Derde LPG, et al. Randomised clinical trials in critical care: past, present and future. Intensive Care Med 2022; 48(2):164–78.

21. Abrams D, Ferguson ND, Brochard L, et al. ECMO for ARDS: from salvage to standard of care? Lancet Respir Med 2019;7(2):108–10.

22. Badulak J, Antonini MV, Stead CM, et al. Extracorporeal membrane oxygenation for COVID-19: updated 2021 guidelines from the extracorporeal life support organization. Asaio j 2021;67(5):485–95.

23. Brodie D, Slutsky AS, Combes A. Extracorporeal life support for adults with respiratory failure and related indications: a review. Jama 2019;322(6): 557–68.

24. Shekar K, Badulak J, Peek G, et al. Extracorporeal life support organization coronavirus disease 2019 interim guidelines: a consensus document from an international group of interdisciplinary extracorporeal membrane oxygenation providers. Asaio j 2020;66(7):707–21.

25. Tonna JE, Abrams D, Brodie D, et al. Management of adult patients supported with venovenous extracorporeal membrane oxygenation (VV ECMO): guideline from the extracorporeal life support organization (ELSO). Asaio j 2021;67(6):601–10.

26. Brodie D, Abrams D, MacLaren G, et al. ECMO during respiratory pandemics: past, present, and future. Am J Respir Crit Care Med 2022;205(12): 1382–90.

27. Mustafa AK, Alexander PJ, Joshi DJ, et al. Extracorporeal membrane oxygenation for patients with COVID-19 in severe respiratory failure. JAMA Surg 2020;155(10):990–2.

28. Creel-Bulos C, Hockstein M, Amin N, et al. Acute cor pulmonale in critically ill patients with covid-19. N Engl J Med 2020;382(21):e70.

29. Salas de Armas IA, Akkanti BH, Janowiak L, et al. Inter-hospital COVID ECMO air transportation. Perfusion 2021;36(4):358–64.

30. Rafiq MU, Valchanov K, Vuylsteke A, et al. Regional extracorporeal membrane oxygenation retrieval service during the severe acute respiratory syndrome coronavirus 2 (SARS-CoV-2) pandemic: an interdisciplinary team approach to maintain service provision despite increased demand. Eur J Cardiothorac Surg 2020;58(5):875–80.

31. Extracorporeal life support organization (ELSO). Resources > guidelines. Available at: https://www.elso.org/Resources/Guidelines.aspx. Accessed April 1, 2022.

32. Mang S, Reyher C, Mutlak H, et al. Awake extracorporeal membrane oxygenation for COVID-19-induced acute respiratory distress syndrome. Am J Respir Crit Care Med 2022;205(7):847–51.

33. Garcia B, Cousin N, Bourel C, et al. Prone positioning under VV-ECMO in SARS-CoV-2-induced acute respiratory distress syndrome. Crit Care 2020;24(1):428.

34. Giani M, Martucci G, Madotto F, et al. Prone positioning during venovenous extracorporeal membrane oxygenation in acute respiratory distress syndrome. A multicenter cohort study and propensity-matched analysis. Ann Am Thorac Soc 2021;18(3):495–501.

35. Rosano A, Martinelli E, Fusina F, et al. Early percutaneous tracheostomy in coronavirus disease 2019: association with hospital mortality and factors associated with removal of tracheostomy tube at ICU discharge. A cohort study on 121 patients. Crit Care Med 2021;49(2):261–70.

36. Dres M, Burrel S, Boutolleau D, et al. SARS-CoV-2 does not spread through extracorporeal membrane oxygenation or dialysis membranes. Am J Respir Crit Care Med 2020;202(3):458–60.

37. Supady A, Weber E, Rieder M, et al. Cytokine adsorption in patients with severe COVID-19 pneumonia requiring extracorporeal membrane oxygenation (CYCOV): a single centre, open-label, randomised, controlled trial. Lancet Respir Med 2021;9(7):755–62.

38. Barnes GD, Burnett A, Allen A, et al. Thromboembolism and anticoagulant therapy during the COVID-19 pandemic: interim clinical guidance from the anticoagulation forum. J Thromb Thrombolysis 2020;50(1): 72–81.

39. Yusuff H, Zochios V, Brodie D. Thrombosis and coagulopathy in COVID-19 patients requiring extracorporeal membrane oxygenation. Asaio j 2020;66(8): 844–6.

40. Bemtgen X, Zotzmann V, Benk C, et al. Thrombotic circuit complications during venovenous extracorporeal membrane oxygenation in COVID-19. J Thromb Thrombolysis 2021;51(2):301–7.

41. Guo Z, Sun L, Li B, et al. Anticoagulation management in severe coronavirus disease 2019 patients on extracorporeal membrane oxygenation. J Cardiothorac Vasc Anesth 2021;35(2): 389–97.

42. Masur J, Freeman CW, Mohan S. A double-edged sword: neurologic complications and mortality in extracorporeal membrane oxygenation therapy for COVID-19-related severe acute respiratory distress syndrome at a tertiary care center. AJNR Am J Neuroradiol 2020;41(11):2009–11.

43. Usman AA, Han J, Acker A, et al. A case series of devastating intracranial hemorrhage during venovenous extracorporeal membrane oxygenation for COVID-19. J Cardiothorac Vasc Anesth 2020; 34(11):3006–12.

44. Zahid MJ, Baig A, Galvez-Jimenez N, et al. Hemorrhagic stroke in setting of severe COVID-19 infection requiring Extracorporeal Membrane Oxygenation (ECMO). J Stroke Cerebrovasc Dis 2020;29(9): 105016.

45. Heman-Ackah SM, Su YS, Spadola M, et al. Neurologically devastating intraparenchymal hemorrhage in COVID-19 patients on extracorporeal membrane oxygenation: a case series. Neurosurgery 2020; 87(2). E147-e151.

46. McMichael ABV, Ryerson LM, Ratano D, et al. 2021 ELSO adult and pediatric anticoagulation guidelines. Asaio j 2022;68(3):303–10.

47. Ramanathan K, MacLaren G, Combes A, et al. Blood transfusion strategies and ECMO during the COVID-19 pandemic - authors' reply. Lancet Respir Med 2020;8(5):e41.

48. Bharat A, Machuca TN, Querrey M, et al. Early outcomes after lung transplantation for severe COVID-19: a series of the first consecutive cases from four countries. Lancet Respir Med 2021;9(5):487–97.

49. Roach A, Chikwe J, Catarino P, et al. Lung transplantation for covid-19-related respiratory failure in the United States. N Engl J Med 2022;386(12):1187–8.

50. Bermudez CA, Crespo MM. The case for prolonged ECMO for COVID-19 ARDS as a bridge to recovery or lung transplantation. Transplantation 2022;106(4): e198–9.

51. Cypel M, Keshavjee S. When to consider lung transplantation for COVID-19. Lancet Respir Med 2020; 8(10):944–6.

52. Combes A, Brodie D, Bartlett R, et al. Position paper for the organization of extracorporeal membrane oxygenation programs for acute respiratory failure in adult patients. Am J Respir Crit Care Med 2014; 190(5):488–96.

53. Supady A, Badulak J, Evans L, et al. Should we ration extracorporeal membrane oxygenation during the COVID-19 pandemic? Lancet Respir Med 2021; 9(4):326–8.

54. Supady A, Brodie D, Curtis JR. Ten things to consider when implementing rationing guidelines during a pandemic. Intensive Care Med 2021; 47(5):605–8.

55. Supady A, Curtis JR, Abrams D, et al. Allocating scarce intensive care resources during the COVID-19 pandemic: practical challenges to theoretical frameworks. Lancet Respir Med 2021;9(4):430–4.

56. Abrams D, Lorusso R, Vincent JL, et al. ECMO during the COVID-19 pandemic: when is it unjustified? Crit Care 2020;24(1):507.

57. Agerstrand C, Dubois R, Takeda K, et al. Extracorporeal membrane oxygenation for coronavirus disease 2019: crisis standards of care. Asaio j 2021; 67(3):245–9.

58. Lebreton G, Schmidt M, Ponnaiah M, et al. Extracorporeal membrane oxygenation network organisation and clinical outcomes during the COVID-19 pandemic in Greater Paris, France: a multicentre cohort study. Lancet Respir Med 2021;9(8):851–62.

59. Levy D, Lebreton G, Pineton de Chambrun M, et al. Outcomes of patients denied extracorporeal membrane oxygenation during the COVID-19 pandemic in greater Paris, France. Am J Respir Crit Care Med 2021;204(8):994–7.

60. Diaz RA, Graf J, Zambrano JM, et al. Extracorporeal membrane oxygenation for COVID-19-associated severe acute respiratory distress syndrome in Chile: a nationwide incidence and cohort study. Am J Respir Crit Care Med 2021;204(1):34–43.

61. Camporota L, Meadows C, Ledot S, et al. Consensus on the referral and admission of patients with severe respiratory failure to the NHS ECMO service. Lancet Respir Med 2021;9(2):e16–7.

62. Extracorporeal Life Support Organization (ELSO). Membership > ECMO availability Map. Available at: https://www.elso.org/Membership/ECMOAvailabilityMap. aspx. Accessed April 1, 2022.

63. Bartlett RH, Ogino MT, Brodie D, et al. Initial ELSO guidance document: ECMO for COVID-19 patients with severe cardiopulmonary failure. Asaio j 2020; 66(5):472–4.

64. MacLaren G, Fisher D, Brodie D. Treating the most critically ill patients with COVID-19: the evolving role of extracorporeal membrane oxygenation. Jama 2022;327(1):31–2.

65. White DB, Angus DC. A proposed lottery system to allocate scarce COVID-19 medications: promoting fairness and generating knowledge. Jama 2020; 324(4):329–30.

66. Lu X, Zhang L, Du H, et al. SARS-CoV-2 infection in children. N Engl J Med 2020;382(17):1663–5.

67. Feldstein LR, Rose EB, Horwitz SM, et al. Multisystem inflammatory syndrome in U.S. Children and adolescents. N Engl J Med 2020;383(4): 334–46.

68. Feldstein LR, Tenforde MW, Friedman KG, et al. Characteristics and outcomes of US children and adolescents with Multisystem inflammatory syndrome in children (MIS-C) compared with severe acute COVID-19. JAMA 2021;325(11): 1074–87.

69. Gerall C, Cheung EW, Klein-Cloud R, et al. Allocation of resources and development of guidelines for extracorporeal membrane oxygenation (ECMO): experience from a pediatric center in the epicenter of the COVID-19 pandemic. J Pediatr Surg 2020; 55(12):2548–54.

70. DeFazio JR, Kahan A, Fallon EM, et al. Development of pediatric surgical decision-making guidelines for COVID-19 in a New York City children's hospital. J Pediatr Surg 2020;55(8):1427–30.

71. Cho HJ, Ogino MT, Jeong IS, et al. Pediatric intensive care preparedness and ECMO availability in children with COVID-19: an international survey. Perfusion 2021;36(6):637–9.

72. Lemmon ME, Truog RD, Ubel PA. Allocating resources across the life span during COVID-19-integrating neonates and children into crisis

standards of care protocols. JAMA Pediatr 2021; 175(4):347–8.

73. Cleary A, Chivers S, Daubeney PE, et al. Impact of COVID-19 on patients with congenital heart disease. Cardiol Young 2021;31(1):163–5.

74. Yager PH, Whalen KA, Cummings BM. Repurposing a pediatric ICU for adults. N Engl J Med 2020; 382(22):e80.

75. Emanuel EJ, Persad G, Upshur R, et al. Fair allocation of scarce medical resources in the time of covid-19. N Engl J Med 2020;382(21): 2049–55.

76. Myran DT, Cantor N, Rhodes E, et al. Physician health care visits for mental health and substance use during the COVID-19 Pandemic in Ontario, Canada. JAMA Netw Open 2022;5(1):e2143160.

77. Pfefferbaum B, North CS. Mental health and the Covid-19 pandemic. N Engl J Med 2020;383(6): 510–2.

Lung Transplantation in Coronavirus-19 Patients
What We Have Learned So Far

Emily Cerier, MD, Kalvin Lung, MD, Chitaru Kurihara, MD, Ankit Bharat, MD*

KEYWORDS

• Lung transplantation evaluation • COVID-19 • Acute respiratory distress syndrome

KEY POINTS

• Lung transplantation is the only viable treatment option for patients with severe irrecoverable coronavirus-19 (COVID-19)-associated acute respiratory distress syndrome or life-debilitating post-COVID fibrosis and shows promising short-term outcomes.
• COVID-19-related respiratory failure lung transplantation requires strict patient selection and extensive lung transplant evaluation must be done.
• COVID-19-related respiratory failure lung transplants are complex and should be done at high-volume centers with multidisciplinary teams.

INTRODUCTION

The novel coronavirus-19 (COVID-19) has infected more than 490 million people since the start of the pandemic in March 2020, causing over 6.1 million deaths.[1] Although some patients remain asymptomatic, COVID-19 infection has been shown to cause anywhere from common cold manifestations to severe illness, characterized by respiratory and multi-organ failure.[2] In fact, 15.7% of COVID-19 patients are noted to have severe illness manifestations.[3] Although several organs may be affected by COVID-19, the lungs are the primary site of disease, with 6% to 10% of patients with COVID-19 ultimately developing severe acute respiratory distress syndrome (ARDS), requiring mechanical ventilation and extracorporeal membrane oxygenation (ECMO).[4,5] Subsequently, the mortality of patients with COVID-19-associated ARDS requiring mechanical ventilation can exceed 20% to 40%.[6,7] Furthermore, there is a subset of survivors from COVID-19 acute lung injury who are left with chronic lung disease necessitating supplemental oxygen and impairing their mobility.[8] This review article discusses the emerging role of lung transplantation in treatment of patients with COVID-19-associated respiratory failure, both acute and chronic.

NATURE OF THE PROBLEM

With the continuously increasing number of COVID-19 cases due to multiple waves of the pandemic, the number of patients developing COVID-19-associated ARDS, requiring prolonged mechanical ventilation and extracorporeal support, or significant morbidity from COVID-19-related chronic lung disease is expected to rise or remain high. Therefore, when medical therapy fails, it is important to consider lung transplantation as a life-saving and life-altering treatment of patients with COVID-19-associated ARDS and post-COVID chronic lung disease, respectively.

Lung transplantation is a well-established therapy for a variety of end-stage lung diseases, such as idiopathic pulmonary fibrosis, chronic obstructive pulmonary disease, cystic fibrosis, and pulmonary hypertension.[9] Currently, over

Department of Thoracic Surgery, Northwestern University Feinberg School of Medicine, 676 North Saint Clair Street, Suite 650, Chicago, IL 60611, USA
* Corresponding author.
E-mail address: ankit.bharat@nm.org

Clin Chest Med 44 (2023) 347–357
https://doi.org/10.1016/j.ccm.2022.11.017

4000 lung transplants occur annually worldwide, with a median survival of 6.7 years.[10,11] However, before the COVID-19 pandemic, lung transplantation was rarely considered for patients with ARDS.[9] There are multiple concerns raised when considering COVID-19-associated lung disease patients for lung transplantation. First, there is a concern that COVID-19 or superinfecting pathogens associated with viral or ventilator-associated pneumonia in the native lung may recur in the newly transplanted lungs. Second, due to severe damage caused by COVID-19 infection, there are technical challenges to transplantation, which may increase ischemic times and worsen transplant outcomes. Third, there is a concern regarding transplant recovery as COVID-19 patients are severely deconditioned from prolonged mechanical ventilation, sedation, and neuromuscular blockade. Finally, there is an uncertainty as to whether the native lung may recover, which could result in long-term outcomes preferable to lung transplantation.[12]

Despite these concerns, lung transplantation was pursued as treatment of irrecoverable COVID-19-associated ARDS and post-COVID fibrosis, which allowed further insight into COVID-19-associated respiratory failure. By examining explanted native lung tissue from COVID-19-associated ARDS transplant recipients and postmortem lung tissue from patients who died of COVID-19-associated ARDS, Bharat and colleagues showed that COVID-19 caused severe and irreversible lung parenchymal damage that is molecularly and pathologically similar to end-stage pulmonary fibrosis.[12] When comparing the three-dimensional matrix organization of end-stage lung tissue between patients who underwent transplant for COVID-19-associated ARDS to those who underwent transplant for idiopathic pulmonary fibrosis, they found similar disorganized matrix patterns with punctate islands of cells surrounding fibrotic airway regions. Furthermore, when comparing single-cell Ribonucleic Acid sequencing of COVID-19-associated ARDS lungs to lungs in the end stages of idiopathic pulmonary fibrosis, there were many similarities across cell lineages. Of note, they observed an abnormal population of basaloid-like epithelial cells expressing Keratin-17 (KRT17) in the explanted lung from patients transplanted for COVID-19-associated ARDS, which had previously been observed lining fibroblastic foci in idiopathic pulmonary fibrosis patients.[12–15] In explanted lung tissue from patients transplanted for COVID-19-associated ARDS, Bharat and colleagues found these KRT17-positive cells localized near collagen (COL) 1A1-positive cells, which they report is a potential marker for irrecoverable fibrosis.[12]

Therefore, like other end-stage lung diseases, lung transplantation is the only solution for patients who develop severe COVID-19 irreversible lung injury, despite optimal medical therapy. Currently, over 200 lung transplants have been performed for COVID-19-related respiratory failure in the United States.[16] With the ongoing pandemic, the need for COVID-19 transplants may remain, making it critically important to ensure appropriate patient selection. In addition to patients who have severe COVID-19-associated ARDS, there is a cohort of patients who develop respiratory insufficiency after initially recovering. The acutely ill and those suffering from chronic respiratory failure from COVID-19 should be considered distinct subsets. Although the acutely ill patients should be generally considered for double lung transplantation, those in the latter group may benefit from either double of single, especially if there is no pulmonary hypertension or opportunistic infections in the damage native lungs. As there are several reports describing the acutely ill patients, we discuss a patient in the latter group.[12,17,18]

CASE REPORT

A 59-year-old woman with history of obstructive sleep apnea, hypertension, and hyperlipidemia presented to an outside hospital 3 days after testing positive for COVID-19 with shortness of breath and bilateral pulmonary infiltrates on chest X-ray (CXR) (**Fig. 1**A). She was admitted to the Intensive Care Unit for 30 days of high-flow oxygen, with an overall 40-day hospitalization. During her hospital course, she was never intubated and received convalescent plasma, tocilizumab, and intravenous steroids for COVID-19 treatment. Following her discharge, she had shortness of breath with minimal activity and was started on continuous oxygen supplementation.

She presented to our institution as an outpatient for lung transplant evaluation for her post-COVID fibrosis 11 months from her initial COVID-19 infection. Her echocardiogram showed mild concentric left ventricular hypertrophy (ejection fraction: 69%) and normal size left atrium, right atrium, and right ventricle, with normal right ventricular systolic function. Her right heart catheterization was notable for moderate nonobstructive coronary artery disease, but normal pulmonary capillary wedge pressure and cardiac output with a pulmonary artery pressure of 34/16. Computed tomography (CT) of her chest showed poorly defined areas of ground glass with associated mild bronchiectasis and significant fibrosis in the upper lobes, with traction bronchiectasis and volume loss (**Fig.** 1C). Her lung ventilation perfusion scan

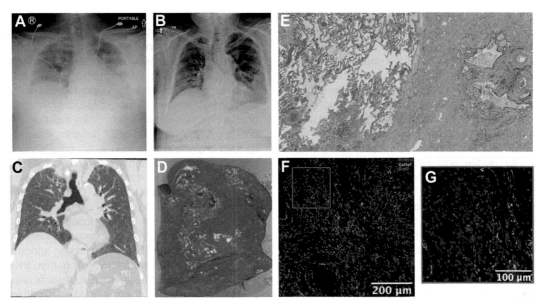

Fig. 1. Patient's chest x-ray (*A*) in the emergency department, 3 days after testing positive for COVID-19 and (*B*) in outpatient clinic, POD22 following left single lung transplant. Patient's computed tomography of chest (*C*) coronal section. Patient's explanted left lung (*D*) with histology using hematoxylin and eosin stain (*E*) showing relatively uninvolved lung parenchyma directly next to fibrotic lung. (*F, G*) Immunofluorescence microscopy showing KRT17 positive staining (*magenta*) cells next to COL1A1 positive cells (*green*).

showed grossly equal perfusion to both lungs (right 54.7% vs left 45.3%), without significant segmental or subsegmental perfusion defects. She was listed for left, right, and bilateral lungs with a Lung Allocation Score of 42.

After 39 days of listing, she received an organ offer for a single left lung with a positive virtual crossmatch. She underwent plasma exchange preoperatively before undergoing her left single lung transplant, which was uneventful with a total ischemic time of 3.75 hours for the transplanted left lung. Final pathology of her explanted lung (**Fig. 1**D) showed uninvolved lung parenchyma next to areas of interstitial fibrosis and capillary congestion (**Fig. 1**E). Immunofluorescence microscopy showed KRT17-positive cells localized near COL1A1-positive cells (**Fig. 1**F, G), suggestive of irrecoverable fibrosis. Postoperatively, her hospital course was unremarkable. Given her positive retrospective crossmatch, she completed antibody-mediated rejection treatment with multiple plasmapheresis treatments, antithymocyte globulin, intravenous immunoglobulin, and eculizumab. Postoperative day (POD) 1, she was extubated to high-flow nasal cannula, which was weaned to nasal cannula on POD 3 and to room air on POD12. She did not have primary graft dysfunction. On POD 4, she was transferred out of the Intensive Care Unit. Her last chest tube was removed on POD 18 and she was discharged home with home health services on POD 19. She

was first seen in outpatient clinic on POD 22 and was noted to be doing well with no need for supplemental oxygen and improving CXR (**Fig. 1**B).

PREOPERATIVE LUNG TRANSPLANT EVALUATION

Currently, there are two main indications for lung transplantation in the setting of COVID-19-related diseases: irrecoverable COVID-19-associated ARDS and post-COVID fibrosis. The former patients will require an expedited inpatient lung transplant work up due to the nature of their disease and inability to leave the intensive care unit, whereas the latter patients may be evaluated as an inpatient versus outpatient setting. Here, the authors discuss the approaches to inpatient versus outpatient evaluations of patients with COVID-19-related indications for lung transplantation.

Outpatient Lung Transplant Evaluation for Post-Coronavirus Fibrosis

As the COVID-19 pandemic continues, the number of patients with post-COVID fibrosis may continue to increase. In fact, King *and colleagues* states that history of severe COVID-19 infection should be added to the differential diagnosis or contributory exposure for all fibrotic interstitial lung disease (ILD) and a part of standard history taking when working up ILD patients.[8] Thus, this prompts the question, "should post-COVID fibrosis be treated similarly to those patients with ILD?" The most critical branch point when deciding to list patients for lung transplantation involves weighing the current morbidity and mortality of the underlying lung disease against the risk of lung transplantation. Multidisciplinary transplant teams, consisting of pulmonologist, surgeons, and others, must decide where the balance falls between the natural history course of the patient's lung disease and the likeliness for transplantation to improve a patient's quality of life and longevity. To assist in this decision-making, in 2014, the International Society of Heart and Lung Transplantation provided consensus guidelines on the appropriate timing of referral and listing of lung transplant candidates.[19] However, as the ISHLT criteria predominantly pertain to progressive fibrotic ILD, and the rate of progression and potential for improvement in post-COVID fibrosis is unknown, it remains questionable whether these criteria can be applied to post-COVID fibrosis patients.

Data regarding the progression or improvement of post-COVID fibrosis are limited. From the case report detailed previously, the co-localization of KRT17-postive cells near COL1A1-positive cells on immunofluorescence microscopy from the explanted post-COVID fibrotic lung suggest that the fibrosis seen in some cases of post-COVID fibrosis is, in fact, irrecoverable. However, the pathogenesis of post-COVID pulmonary fibrosis is incompletely understood. Multiple fibrogenic mechanisms have been demonstrated to be engaged by COVID-19 and include viral activation of profibrotic pathways, such as alterations in the renin–angiotensin system and activation of growth factors, direct cellular injury of macrophages, endothelial cells, and alveolar epithelial cells, cytokine-induced injury through immune recruitment, and mechanical injury from barotrauma and extracellular matrix dysregulation.[20]

Although the previous case report demonstrates sustained irrecoverable post-COVID fibrosis, there are other studies which have reported anywhere from persistent fibrotic abnormalities to complete radiographic resolution of fibrotic changes on chest CT following COVID-19 infection. Han and colleagues prospectively followed 114 patients with severe COVID-19 pneumonia for 6 months following infection where they found that 35% of patients continued to have fibrotic-like changes on chest CT, whereas 38% of patients had complete radiologic resolution, and 27% of patients had residual ground-glass opacifications or interstitial thickening.[21] In a study analyzing 3 month follow-up in 52 patients who had COVID-19 with an initial abnormal CT chest, 42% of patients continued to have residual CT chest abnormalities.

Although those with residual radiographic abnormalities were also more likely to be symptomatic, with shortness of breath, chest pain, or cough, 33% of those patients with complete radiographic resolution were also symptomatic.[22] The persistence of symptoms despite radiographic findings highlights the need to not only consider radiographic findings but also pulmonary function tests (PFT). In fact, in a group of 57 patients who experienced anywhere from mild to severe COVID-19 infection, 75% of patients had abnormalities on PFTs 30 days after discharge.[23] Furthermore, Guler and colleagues found that 4 months following mild/moderate COVID-19 infection, average PFT was normal, as opposed to 4 months following severe COVID-19 infection where patients averaged lower lung volumes and abnormal and reduced diffusion capacity.[24] Together, these studies show that although there is a subset of patients who will recover, there is a subset of patients who continue to remain symptomatic with clear radiologic lung fibrosis, who are candidates for lung transplantation. Risk factors for the development of those in the latter group are older age, history of smoking or alcohol abuse, severe COVID-19 infection, longer Intensive Care Unit admissions, and need for mechanical ventilation.[25]

When deciding whether or not those patients with symptomatic post-COVID should be worked up for transplant, one should first carefully assess for previously unrecognized fibrotic lung disease, as an estimated 2% to 7% of nonsmokers and 4% to 9% of smokers have interstitial lung abnormalities which often go undetected in the absence of CT chest imaging.[26] This can be done by reviewing any available chest imaging done before COVID-19 infection and by obtaining a thorough history (symptoms before COVID-19 infection, occupational or other exposures associated with ILD, family history of ILD, and associated signs and symptoms of connective tissue disorder). Following, baseline PFT, chest CT, and 6-min walk test (6MWT) should be performed. Those patients who have residual pulmonary sequelae, especially those with significant morbidity, should then subsequently be referred to pulmonary rehabilitation. Furthermore, a trial of corticosteroids should be considered as preliminary studies document a benefit in those patients with radiographic findings of organizing pneumonia.[27–29] Patients should be serially followed with repeat PFT, CT chest, and 6MWT. Those patients who demonstrate disease progression should then be considered for a trial of anti-fibrotic therapy, with either pirfenidone or nintedanib. However, clinical trials investigating the effects of these interventions are ongoing.[30–32] Lung transplantation should then be considered for those patients with progressive or residual disease with substantial morbidity related to the lung disease. These patients undergoing transplant work up should subsequently undergo screening for anxiety, depression, and other mental health disorders which may have developed since their COVID-19 infection, given the substantial and diverse mental health burden noted in COVID-19 patients after hospitalization.[33] If any mental health disorders are newly identified, patients should be referred for appropriate treatment before transplant. Of note, for those patients with nonprogressive disease, all efforts for optimal medical management and rehabilitation should be trialed with enough time for recovery before considering lung transplantation. Although it remains uncertain what a sufficient amount of time for recovery for these static post-COVID fibrosis patients would be, the authors of this article suggest a minimum of 6 months to 1 year based off a recent review article investigating treatments for post-COVID fibrosis, recommending medical treatment for 6 months, and historic data of SARS patients with fibrotic lung damage showing recovery within 1 year.[34–36]

Inpatient Lung Transplant Evaluation for Coronavirus-19 Patients

In general, there are two types of patients undergoing inpatient lung transplant evaluation for COVID-19-related illness: those with COVID-19-associated ARDS, either on mechanical ventilation or ECMO with inability to wean, or those who have cleared their initial COVID-19 infection, but have high supplemental oxygen requirements, prohibiting them from a safe discharge. Timing of transplant evaluation in these patients is even more critical than those with post-COVID fibrosis patients discussed previously. Clinicians must identify those patients with COVID-19-associated ARDS who are likely to recover, without transplant, while simultaneously not waiting too long to see if a patient will recover allowing time for the patient to develop severe complications and deconditioning which would then preclude them from transplantation.

The first question to ask when evaluating any inpatient COVID-19 patient is, "Do they have any contraindications to lung transplantation?" This serves as an appropriate initial screening question for this population as if the patient already has a well-known contraindication to lung transplantation, the option of salvage lung transplantation can be taken out of consideration. Currently accepted general criteria for the selection of COVID-19 patients for lung transplantation are

outlined in **Box 1**. Of note, with regard to malignancy, patients should not have an active or recent malignancy. Patients should have a minimum of 2-year disease-free interval from cancer with a low likelihood of cancer recurrence.[8] In addition, the last criteria listed in **Table 1** brings up another critical issue: "Is the patient agreeable to lung transplantation?" This would require the patient to be off sedation and have the capacity to provide informed consent. However, in many cases of COVID-19-associated ARDS, the patient cannot be taken off sedation without severe hypoxemia and hemodynamic instability. In these instances, every effort should be made to safely wake patients up to discuss lung transplantation, provide education, assess patient interest in the procedure, and obtain informed consent. If sedation is unable to be safely held, it is recommended for clinicians to demonstrate the absence of irreversible brain injury through either physical assessment and brain imaging (ie, CT) or neuropsychological consultation.

Box 1
General criteria for lung transplantation in coronavirus-19 patient

Age less than 65 year old, with extension to less than 70 year old in exceptionally fit patients

Isolated lung failure (single-organ failure), however, in certain cases multi-organ transplantation can be considered

Absence of malignancy

No disabling comorbidities

No substance dependence (alcohol, drugs, and so forth)

Not an active smoker

Body mass index between 17 and 32 kg/m^2 (exceptions allowed on case-by-case basis)

Reliable postoperative social support (at minimum: one primary and one secondary caregiver)

Insurance approval and/or financial support identified for transplant associated care

Patient is participating in physical therapy while hospitalized (exceptions allowed for select cases undergoing urgent transplant evaluation, with a high potential for posttransplant recovery, and rehabilitation is hindered predominantly due to pulmonary failure from COVID-19)

Patient and social support in agreement to lung transplantation and willing to relocate close to transplant center for a period established by the transplant center

Table 1
Summary of published literature on coronavirus-19-related lung transplantation

Authors	Title	Month-Year Published	Summary
King et al,[8] 2010	Lung transplantation for patients with COVID-19	Aug-21	Review paper discussing approaches to lung transplantation in the setting of post-COVID fibrosis or COVID-19-associated ARDS by high-volume lung transplant providers.[8]
Bharat et al,[12] 2020	Lung transplantation for patients with severe COVID-19	Nov-20	Case series detailing the approach to/outcomes of three patients with COVID-19-associated ARDS and additional investigation of explanted lung tissue from the transplants and comparison to control lung samples.[12]
Roach et al,[16] 2022	Lung transplantation for COVID-19-related respiratory failure in the United States	Mar-22	A retrospective review of lung transplants performed between August 2020 and September 2021 reported in the United Network for Organ Sharing (UNOS) registry, investigating the survival and clinical outcomes of those transplants performed for COVID-19 respiratory failure.[8]
Bharat et al,[17] 2021	Early outcomes after lung transplantation for severe COVID-19: a series of the first consecutive cases from four countries	Mar-21	International, multicenter case series of 12 patients who underwent bilateral lung transplantation for COVID-19-associated ARDS from May to September 2020.[17]
Kurihara et al,[18] 2022	Clinical characteristics and outcomes of patients with COVID-19-associated acute respiratory distress syndrome who underwent lung transplant	Jan-22	A retrospective, single-center, case series of 102 consecutive lung transplants, from January 2020 to September 2021, which analyzed the clinical outcomes of patients undergoing lung transplantation for COVID-19-associated ARDS and compared them with the outcomes of lung transplant patients without COVID during that time.[18]

Furthermore, clinicians then must discuss lung transplantation with the patient's medical power of attorney who can provide informed decisions in line with the patient's wishes.[17]

Once patients have passed these first screening criteria, the next question to ask is: "Will the patient's lungs recover?" As much is still unknown regarding the timeline or possibility of recovery following acute lung injury from COVID-19, this question requires the best judgment of a multidisciplinary lung transplant team. Patients should undergo an appropriate trial of standard-of-care medical therapy for their COVID-19 infection to optimize any possibility of lung recovery. Although pharmaceutical approaches to COVID-19 are evolving, this trial should otherwise include lung-protective ventilation and negative fluid balance as these clinical practices are critical to prevent worsening lung injury.[8] Currently, the literature supports a minimum of 4 to 6 weeks' time to allow for lung recovery from the onset of COVID-19-associated ARDS before lung transplantation; however, many centers wait for ≥8 weeks.[8,12,17] Specifically for COVID-19-associated ARDS patients supported on ECMO, Kurihara *and colleagues* showed that patients should be supported for at least 4 weeks before consideration of lung transplantation.[18] Exceptions can be made to the minimum 4 week wait period if a life-threatening pulmonary complication arises first, which cannot be managed medically or with extracorporeal life support (ECMO) and requires lung transplantation. Furthermore, it is recommended that two physicians, from two different specialties (surgery, critical care, or pulmonology), agree that lung recovery is unlikely despite optimal medical management. Of note, lung transplantation should not be considered in cases where patients are showing ongoing lung improvement, regardless of time elapsed in COVID-19-associated ARDS.[17]

CT imaging may have a possible role in aiding physicians in assessing the progression/recovery of lung injury in COVID-19 patients and distinguishing patients who have irrecoverable lung damage. King *and colleagues* report that CT chest findings such as traction bronchiectasis and subpleural fibrosis are suggestive of irreversible injury in COVID-19 patients, whereas ground-glass infiltrates are potentially reversible.[8] Furthermore, we have previously discussed how other studies have seen resolution of fibrotic changes on CT scan following COVID-19 infection, showing the potential utility for CT imaging to discern these two patient populations.[21,22] CT chest imaging can additionally assist in defining potentially treatable causes of lung dysfunction, such as organizing pneumonia, pulmonary edema, or pleural disease.[8]

The final essential question to ask when working up inpatient COVID-19 patients for lung transplantation is, "Has the patient cleared their COVID-19 infection?" Current literature states that immunocompetent patients with severe COVID-19 infection have cleared all active virus by 20 days from symptom onset, whereas severely immunocompromised patients may continue to have active virus for significantly longer.[37,38] As transplantation will require immunosuppression, especially in the early posttransplant period, any residual active virus is a major threat to the transplant patient. Therefore, experts in COVID-19-related lung transplantation suggest a very conservative approach when proving clearance of the virus. Most patients are initially diagnosed with COVID-19 through real-time polymerase chain reaction (RT-PCR) testing, which detects COVID-19 Ribonucleic Acid on upper respiratory tract samples, although lower respiratory tract samples have

higher viral loads and are therefore less likely to have a false negative result.[39] However, positive RT-PCR results are limited as this does not necessarily indicate actively replicating virus as the Ribonucleic Acid from viral fragments can cause persistent positive RT-PCR results. Viral culture is the gold standard test to establish active virus; however, given the potential infectious control issues with performing viral cultures, these are not widely available.[40] Therefore, to prove clearance of COVID-19 infection in lung transplantation evaluation, expert consensus recommends two negative RT-PCR tests, obtained at least 24 hours apart from bronchial alveolar lavage samples. In cases where patients are not on the ventilator and without tracheostomy, the two negative RT-PCR tests may be obtained from a nasopharyngeal swab.[17] Although this approach may delay lung transplantation unnecessarily in those patients who have persistent positive testing, given the severe potential morbidity of transplanting patients with active infection, this conservative approach has been accepted.

Single Versus Bilateral Lung Transplant Listing

Initially, only bilateral lung transplantation was recommended for COVID-19-related lung transplantation as many COVID-19 patients being evaluated for lung transplant had developed significant pulmonary hypertension, which would only be addressed by bilateral lung transplantation.[39,40] Furthermore, as explants from the initial COVID-19 lung transplant recipients had cavitary areas of pneumonia, there was concern that these could serve as nidus of future infection if single lung transplantation was pursued, especially once postoperative immunosuppression was started.[40] However, as more lung transplants are performed for post-COVID fibrosis, we believe that there will be a utility for single lung transplantation with careful patient selection, as highlighted in our previously discussed case report. We propose if when patients undergo extensive outpatient lung transplant workup, there is no pulmonary hypertension, and only mild–moderate, but not severe fibrosis, on CT chest, single lung transplantation may be considered. A lung ventilation perfusion scan would subsequently be needed to assess the ideal side for single lung transplantation, and if even, the patient may receive either laterality.

OPERATIVE APPROACH

Performing lung transplantation in patients with COVID-19-related ARDS is not the same as performing lung transplants in those with non-

COVID-19-related indications. Kurihara *and colleagues* performed a study comparing clinical characteristics and outcomes of patients undergoing lung transplant for COVID-19-associated ARDS to those undergoing lung transplant for chronic end-stage lung disease without COVID-19, where they demonstrated the complexity and challenges associated with COVID-19-associated ARDS lung transplants. They noted patients undergoing lung transplantation for COVID-19-associated ARDS had nearly double the lung allocation scores compared with those with chronic end-stage lung disease without COVID-19 (85.8 vs 46.7). Furthermore, they reported that 56.7% of COVID-19-associated ARDS lung transplant recipients were on preoperative ECMO, compared with 1.4% of non-COVID-19 transplants, highlighting just how sicker the COVID-19-associated ARDS lung transplant patient is compared with standard lung transplant recipient. Intraoperatively, they found COVID-19-associated ARDS lung transplants had higher rates of veno-arterial ECMO use (96.7% vs 62.5%) and required more intraoperative red blood cell transfusions (6.5 units vs 0 units) and longer operative time (8.5 vs 7.4 hours), demonstrating the technical challenges associated with performing transplants in this population.[18]

When performing lung transplantation for COVID-19-associated ARDS, there are a couple critical operative factors to note. First, surgeons should prepare to perform the lung transplantation on cardiopulmonary bypass or veno-arterial ECMO support.[18] Although the use of cardiopulmonary bypass is potentially associated with worse outcomes in lung transplantation because of the high incidence of pulmonary hypertension, right ventricular dysfunction, and pleural adhesions in patients with COVID-19-associated ARDS, surgeons should use intraoperative cardiopulmonary support when performing these transplants.[17,41] VA-ECMO can be used in place of cardiopulmonary bypass to reduce total blood loss and need for blood transfusion which are anticipated with cardiopulmonary bypass.[42–44] However, in patients that have extensive and thick pleural adhesions, there is a possibility of entraining air in the ECMO circuit during the dissection. Hence, we suggest that either cardiopulmonary bypass be considered in those patients or at least be available for immediate conversion in case of emergency. Second, it is important to expect high intraoperative blood loss and be prepared to give a large number of blood products. This is likely secondary to the increased complexity of lung transplantation in COVID-19-associated ARDS patients due to factors such as pleural adhesions, fragile tissue quality, and platelet dysfunction

form preoperative ECMO support.[40,42] When the blood loss is too extensive, the use of cardiopulmonary bypass may be required, although it would have the attendant risk of disseminating pulmonary pathogens through the systemic circulation.

POSTOPERATIVE MANAGEMENT

Following transplantation, these COVID-19 lung transplant patients must be followed closely. King *and colleagues* report that COVID-19 lung transplant recipients had no different course or risk of specific posttransplantation complications compared with a general transplant population, but they attributed this to the patients being closely monitored and evaluated before transplant.[8] Conversely, Kurihara *and colleagues* report COVID-19-associated ARDS lung transplant patients had higher rates of Primary Graft Dysfunction (grades 1–3) and permanent hemodialysis use and longer postoperative ventilator requirements, Intensive Care Unit stays, and overall hospital admissions compared with non-COVID-19-related transplants. However, they additionally reported that COVID-19 lung transplant recipients had a higher rate of improvement in their Karnofsky Performance Status after lung transplant compared with the non-COVID-19 transplants.[18] Bharat *and colleagues* note that this prolonged ventilation and difficult initial recovery are expected as this COVID-19 patient population are generally deconditioned before transplant and that this highlights the importance of appropriate selection of patients with a healthy baseline status before their COVID-19 infection, so they may safely tolerate the posttransplant rehabilitation.[17] Taken together, the increased complexity of both the lung transplant operation and postoperative management highlights the need for COVID-19 lung transplantation to be performed in high-volume centers with access to many hospital resources.

OUTCOMES

As it has only been 2 years since the first COVID-19-related lung transplant was performed in June 2020, there is no long-term data on COVID-19 lung transplant outcomes (see **Table 1**). However, studies have shown short-term survival greater than 90% at both 3 months and 1 year.[17] Roach *and colleagues* performed a retrospective review of the United Network for Organ Sharing (UNOS) registry, analyzing lung transplants performed between August 2020 and September 2021, where they found COVID-19-related lung transplants made up 7% of all lung transplants. Of the 214

COVID-19-related lung transplants identified, 65% were performed for COVID-19-associated ARDS with the remaining performed for post-COVID fibrosis. This is the largest study analyzing COVID-19-related lung transplant outcomes published and they report a 2.2% 30-day mortality with 95.6% 3-month survival rate, which rivals the survival rate among patients undergoing lung transplantation for non-COVID-19-related indications.[16] Overall, lung transplant for COVID-19-related indications is becoming more common and current outcomes of COVID-19-related lung transplantation are promising.

FUTURE DIRECTIONS

As the COVID-19 pandemic continues with more waves and new subvariants, lung transplantation for COVID-19-related respiratory failure will become increasingly more common. As we get farther out from the initial COVID-19 lung transplants, further studies will be needed to analyze long-term outcomes of these transplant recipients and see how they compare to non-COVID-19-related lung transplants. Further studies will also be needed to investigate the outcomes of COVID-19 single lung transplants and how they compare to those who received bilateral lung transplants. As COVID-19-related lung transplantation demand increases, especially as more patients develop post-COVID fibrosis, expanding the donor pool of lungs through the use of single lung transplantation must be considered. Finally, as we learn more about the COVID-19 virus and the natural course of disease, we must continuously revise our guidelines and criteria for lung transplant evaluation and patient selection.

SUMMARY

COVID-19 can result in severe irrecoverable ARDS or life-limiting fibrosis for which lung transplantation is currently the only viable treatment. COVID-19 lung transplantation has transformed the field of lung transplantation, as before the pandemic, few transplants had ever been performed in the setting of infectious disease or ARDS. Given the complexities associated with COVID-19 lung transplantation, it requires strict patient selection with an experienced multidisciplinary team in a high-resource hospital setting. Current short-term outcomes of COVID-19 lung transplantation are promising; however, further follow-up studies are needed to determine long-term outcomes and whether this subset of lung transplant patients may be predisposed to unique complications.

CLINICS CARE POINTS

- Lung transplantation is the only viable treatment option for patients with severe irrecoverable COVID-19-associated ARDS or life-debilitating post-COVID fibrosis and shows promising short-term outcomes.
- COVID-19-related respiratory failure lung transplantation requires strict patient selection and extensive lung transplant evaluation must be done.
- COVID-19-related respiratory failure lung transplants are complex and should be done at high-volume centers with multidisciplinary teams.

DISCLOSURE

E.J. Cerier is supported by the National Institutes of Health, United States Grant T32AI083216 and Thoracic Surgery Foundation, United States, A. Bharat is supported by the National Institutes of Health Grants: HL145478, HL147290, and HL147575. The authors declare they have no conflict of interest.

REFERENCES

1. WHO COVID-19 dashboard. Available at: https://covid19.who.int/. Accessed April 11, 2022.
2. Mokhtari T, Hassani F, Ghaffari N, et al. COVID-19 and multiorgan failure: a narrative review on potential mechanisms. J Mol Histol 2020;51(6):613–28.
3. Baud D, Qi X, Nielsen-Saines K, et al. Real estimates of mortality following COVID-19 infection. Lancet Infect Dis 2020;20(7):773.
4. Geleris J, Sun Y, Platt J, et al. Observational study of hydroxychloroquine in hospitalized patients with covid-19. N Engl J Med 2020;382(25):2411–8.
5. Richardson S, Hirsch JS, Narasimhan M, et al. Presenting characteristics, comorbidities, and outcomes among 5700 patients hospitalized with COVID-19 in the New York city area. JAMA 2020; 323(20):2052–9.
6. Horby P, Lim WS, Emberson JR, et al. Dexamethasone in hospitalized patients with covid-19. N Engl J Med 2021;384(8):693–704.
7. Beigel JH, Tomashek KM, Dodd LE. Remdesivir for the treatment of covid-19 - preliminary report reply. N Engl J Med 2020;383(10):994.
8. King CS, Mannem H, Kukreja J, et al. Lung transplantation for patients with COVID-19. Chest Jan 2022;161(1):169–78.

9. van der Mark SC, Hoek RAS, Hellemons ME. Developments in lung transplantation over the past decade. Eur Respir Rev 2020;29(157). https://doi.org/10.1183/16000617.0132-2019.

10. Chambers DC, Cherikh WS, Harhay MO, et al. The international thoracic organ transplant registry of the international society for heart and lung transplantation: thirty-sixth adult lung and heart-lung transplantation report-2019; focus theme: donor and recipient size match. J Heart Lung Transplant 2019;38(10):1042–55.

11. Erasmus ME, van der Bij W. Death after lung transplantation: improving long term survival despite perilous early postoperative years. Transpl Int 2020; 33(2):128–9.

12. Bharat A, Querrey M, Markov NS, et al. Lung transplantation for patients with severe COVID-19. Sci Translational Med 2020;12(574):eabe4282.

13. Adams TS, Schupp JC, Poli S, et al. Single-cell RNA-seq reveals ectopic and aberrant lung-resident cell populations in idiopathic pulmonary fibrosis. Sci Adv 2020;6(28):eaba1983.

14. Habermann AC, Gutierrez AJ, Bui LT, et al. Single-cell RNA sequencing reveals profibrotic roles of distinct epithelial and mesenchymal lineages in pulmonary fibrosis. Sci Adv 2020;6(28):eaba1972.

15. Reyfman PA, Walter JM, Joshi N, et al. Single-cell transcriptomic analysis of human lung provides insights into the pathobiology of pulmonary fibrosis. Am J Respir Crit Care Med 2019;199(12):1517–36.

16. Roach A, Chikwe J, Catarino P, et al. Lung transplantation for covid-19–related respiratory failure in the United States. N Engl J Med 2022;386(12):1187–8.

17. Bharat A, Machuca TN, Querrey M, et al. Early outcomes after lung transplantation for severe COVID-19: a series of the first consecutive cases from four countries. Lancet Respir Med 2021;9(5):487–97.

18. Kurihara C, Manerikar A, Querrey M, et al. Clinical characteristics and outcomes of patients with COVID-19–associated acute respiratory distress syndrome who underwent lung transplant. JAMA 2022;327(7):652–61.

19. Weill D, Benden C, Corris PA, et al. A consensus document for the selection of lung transplant candidates: 2014–an update from the pulmonary transplantation council of the international society for heart and lung transplantation. J Heart Lung Transplant 2015;34(1):1–15.

20. McDonald LT. Healing after COVID-19: are survivors at risk for pulmonary fibrosis? Am J Physiol Lung Cell Mol Physiol 2021;320(2):L257–65.

21. Han X, Fan Y, Alwalid O, et al. Six-month follow-up chest CT findings after severe COVID-19 pneumonia. Radiology 2021;299(1):E177–86.

22. Tabatabaei SMH, Rajebi H, Moghaddas F, et al. Chest CT in COVID-19 pneumonia: what are the findings in mid-term follow-up? Emerg Radiol 2020; 27(6):711–9.

23. Huang Y, Tan C, Wu J, et al. Impact of coronavirus disease 2019 on pulmonary function in early convalescence phase. Respir Res 2020;21(1):163.

24. Guler SA, Ebner L, Aubry-Beigelman C, et al. Pulmonary function and radiological features 4 months after COVID-19: first results from the national prospective observational Swiss COVID-19 lung study. Eur Respir J 2021;57(4). https://doi.org/10.1183/13993003.03690-2020.

25. Ojo AS, Balogun SA, Williams OT, et al. Pulmonary fibrosis in COVID-19 survivors: predictive factors and risk reduction strategies. Pulm Med 2020; 2020:6175964.

26. Hatabu H, Hunninghake GM, Richeldi L, et al. Interstitial lung abnormalities detected incidentally on CT: a position paper from the fleischner society. Lancet Respir Med 2020;8(7):726–37.

27. González J, Benítez ID, Carmona P, et al. Pulmonary function and radiologic features in survivors of critical COVID-19: a 3-month prospective cohort. Chest 2021;160(1):187–98.

28. Myall KJ, Mukherjee B, Castanheira AM, et al. Persistent post-COVID-19 interstitial lung disease. An observational study of corticosteroid treatment. Ann Am Thorac Soc 2021;18(5):799–806.

29. Vadász I, Husain-Syed F, Dorfmüller P, et al. Severe organising pneumonia following COVID-19. Thorax 2021;76(2):201–4.

30. National Institutes of Health Clinical Center. Pirfenidone compared to placebo in post-COVID19 pulmonary fibrosis COVID-19 (FIBRO-COVID). National Institutes of health. Available at: https://clinicaltrials.gov/ct2/show/NCT04607928?term=pirfenidone&cond=Covid19&draw=2. Updated 12/30/21. Accessed 05/10/22, 2022.

31. Pirfenidone vs. Nintedanib for fibrotic lung disease after coronavirus disease-19 pneumonia (PINCER). National Institutes of health. Available at: https://clinicaltrials.gov/ct2/show/NCT04856111?term=pirfenidone&cond=Covid19&draw=2. Updated 04/26/22. Accessed 05/10/22, 2022.

32. The study of the use of nintedanib in slowing lung disease in patients with fibrotic or non-fibrotic interstitial lung disease related to COVID-19 (ENDCOV-I). National Institutes of health. Available at: https://clinicaltrials.gov/ct2/show/NCT04619680?term=nintedanib&cond=Covid19&draw=2. Updated 4/14/22. Accessed 05/10/22, 2022.

33. Evans RA, McAuley H, Harrison EM, et al. Physical, cognitive, and mental health impacts of COVID-19 after hospitalisation (PHOSP-COVID): a UK multicentre, prospective cohort study. Lancet Respir Med 2021;9(11):1275–87.

34. Hui DS, Joynt GM, Wong KT, et al. Impact of severe acute respiratory syndrome (SARS) on pulmonary

function, functional capacity and quality of life in a cohort of survivors. Thorax 2005;60(5):401–9.

35. Wong KT, Antonio GE, Hui DS, et al. Severe acute respiratory syndrome: thin-section computed tomography features, temporal changes, and clinicoradiologic correlation during the convalescent period. J Comput Assist Tomogr 2004;28(6):790–5.

36. Bazdyrev E, Rusina P, Panova M, et al. Lung fibrosis after COVID-19: treatment prospects. Pharmaceuticals (Basel) 2021;14(8). https://doi.org/10.3390/ph14080807.

37. Ending isolation and precautions for people with COVID-19: interim guidance. Available at: https://www.cdc.gov/coronavirus/2019-ncov/hcp/duration-isolation.html. Updated 01/14/22. Accessed 05/17/22, 2022.

38. Aydillo T, Gonzalez-Reiche AS, Aslam S, et al. Shedding of viable SARS-CoV-2 after immunosuppressive therapy for cancer. N Engl J Med 2020;383(26):2586–8.

39. Lai CKC, Lam W. Laboratory testing for the diagnosis of COVID-19. Biochem Biophys Res Commun 2021;538:226–30.

40. Jefferson T, Spencer EA, Brassey J, et al. Viral cultures for coronavirus disease 2019 infectivity assessment: a systematic review. Clin Infect Dis 2020;73(11):e3884–99.

41. Weingarten N, Schraufnagel D, Plitt G, et al. Comparison of mechanical cardiopulmonary support strategies during lung transplantation. Expert Rev Med Devices 2020;17(10):1075–93.

42. Bermudez CA, Shiose A, Esper SA, et al. Outcomes of intraoperative venoarterial extracorporeal membrane oxygenation versus cardiopulmonary bypass during lung transplantation. Ann Thorac Surg 2014; 98(6):1936–42. discussion 1942-3.

43. Moreno Garijo J, Cypel M, McRae K, et al. The evolving role of extracorporeal membrane oxygenation in lung transplantation: implications for anesthetic management. J Cardiothorac Vasc Anesth 2019;33(7):1995–2006.

44. Hashimoto K, Hoetzenecker K, Yeung JC, et al. Intraoperative extracorporeal support during lung transplantation in patients bridged with venovenous extracorporeal membrane oxygenation. J Heart Lung Transplant 2018;37(12):1418–24.

SARS-CoV-2 Infection and COVID-19 in Children

Alpana Waghmare, MD[a,b], Diego R. Hijano, MD, MSc[c],*

KEYWORDS

• COVID-19 • Pediatrics • SARS-CoV-2 • Children • MIS-C

KEY POINTS

• Severe acute respiratory syndrome coronavirus-2 (SARS-CoV-2) prevalence is high in pediatric populations, especially during the Omicron variant and subvariant waves.
• Clinical manifestations of coronavirus disease 2019 (COVID-19) are generally less severe than in adults, although severe disease can occur in high-risk individuals.
• Multisystem inflammatory syndrome in children is a unique post-COVID phenomenon that occurs rarely, mostly in children approximately 1 month after acute SARS-CoV-2 infection.
• SARS-CoV-2 vaccination remains crucial to prevent severe disease in children.
• Treatment considerations generally follow recommendations for adults and older adolescents should be managed similarly to adults.

EPIDEMIOLOGY

Several databases are available to determine the burden of severe acute respiratory syndrome coronavirus-2 (SARS-CoV-2) infection and coronavirus disease 2019 (COVID-19) in pediatric populations. The COVerAGE database (COVerAGE-DB), an open-access database from more than 103 countries, recorded 56.9 million COVID-19 cases children and adolescents aged less than 20 years with a prevalence range from 0% to 37% of the national caseload across countries.[1] Of these, 63% occurred among adolescents aged 10 to 19 years, and 37% occurred among children aged 0 to 9 years. The Pediatric COVID-19 case registry, the largest registry in the United States, collected information from 12,917 children with COVID-19 during the first year of the pandemic.[2] Infections were most common among those 12 to 18 years of age (31%), followed by 5 to 11 years of age (24%) with no significant difference in gender. Most cases were in White Caucasians followed by in Blacks. One in 4 cases was in

Hispanic/Latinos. Reported COVID-19 cases in children increased significantly in 2022 during the Omicron surge. In the United States alone, more than 5 million of a total 13 million cases were diagnosed between January 1, 2022 and May 12, 2022, and the percent of total cases occurring in children increased from 10% to 30%.[3–5] As of February 2022, almost 75% of children and adolescents had serologic evidence of previous infection with SARS-CoV-2, with approximately one-third becoming newly seropositive since December 2021 with the highest in the age group with lowest vaccination rates (5–11 years, 28%).[6]

Most children seem to have asymptomatic, mild, or moderate disease and recover within 1 to 2 weeks of disease onset.[7–9] However, children with COVID-19 may develop severe complications, such as respiratory distress syndrome, myocarditis, acute renal failure, and multisystem organ failure.[10–14] Around 0.1% to 1.5% of pediatric COVID-19 patients require hospitalization, representing close to 5% of all pediatric hospitalizations in the United States.[3] Age, race,

[a] Department of Pediatrics, University of Washington, Fred Hutchinson Cancer Research Center Vaccine, 1100 Fairview Avenue North, Seattle, WA 98109, USA; [b] Department of Infectious Diseases, Division Seattle Children's Hospital, Seattle, WA, USA; [c] St. Jude Children's Research Hospital, 262 Danny Thomas Place Mail Stop 230, Memphis, TN 38105, USA
* Corresponding author.
E-mail address: Diego.Hijano@STJUDE.ORG

Clin Chest Med 44 (2023) 359–371
https://doi.org/10.1016/j.ccm.2022.11.014

and ethnicity have been described as risk factors for hospitalization with the highest rates seen in those aged younger than 12 months, Hispanics, and non-Hispanic Black children.[15–20] The annual COVID-19-associated hospitalization rate by age is shown in **Table 1**. Among children hospitalized with COVID-19 in the United States, between 28% and 40% required intensive care unit (ICU), 6% to 18% needed invasive mechanical ventilation, and up to 3% died.[21,22]

SARS-CoV-2-related death in children and adolescents is rare.[23,24] On February 2021, a pooled analysis from Europe and the US estimated COVID-19-associated death in children to be 0.17 per 100,000.[4,25] Among the 4.4 million COVID-19 deaths reported in the COVerAGE-DB, more than 17,200 (0.4%) occurred in children and adolescents aged younger than 20 years, with 53% among adolescents aged 10–19 years, and 47% among children aged 0–9 years.[1] Case fatality ratios (CFRs) have varied among continents over time. Although Asia had the highest CFR initially, Europe, and North America, followed by South America surpassed those of Asia shortly after a pandemic was declared. High-income countries had an exponential increased in their CFRs compared with low-income countries probably due to underreporting and lower testing capacities from low-income countries.[26] Specifically, the percentage of COVID-19 mortality in those aged younger than 20 years, varied among countries based on income: high-income (0.1), upper-middle-income (0.6%), low-middle-income (1.2%), and low-income (0.9%) countries.[1] Cumulative mortality rates for the United States are shown in **Table 1**.

RISK FACTORS FOR SEVERE DISEASE

Our understanding of COVID-19 severity in children has evolved over time. Although children with certain underlying medical conditions are at increased risk for severe illness (hospitalization, need for intensive care or mechanical ventilation, death) evidence associating specific conditions is limited. In addition, children without comorbidities can also experience severe COVID-19.[11,15,17,18,27–32]

In children aged younger than 2 years, chronic lung disease, neurological disorders, cardiovascular disease, prematurity, or airway abnormalities are associated with an increased risk for severe COVID-19.[33] Among children aged 2 to 18 years, obesity, diabetes, and feeding tube dependence carried significant risk for severity (**Box 1**). Individuals with sickle cell disease, due to underlying cardiopulmonary comorbidities, are more likely to be hospitalized, develop pneumonia, and present with hypoxemia due to COVID-19. However, mortality has not been significantly different across studies.[34–37]

There are conflicting reports on whether immunocompromised individuals, including recipients of solid organ or hematopoietic cell transplants, are at higher risk for severe diseases.[38–45] Although some of these differences have been adjudicated to lower threshold for hospital admission in children with these conditions, Mukkada and colleagues[43] showed that cancer is independently associated with severe disease. In their cohort, one-fifth of children and adolescents with cancer experience severe COVID-19, and deaths occurred in a higher proportion than is reported for those without comorbidities. Specifically, in patients aged 15 to 18 years, severe lymphopenia and intensive chemotherapy were independently associated with disease severity.[43]

Lack of vaccination is the most important modifiable risk factor for severe disease. Among 400 children hospitalized for COVID-19 during the Omicron wave, 9 in 10 were unvaccinated COVID-19-associated hospitalization rates among unvaccinated children aged 5 to 11 years were twice as high as rates in children vaccinated with a primary series (19 vs 9 per 100,000).[46] Similar results have been reported for those aged 12 to

Table 1
Clinical outcomes by age in pediatric patients with coronavirus disease 2019

Age	Annual Hospitalization Rate per 100,000[4,133]	Overall Cumulative Mortality per Million[134]
Overall (<18 y)	48.2	18.4[a]
0–4 y	66.8	<12 mon: 80.6 1–4 y: 9.1
5–11 y	25	6.9
12–17 y	59.9	17.8
18–19 y		48.5

[a] Range 0–19 y.

Box 1
Risk factors for severe coronavirus disease 2019 disease in children

Risk factors

  Asthma or other chronic pulmonary diseases

  Obesity[a]

  Diabetes mellitus

  Congenital heart disease/cardiovascular disease

  Sickle cell disease

  Neurologic conditions

  Metabolic conditions

  Genetic conditions

  Medical complexity

  Immunosuppression

[a]Body mass index [BMI] greater than 95th percentile for age and sex.

---

17 years, in whom the rates of hospitalization among unvaccinated were 2.5× higher when compared with vaccinated teens.[47] This data is further supported by studies from adults showing the impact of vaccination in preventing severe disease, hospitalization, and death.

CLINICAL MANIFESTATIONS

The clinical presentation of COVID-19 in children is diverse and varies by age. Asymptomatic infection in children ranges from 10% to 42%.[8] The most common symptoms in children are fever and cough, followed by shortness of breath, sore throat, headache, myalgia, fatigue, and, less frequently, rhinorrhea.[38,48–50] Studies limited to infants have shown that poor feeding with fever in the absence of obvious signs can be part of the clinical presentation. In addition, several groups have described SASR-CoV-2-associated bronchiolitis.[51] There is less evidence on the clinical presentation of COVID-19 in immunocompromised children. The Pediatric COVID-19 case registry has 614 immunocompromised patients and 12,309 immunocompetent children.[2] Asymptomatic infection was seen in almost 40% of immunocompromised children compared with around 20% in immunocompetent children (**Table 2**).

Box 1
In an international registry of 1500 children with cancer, asymptomatic infection was reported in one-third, with fever and cough being the most common symptoms in those who became sick.[43]

Rhinorrhea and stuffy nose and gastrointestinal (GI) symptoms were reported in 10% of cases and tachypnea, sore throat, body aches, and headaches in 5% to 7%. Anosmia, ageusia, chills, and cutaneous manifestations were seen in less than 3% of the patients. Similar results have been reported by others.[40–44,52]

SARS-CoV-2 produces heterogeneous respiratory involvement in children. The vast majority has mild upper respiratory tract symptoms. However, progression to the lower respiratory tract has been well described, with pneumonia being the most frequent manifestations and acute respiratory distress syndrome the most severe one.[27,49,53,54] Chest radiograph imaging is the first preferred method to assess children with suspected pneumonia. Radiologic abnormalities can be present in about half of the patients with dyspnea and differ from that observed in adults. They can be unilateral or bilateral, single, or multiple, and most seen in the lower lobes. Unilateral increased density and bilateral peribronchial changes are commonly seen. Ground-glass opacities and patchy shadowing on a chest computerized tomography (CT) scan are the most recognized signs in children.[55–64] Less common manifestations including single-round consolidation, pleural effusion, small nodules, or lymphadenopathy have been reported. According to the US COVID-19 pediatric registry, abnormal findings on pulmonary imaging. (**Table 3**) during the first week of disease were most seen in immunocompromised children, with the most common radiologic findings being multifocal or patchy opacities, followed by interstitial infiltrates and bronchial thickening.[2]

Although COVID-19 affects mainly the lungs, extrapulmonary manifestations affecting several systems have been described in adults as well as in children. Myocarditis, pericarditis, heart failure, and arrhythmias have been described in children and adolescents.[65] The risk of myocarditis and myocarditis or pericarditis associated with SARS-CoV-2 infection varies by age and gender but is overall low and higher than after mRNA vaccination. The highest incidence is seen in boys aged 12 to 17 years (50.1–64.9 cases per 100,000) followed by boys 5 to 11 years (12.6–17.6 cases per 100,000).[66–68] Cardiac manifestations in children with preexisting heart conditions do not significantly differ from those without cardiac disease; however, SARS-CoV-2 can worsen the basal status of this population.[69]

Neurological manifestations are frequent and vary in severity. Between 20% and 40% of children hospitalized with COVID-19 had one or more neurological symptom, affecting the central and/or peripheral nervous system.[70–72] As with cardiac

Table 2
Frequency of symptoms in immunocompetent and immunocompromised children in the US COVID-19 pediatric registry[2]

		Day 0			
		General Pediatric, n = 12309		Immunocompromised, n = 614	
Symptoms	Yes	9554	77.62%	383	62.38%
	No	2670	21.69%	229	37.30%
Fever		5362	43.56%	227	36.97%
Cough		4590	37.29%	186	30.29%
Rhinorrhea		2983	24.23%	105	17.10%
Headache		2584	20.99%	74	12.05%
Sore throat		2223	18.06%	48	7.82%
Decreased oral intake		1784	14.49%	74	12.05%
Myalgia		1612	13.10%	61	9.93%
Vomiting		1528	12.41%	61	9.93%
Lethargy		1346	10.94%	56	9.12%
Shortness of breath		1239	10.07%	71	11.56%
Diarrhea		1181	9.59%	66	10.75%
Abdominal pain		1167	9.48%	49	7.98%
Nausea		1082	8.79%	55	8.96%
Loss of smell/taste		958	7.78%	35	5.70%
Chest pain		558	4.53%	27	4.40%
Rash		472	3.83%	6	0.98%
Conjunctivitis		337	2.74%	6	0.98%
Wheezing		259	2.10%	8	1.30%
Seizure		172	1.40%	5	0.81%
Apnea		54	0.44%	1	0.16%
Hypothermia		32	0.26%	4	0.65%
Hemoptysis		19	0.15%	1	0.16%

Data from Pediatric COVID-19 Case Registry. Accessed June 28th, 2022. https://www.pedscovid19registry.com.

manifestations, CNS involvement can be seen in the acute phase or as part of multisystem inflammatory syndrome in children (MIS-C).[70] The vast majority of these are transient and fully resolve over time. In addition to anosmia and ageusia, common manifestations are headache, encephalopathy, seizures, and weakness. Children with preexisting neurological disease could experience exacerbation and/or progression of their underlying condition, especially those with neuromuscular disease.

Dermatologic manifestations include the vasculitic chilblain-like acral pattern of the distal toes, consisting of reddish-purple nodules on the distal digits and often refer as "COVID toes" and have been described more frequently in children and young adults.[73]

The most common GI symptoms in children with COVID-19 are vomiting and diarrhea, followed by anorexia, abdominal pain, and poor appetite.[48,74–76] GI symptoms can be the first manifestation of COVID-19 and can occur with or without respiratory symptoms.[77,78] Although most of these are self-limited, a Spanish multicenter study showed that children with COVID-19 and GI symptoms had more severe disease than those without GI symptoms.[79] Of note, children with GI symptoms required careful monitoring given that vomiting, abdominal pain, and/or diarrhea can be a manifestation of MIS-C.

MULTISYSTEM INFLAMMATORY SYNDROME IN CHILDREN

MIS-C has been most frequently described in children aged from 1 to 14 years and is most prevalent in children aged older than 5 years.[80] Since first reported in England in April 2020, several studies have reported cases of MIS-C with peaks that lag the peak of acute COVID-19.[81–86] These have led

Table 3
Pulmonary findings during the first week of diagnosis with coronavirus disease 2019 in immunocompetent and immunocompromised children in the US COVID-19 pediatric registry[2]

| | Day 0 | | | |
| | General Pediatric, n = 12309 | | Immunocompromised, n = 614 | |
Finding				
Abnormal XR	911	7.40%	82	13.36%
Bronchial or peribronchial thickening/cuffing	270	2.19%	10	1.63%
Interstitial infiltrates	188	1.53%	14	2.28%
Lobar consolidation	86	0.70%	10	1.63%
Multifocal or patchy opacity	456	3.70%	52	8.47%
Abnormal CT	82	0.67%	21	3.42%
Bronchial or peribronchial thickening/cuffing	4	0.03%	1	0.16%
Interstitial infiltrates	4	0.03%	2	0.33%
Lobar consolidation	13	0.11%	2	0.33%
Multifocal or patchy opacity or ground glass opacity	53	0.43%	12	1.95%
Nodule(s)	9	0.07%	4	0.65%
Tree-in-bud opacities	1	0.01%	0	0.00%

Data from Pediatric COVID-19 Case Registry. Accessed June 28th, 2022. https://www.pedscovid19registry.com.

to the hypothesis that MIS-C is an immune-mediated port infectious complication of SARS-CoV-2. The incidence of MIS-C early in the pandemic was 1 case per 3000 infections in individuals aged younger than 21 years.[87] To date, more than 8525 cases and 69 deaths have been reported in the United States. The median age of patients with MIS-C was 9 years. Half of children with MIS-C were aged between 5 and 13 years and 61% were boys.[80] Almost 60% of the reported patients with race/ethnicity information available (N = 8038) occurred in children who are Hispanic/Latino or Black, non-Hispanic.[80,88] The most common manifestations are persistent fever and GI symptoms such as abdominal pain, vomiting, and diarrhea. Individuals can also have mild-to-moderate respiratory symptoms, rash, conjunctivitis, mucous membrane involvement, and neurocognitive impairment. Respiratory failure, as seen in acute COVID-19, is not a common characteristic of MIS-C.[83,84,89–91] Cardiac involvement is commonly and can include acute myocardial dysfunction, arrhythmias or conduction abnormalities, and coronary artery dilation.[92–94] Several laboratory abnormalities have been associated with MIS-C including increased in inflammatory markers such as c-reactive protein (CRP), erythrocyte sedimentation rate (ESR), ferritin, fibrinogen, and D-dimer. Troponin and brain natriuretic peptide are often elevated. Both The Centers for Disease Control and Prevention (CDC) and The World

Health Organization (WHO) have defined criteria to diagnose MIS-C that includes clinical presentation, laboratory finding, and organ involvement.[89,90] MIS-C shares characteristics with Kawasaki disease (KD); however, MIS-C affects older children and disproportionally affects Black and Hispanic with very few cases described in Asian children. In addition, GI symptoms are more common and prominent in MIS-C, and inflammatory markers tend to be higher when compared with KD.[95–97] Although these distinctions can be helpful, ultimately, a previous history of SARS-CoV-2 infection or known COVID-exposure will aid in determining MIS-C or KD.[89,90] Although the course of MIS-C can be severe, requiring intensive care support, outcomes are overall good with most children recovering. However, deaths have been reported, and long-term outcomes in those who have recovered have not been properly studied.[80,83,84,98,99]

Post-COVID Conditions

The phenomenon of persistent symptoms following COVID-19 has been variably termed long COVID, long-haul COVID, postacute sequelae of COVID-19, post-COVID, and COVID syndrome. The WHO defines post-COVID-19 conditions as occurring in individuals with a history of probable or confirmed SARS-CoV-2 infection, usually 3 months from the onset of COVID-19 with symptoms and that last for at least 2 months and cannot be explained by an alternative diagnosis.[100] Importantly, the WHO specifies that a separate definition may be applicable to children. The CDC definition of post-COVID-19 conditions includes a wide range of health consequences that are present 4 or more weeks after infection with SARS-CoV-2.[101] Overall, post-COVID-19 conditions in children seem to be less common than in adults. An early publication from a national survey in the United Kingdom estimates that 7% to 8% of children may experience continued symptoms for over 12 weeks. The most common symptoms are fatigue, headache, insomnia, trouble concentrating, muscle and joint pain, and cough and can occurred after infection, irrespective of its severity, or MIS-C. These symptoms can limit physical activity, cause distress about symptoms, decrease school attendance/participation, and become mental health challenges.[102,103] A systematic review of 21 studies that included children and adolescents found a 25.24% prevalence of long-COVID, with mood symptoms, fatigue, and sleep disorders most commonly reported.[104] Other studies have reported varying ranges of persistent symptoms after COVID. A Danish study reported higher rates of symptoms at 2 months postinfection in children aged 0 to 14 years compared with controls in a cross-sectional case-control study,[105] whereas an international study of ~1800 children demonstrated very low prevalence of symptoms at day 90.[106]

Several factors may influence the reported prevalence of prolonged symptoms in children and the apparent discrepancy among various studies. Namely, stratification by age, gender, vaccination status, and viral variant are likely needed to fully characterize the effect. Initial data has suggested that the risk of long COVID is reduced in individuals that had received 2 doses of vaccine[107,108]; however, data specific to children and with newer variants are currently lacking. Infection with different viral variants, especially Omicron, is likely to influence the risk of long COVID[109]; however, data in children are not yet available.

Treatment

Systematic data on the use of specific treatments for COVID-19 in pediatric patients remain limited. Through some clinical trials of COVID-19 therapeutics allowed inclusion of adolescents, adolescent enrollment in most trials was low and sometimes nonexistent. Nonetheless, several agents are now approved and/or have emergency use authorization for use in children and adolescents. As the landscape of therapeutics continues to change and new data become available,

recommendations are likely to also change. Guidelines from the Infectious Diseases Society of America (https://www.idsociety.org/practice-guideline/covid-19-guideline-treatment-and-management/) and the National Institutes of Health (https://www.covid19treatmentguidelines.nih.gov/) are updated regularly and provide up-to-date reviews of currently available data.

Remdesivir

Remdesivir is approved by the FDA for use in hospitalized and nonhospitalized pediatric patients aged 28 days or older and weighing 3.0 kg or greater.[110] Remdesivir for use in early infection was evaluated in nonhospitalized, high-risk adults with mild-to-moderate disease, where a 3-day infusion was associated with an 87% risk reduction of hospitalization or death.[111] Only 8 adolescents aged younger than 18 years were included in the trial; however, current guidelines recommend consideration of use in nonhospitalized children or hospitalized children not on oxygen, aged 12 years or older who are at high risk of progression to severe COVID-19.[112] Children aged younger than 12 years can be considered for remdesivir as well, although data are lacking. The efficacy of remdesivir in hospitalized individuals is limited to trials involving adult subjects.[113–116] Interim results of a phase 2/3, single-arm, open-label study aimed at evaluating the safety, tolerability, and pharmacokinetics of remdesivir in children demonstrated overall acceptable safety profile,[117] although the lack of a placebo group in this trial limits the evaluation of efficacy. Remdesivir thus is recommended for pediatric patients who have a new or increasing oxygen need.

Ritonavir-boosted nirmatrelvir (paxlovid)

The FDA issued an emergency use authorization (EUA) for ritonavir-boosted nirmatrelvir for nonhospitalized individuals with mild to moderate COVID-19 aged ≥12 years and at high risk for progression to severe disease.[118] Efficacy, however, has only been demonstrated in adults, where an 89% relative risk reduction was found compared to placebo.[119] Given the efficacy data in adults, ritonavir-boosted nirmatrelvir is recommended for adolescents aged 12 years or older who are at high risk of progressing to severe disease.[112] Importantly, drug interactions must be considered when administering ritonavir-boosted nirmatrelvir, which may prevent use in certain high-risk populations such as immunocompromised children.

Monoclonal antibodies

Several monoclonal antibodies (mAbs) have been developed and received EUAs for adults and children aged 12 years or older; however, emergence of SARS-CoV-2 variants has rendered most mAbs ineffective for use as treatment. Currently, bebtelovimab is the only mAb available for use that has maintained in vitro activity against Omicron subvariants.[120] No clinical data is available in either adults or children demonstrating efficacy, thus, despite the EUA for use in nonhospitalized patients, current guidelines do not recommend for or against use in children aged 12 years or older who have mild-to-moderate COVID-19 with high risk of progression to severe COVID-19. Up-to date guidance on activity of different mAbs against circulating SARS-CoV-2 variants can be found at https://www.covid19treatmentguidelines.nih.gov/ therapies/anti-sars-cov-2-antibody-products/ anti-sars-cov-2-monoclonal-antibodies/. The use of mAbs for prophylaxis is discussed below.

Corticosteroids and other immunomodulators
In general, despite lack of systematic data on use, recommendations for corticosteroid use in children with COVID-19 follow recommendations in adults. The benefits of corticosteroids have been demonstrated in several clinical trials, including the Randomised Evaluation of COVID-19 Therapy (RECOVERY) trial where a mortality benefit was observed in adults with COVID-19 on supplemental oxygen receiving dexamethasone.[121] Given overall lower mortality in children, and that the strongest effect was seen in patients on higher levels of oxygen support, dexamethasone is reserved for children requiring high flow or more supplemental oxygen.[112] Several other immunomodulators have been evaluated in adults with moderate to severe COVID-19, including baricitinib, tofacitinib, and tocilizumab.[122–127] Without pediatric efficacy data, potential benefits of these therapies must be extrapolated from adult studies, and therefore, the use is limited to patients with severe COVID-19 (noninvasive and invasive mechanical ventilation).[112]

Prevention and Prophylaxis

Vaccination
The mainstay of prevention of severe COVID-19 in children is vaccination. Currently 2 mRNA vaccines (Pfizer/BioNTech, Moderna) and 1 protein subunit vaccine (Novavax) are either approved or hold EUA status for children in the United States. Both the Pfizer-BioNTech and Moderna vaccines are authorized down to 6 months of age, whereas the Novavax vaccine is authorized down to 12 years of age. Up to date dosing schedules for primary series and booster doses can be found at https://www.cdc.gov/coronavirus/2019-ncov/vaccines/stay-up-to-date.html#recommendations. Vaccine effectiveness estimates for children have varied by vaccine dosing regimens, history of prior infection, and SARS-CoV-2 variant predominance[128]; however, protection against severe disease remains an important clinical endpoint. The American Academy of Pediatrics and the Advisory Committee on Immunization Practices recommend vaccination (including booster doses) for all children aged 6 months or older.[129,130]

Monoclonal antibodies for preexposure and postexposure prophylaxis
As outlined above, emergence of SARS-CoV-2 variants has resulted in several mAbs being no longer effective for both treatment and prophylaxis. Prophylaxis with mAb is generally reserved for those that are unable to mount an adequate response to vaccination, namely individuals that are moderately to severely immunocompromised. Tixagevimab 300 mg plus cilgavimab 300 mg (Evusheld) is the only available mAb combination currently available for use as preexposure prophylaxis against SARS-CoV-2 for adults and adolescents aged 12 years or older with moderate-to-severe immunocompromise or in individuals unable to be fully vaccinated due to history of severe adverse reactions to COVID vaccines.[112] Of note, current dosing guidance, including repeat dosing at 6 months, are not based on clinical trial data therefore data on efficacy is limited, especially in pediatrics.[131,132] No mAbs are currently approved for postexposure prophylaxis; however, this may change as new variants and mAbs emerge.

SUMMARY

Although our knowledge of COVID-19 has significantly evolved over the course of the pandemic, COVID-19 continues to be an important health problem around the world. We have a better understanding of the various clinical presentations and risks factors for severe disease. We have access to accurate diagnostics tests and limited, yet effective therapies targeting the virus or modulating the immune response to it. Vaccines, which continue to prove safe and effective, are now available for anyone aged 6 month and older. However, lack of access, inequity, disinformation, and vaccine hesitancy have led to disparities in vaccination rates among countries, enabling the virus to mutate and leaving all of us vulnerable to new surges. Particularly vulnerable, are children, who have the lowest vaccination rates and have been increasingly affected with each new wave driven by a different variant of concern. Scientifically we have made remarkable and unprecedented progress and while many answers lay ahead, we will undoubtedly be able to answer them. However, the biggest questions, is whether we will be able to bring drown the social and economic disparities needed to overcome this pandemic.

CLINICS CARE POINTS

- Although severe COVID-19 is less frequent in children, the direct and indirect effects of COVID-19 on children's health continues to be substantial.
- Vaccines against SARS-CoV-2 are available for everyone 6 months of age and older. They have been proven to be safe and effective in reducing the risk of severe disease.

FINANCIAL DISCLOSURES

A. Waghmare receives grant support from Ansun Biopharma, Allovir and Pfizer and is an Advisory Board Member for Kyorin Pharmaceutical. D.R. Hijano has no financial disclosures.

REFERENCES

1. COVID-19 confirmed cases and deaths. the United Nations Children's Fund (UNICEF). Available at: https://data.unicef.org/resources/covid-19-confirmed-cases-and-deaths-dashboard/. Accessed June 28th, 2022.
2. Pediatric COVID-19 case registry. Available at: https://www.pedscovid19registry.com. Accessed June 28th, 2022.
3. Children and COVID-19: state-level data report. American Academy of pediatrics. Available at: https://www.aap.org/en/pages/2019-novel-coronavirus-covid-19-infections/children-and-covid-19-state-level-data-report/. Accessed June 24, 2022.
4. COVID data tracker/demographics. Centers for Disease Control and Prevention. Available at: https://covid.cdc.gov/covid-data-tracker/#datatracker-home. Accessed June 28, 2022.
5. COVID-19 dashboard by the center for systems science and engineering (CSSE) at johns hopkins university (JHU). Johns hopkins university, center for systems science and engineering. 2022. Available at: https://coronavirus.jhu.edu/map.html. Accessed June 28, 2022.
6. Clarke KEN, Jones JM, Deng Y, et al. Seroprevalence of infection-induced SARS-CoV-2 antibodies - United States, september 2021-february 2022. MMWR Morb Mortal Wkly Rep 2022;71(17):606–8.
7. Badal S, Thapa Bajgain K, Badal S, et al. Prevalence, clinical characteristics, and outcomes of pediatric COVID-19: a systematic review and meta-analysis. J Clin Virol 2021;135:104715.
8. Milani GP, Bottino I, Rocchi A, et al. Frequency of children vs adults carrying severe acute respiratory syndrome coronavirus 2 asymptomatically. JAMA Pediatr 2021;175(2):193–4.
9. Yasuhara J, Kuno T, Takagi H, et al. Clinical characteristics of COVID-19 in children: a systematic review. Pediatr Pulmonol 2020;55(10):2565–75.
10. Dong Y, Mo X, Hu Y, et al. Epidemiology of COVID-19 among children in China. Pediatrics 2020;145(6). https://doi.org/10.1542/peds.2020-0702.
11. Drouin O, Hepburn CM, Farrar DS, et al. Characteristics of children admitted to hospital with acute SARS-CoV-2 infection in Canada in 2020. CMAJ 2021;193(38):E1483–93.
12. Forrest CB, Burrows EK, Mejias A, et al. Severity of acute COVID-19 in children <18 Years old march 2020 to december 2021. Pediatrics 2022;149(4). https://doi.org/10.1542/peds.2021-055765.
13. Irfan O, Muttalib F, Tang K, et al. Clinical characteristics, treatment and outcomes of paediatric COVID-19: a systematic review and meta-analysis. Arch Dis Child 2021;106(5):440–8.
14. Kainth MK, Goenka PK, Williamson KA, et al. Early experience of COVID-19 in a US children's hospital. Pediatrics 2020;146(4). https://doi.org/10.1542/peds.2020-003186.
15. Bellino S, Punzo O, Rota MC, et al. COVID-19 disease severity risk factors for pediatric patients in Italy. Pediatrics 2020;146(4). https://doi.org/10.1542/peds.2020-009399.
16. Butt AA, Dargham SR, Loka S, et al. COVID-19 disease severity in children infected with the omicron variant. Clin Infect Dis 2022. https://doi.org/10.1093/cid/ciac275.
17. Campbell JI, Dubois MM, Savage TJ, et al. Comorbidities associated with hospitalization and progression among adolescents with symptomatic coronavirus disease 2019. J Pediatr 2022;245:102–10.e2.
18. Choi JH, Choi SH, Yun KW. Risk factors for severe COVID-19 in children: a systematic review and meta-analysis. J Korean Med Sci 2022;37(5):e35.
19. Martin B, DeWitt PE, Russell S, et al. Characteristics, outcomes, and severity risk factors associated with SARS-CoV-2 infection among children in the US National COVID cohort collaborative. JAMA Netw Open 2022;5(2):e2143151. https://doi.org/10.1001/jamanetworkopen.2021.43151.
20. O'Neill L, Chumbler NR. Risk factors for COVID-19 hospitalization in school-age children. Health Serv Res Manag Epidemiol 2022;9. 23333928221104677.
21. American Academy of Pediatrics. Coronaviruses, Including SARS-CoV-2 and MERS-CoV. In:

Kimberlin DW, Barnett ED, Lynfield R, Sawyer MH, eds. Red Book: 2021 Report of the Comittee on Infectious Diseases. Itasca, IL: American Academy of Pediatrics: 2021, 280–285.

22. COVID Data Tracker. Centers for disease control and prevention. Available at: https://covid.cdc.gov/covid-data-tracker/?utm_campaign=Private%20Equity%20Newsletter&utm_source=hs_email&utm_medium=email&_hsenc=p2ANqtz-_M9OSt7jgR0ag2vPQVMdjmHOJhtBfAKqb3OsXS0Pr1RdsT3Wm9YvOe0XcLivUaeChn93xw#cases-deaths-testing-trends. Accessed June 20, 2022.

23. Bixler D, Miller AD, Mattison CP, et al. SARS-CoV-2-Associated deaths among persons aged <21 Years - United States, february 12-july 31, 2020. MMWR Morb Mortal Wkly Rep 2020;69(37):1324–9.

24. Smith C, Odd D, Harwood R, et al. Deaths in children and young people in England after SARS-CoV-2 infection during the first pandemic year. Nat Med 2022;28(1):185–92.

25. Bhopal SS, Bagaria J, Olabi B, et al. Children and young people remain at low risk of COVID-19 mortality. Lancet Child Adolesc Health 2021;5(5):e12–3.

26. Abou Ghayda R, Lee KH, Han YJ, et al. The global case fatality rate of coronavirus disease 2019 by continents and national income: a meta-analysis. J Med Virol 2022;94(6):2402–13.

27. Chao JY, Derespina KR, Herold BC, et al. Clinical characteristics and outcomes of hospitalized and critically ill children and adolescents with coronavirus disease 2019 at a tertiary care medical center in New York city. J Pediatr 2020;223:14–9.e2.

28. Graff K, Smith C, Silveira L, et al. Risk factors for severe COVID-19 in children. Pediatr Infect Dis J 2021;40(4):e137–45.

29. Kompaniyets L, Agathis NT, Nelson JM, et al. Underlying medical conditions associated with severe COVID-19 illness among children. JAMA Netw Open 2021;4(6):e2111182.

30. Tsabouri S, Makis A, Kosmeri C, et al. Risk factors for severity in children with coronavirus disease 2019: a comprehensive literature review. Pediatr Clin North Am 2021;68(1):321–38.

31. Ward JL, Harwood R, Smith C, et al. Risk factors for PICU admission and death among children and young people hospitalized with COVID-19 and PIMS-TS in England during the first pandemic year. Nat Med 2022;28(1):193–200.

32. Zhou B, Yuan Y, Wang S, et al. Risk profiles of severe illness in children with COVID-19: a meta-analysis of individual patients. Pediatr Res 2021;90(2):347–52.

33. Woodruff RC, Campbell AP, Taylor CA, et al. Risk factors for severe COVID-19 in children. Pediatrics 2021. https://doi.org/10.1542/peds.2021-053418.

34. Heilbronner C, Berteloot L, Tremolieres P, et al. Patients with sickle cell disease and suspected COVID-19 in a paediatric intensive care unit. Br J Haematol 2020;190(1):e21–4.

35. Martin OY, Darbari DS, Margulies S, et al. Pediatric sickle cell disease and the COVID-19 pandemic: a year in review at children's national hospital. Blood 2021;138(Supplement 1):3036.

36. Sayad B, Karimi M, Rahimi Z. Sickle cell disease and COVID-19: susceptibility and severity. Pediatr Blood Cancer 2021;68(8):e29075.

37. Singh A, Brandow AM, Panepinto JA. COVID-19 in individuals with sickle cell disease/trait compared with other Black individuals. Blood Adv 2021;5(7):1915–21.

38. Bisogno G, Provenzi M, Zama D, et al. Clinical Characteristics and Outcome of Severe Acute Respiratory Syndrome Coronavirus 2 Infection in Italian Pediatric Oncology Patients: a Study From the Infectious Diseases Working Group of the Associazione Italiana di Oncologia e Ematologia Pediatrica. J Pediatr Infect Dis Soc 2020;9(5):530–4.

39. Goss MB, Galván NTN, Ruan W, et al. The pediatric solid organ transplant experience with COVID-19: an initial multi-center, multi-organ case series. Pediatr Transplant 2021;25(3):e13868.

40. Haeusler GM, Ammann RA, Carlesse F, et al. SARS-CoV-2 in children with cancer or after haematopoietic stem cell transplant: an analysis of 131 patients. Eur J Cancer 2021;159:78–86.

41. Kebudi R, Kurucu N, Tuğcu D, et al. COVID-19 infection in children with cancer and stem cell transplant recipients in Turkey: a nationwide study. Pediatr Blood Cancer 2021;68(6):e28915.

42. Millen GC, Arnold R, Cazier JB, et al. COVID-19 in children with haematological malignancies. Arch Dis Child 2022;107(2):186–8.

43. Mukkada S, Bhakta N, Chantada GL, et al. Global characteristics and outcomes of SARS-CoV-2 infection in children and adolescents with cancer (GRCCC): a cohort study. Lancet Oncol 2021;22(10):1416–26.

44. Nicastro E, Verdoni L, Bettini LR, et al. COVID-19 in immunosuppressed children. Front Pediatr 2021;9:629240.

45. Rüthrich MM, Giessen-Jung C, Borgmann S, et al. COVID-19 in cancer patients: clinical characteristics and outcome-an analysis of the LEOSS registry. Ann Hematol 2021;100(2):383–93.

46. Shi DS, Whitaker M, Marks KJ, et al. Hospitalizations of children aged 5-11 Years with laboratory-confirmed COVID-19 - COVID-NET, 14 states, march 2020-february 2022. MMWR Morb Mortal Wkly Rep 2022;71(16):574–81.

47. Havers FP, Whitaker M, Self JL, et al. Hospitalization of adolescents aged 12-17 Years with

laboratory-confirmed COVID-19 - COVID-NET, 14 states, march 1, 2020-april 24, 2021. MMWR Morb Mortal Wkly Rep 2021;70(23):851–7.

48. Bailey LC, Razzaghi H, Burrows EK, et al. Assessment of 135 794 pediatric patients tested for severe acute respiratory syndrome coronavirus 2 across the United States. JAMA Pediatr 2021; 175(2):176–84.

49. Derespina KR, Kaushik S, Plichta A, et al. Clinical manifestations and outcomes of critically ill children and adolescents with coronavirus disease 2019 in New York city. J Pediatr 2020;226:55–63. e2.

50. Hoang A, Chorath K, Moreira A, et al. COVID-19 in 7780 pediatric patients: a systematic review. Eclinicalmedicine 2020;24:100433.

51. Di Nardo M, van Leeuwen G, Loreti A, et al. A literature review of 2019 novel coronavirus (SARS-CoV2) infection in neonates and children. Pediatr Res 2021;89(5):1101–8.

52. Liang W, Guan W, Chen R, et al. Cancer patients in SARS-CoV-2 infection: a nationwide analysis in China. Lancet Oncol Mar 2020;21(3):335–7.

53. Chen T, Wu D, Chen H, et al. Clinical characteristics of 113 deceased patients with coronavirus disease 2019: retrospective study. BMJ 26 2020;368: m1091.

54. Jurado Hernández JL, Álvarez Orozco IF. COVID-19 in children: respiratory involvement and some differences with the adults. Front Pediatr 2021;9: 622240.

55. Li B, Shen J, Li L, et al. Radiographic and clinical features of children with coronavirus disease (COVID-19) pneumonia. Indian Pediatr 2020; 57(5):423–6.

56. Nino G, Zember J, Sanchez-Jacob R, et al. Pediatric lung imaging features of COVID-19: a systematic review and meta-analysis. Pediatr Pulmonol 2021;56(1):252–63.

57. Caro-Dominguez P, Shelmerdine SC, Toso S, et al. Thoracic imaging of coronavirus disease 2019 (COVID-19) in children: a series of 91 cases. Pediatr Radiol 2020;50(10):1354–68.

58. Chen Z, Fan H, Cai J, et al. High-resolution computed tomography manifestations of COVID-19 infections in patients of different ages. Eur J Radiol 2020;126:108972.

59. Duan YN, Zhu YQ, Tang LL, et al. CT features of novel coronavirus pneumonia (COVID-19) in children. Eur Radiol 2020;30(8):4427–33.

60. Kurian J, Blumfield E, Levin TL, et al. Imaging findings in acute pediatric coronavirus disease 2019 (COVID-19) pneumonia and multisystem inflammatory syndrome in children (MIS-C). Pediatr Radiol 2022;1–13. https://doi.org/10.1007/s00247-022-05393-9.

61. Li W, Cui H, Li K, et al. Chest computed tomography in children with COVID-19 respiratory infection. Pediatr Radiol 2020;50(6):796–9.

62. Lu Y, Wen H, Rong D, et al. Clinical characteristics and radiological features of children infected with the 2019 novel coronavirus. Clin Radiol 2020; 75(7):520–5.

63. Palabiyik F, Kokurcan SO, Hatipoglu N, et al. Imaging of COVID-19 pneumonia in children. Br J Radiol Sep 1 2020;93(1113):20200647.

64. Xia W, Shao J, Guo Y, et al. Clinical and CT features in pediatric patients with COVID-19 infection: different points from adults. Pediatr Pulmonol 2020;55(5):1169–74.

65. Jone PN, John A, Oster ME, et al. SARS-CoV-2 infection and associated cardiovascular manifestations and complications in children and young adults: a scientific statement from the american heart association. Circulation 2022;145(19): e1037–52.

66. Block JP, Boehmer TK, Forrest CB, et al. Cardiac complications after SARS-CoV-2 infection and mRNA COVID-19 vaccination - PCORnet, United States, january 2021-january 2022. MMWR Morb Mortal Wkly Rep 2022;71(14):517–23.

67. Boehmer TK, Kompaniyets L, Lavery AM, et al. Association between COVID-19 and myocarditis using hospital-based administrative data - United States, march 2020-january 2021. MMWR Morb Mortal Wkly Rep 2021;70(35):1228–32.

68. Patone M, Mei XW, Handunnetthi L, et al. Risks of myocarditis, pericarditis, and cardiac arrhythmias associated with COVID-19 vaccination or SARS-CoV-2 infection. Nat Med 2022;28(2):410–22.

69. Alsaied T, Aboulhosn JA, Cotts TB, et al. Coronavirus disease 2019 (COVID-19) pandemic implications in pediatric and adult congenital heart disease. J Am Heart Assoc 2020;9(12):e017224.

70. Fink EL, Robertson CL, Wainwright MS, et al. Prevalence and risk factors of neurologic manifestations in hospitalized children diagnosed with acute SARS-CoV-2 or MIS-C. Pediatr Neurol 2022; 128:33–44.

71. LaRovere KL, Riggs BJ, Poussaint TY, et al. Neurologic involvement in children and adolescents hospitalized in the United States for COVID-19 or multisystem inflammatory syndrome. JAMA Neurol 2021;78(5):536–47.

72. Lin JE, Asfour A, Sewell TB, et al. Neurological issues in children with COVID-19. Neurosci Lett 2021;743:135567.

73. Andina D, Belloni-Fortina A, Bodemer C, et al. Skin manifestations of COVID-19 in children: Part 1. Clin Exp Dermatol 2021;46(3):444–50.

74. Assa A, Benninga MA, Borrelli O, et al. Gastrointestinal perspective of coronavirus disease 2019 in

children-an updated review. J Pediatr Gastroenterol Nutr 2021;73(3):299–305.

75. Cheung KS, Hung IFN, Chan PPY, et al. Gastrointestinal manifestations of SARS-CoV-2 infection and virus load in fecal samples from a Hong Kong cohort: systematic review and meta-analysis. Gastroenterology 2020;159(1):81–95.

76. Dipasquale V, Passanisi S, Cucinotta U, et al. Implications of SARS-COV-2 infection in the diagnosis and management of the pediatric gastrointestinal disease. Ital J Pediatr 2021;47(1):71.

77. Moradveisi B, Ataee P, Ghaffarieh A, et al. Diarrhea as a presenting symptom of coronavirus disease 2019 in children. Adv Biomed Res 2020;9:35.

78. Wang J, Yuan X. Digestive system symptoms and function in children with COVID-19: a meta-analysis. Medicine (Baltimore) 19 2021;100(11): e24897.

79. Gonzalez Jimenez D, Velasco Rodríguez-Belvís M, Ferrer Gonzalez P, et al. COVID-19 gastrointestinal manifestations are independent predictors of PICU admission in hospitalized pediatric patients. Pediatr Infect Dis J 2020;39(12):e459–62.

80. Health department-reported cases of multisystem inflammatory syndrome in children (MIS-C) in the United States. Centers for disease control and prevention. Available at: https://covid.cdc.gov/covid-data-tracker/#mis-national-surveillance. Accessed June 29, 2022.

81. Antúnez-Montes OY, Escamilla MI, Figueroa-Uribe AF, et al. COVID-19 and multisystem inflammatory syndrome in Latin American children: a multinational study. Pediatr Infect Dis J 2021; 40(1):e1–6.

82. Belay ED, Abrams J, Oster ME, et al. Trends in geographic and temporal distribution of US children with multisystem inflammatory syndrome during the COVID-19 pandemic. JAMA Pediatr 2021; 175(8):837–45.

83. Dufort EM, Koumans EH, Chow EJ, et al. Multisystem inflammatory syndrome in children in New York state. N Engl J Med 2020;383(4):347–58.

84. Feldstein LR, Rose EB, Horwitz SM, et al. Multisystem inflammatory syndrome in U.S. Children and adolescents. N Engl J Med 2020;383(4): 334–46.

85. Feldstein LR, Tenforde MW, Friedman KG, et al. Characteristics and outcomes of US children and adolescents with multisystem inflammatory syndrome in children (MIS-C) compared with severe acute COVID-19. JAMA 2021;325(11):1074–87.

86. Miller AD, Zambrano LD, Yousaf AR, et al. Multisystem inflammatory syndrome in children-United States, February 2020-July 2021. Clin Infect Dis 2021. https://doi.org/10.1093/cid/ciab1007.

87. Payne AB, Gilani Z, Godfred-Cato S, et al. Incidence of multisystem inflammatory syndrome in children among US persons infected with SARS-CoV-2. JAMA Netw Open 2021;4(6):e2116420.

88. Stierman B, Abrams JY, Godfred-Cato SE, et al. Racial and ethnic disparities in multisystem inflammatory syndrome in children in the United States, march 2020 to february 2021. Pediatr Infect Dis J 2021;40(11):e400–6.

89. Information for healthcare providers about multisystem inflammatory syndrome in children (MIS-C). Center for disease control and prevention. Available at: https://www.cdc.gov/mis/mis-c/hcp/index.html?CDC_AA_refVal=https%3A%2F%2Fwww.cdc.gov%2Fmis%2Fhcp%2Findex.html. Accessed June 27, 2022.

90. Multisystem inflammatory syndrome in children and adolescents temporally related to COVID-19. World Health Organization. Available at: https://www.who.int/news-room/commentaries/detail/multisystem-inflammatory-syndrome-in-children-and-adolescents-with-covid-19. Accessed June 21, 2022.

91. Cheung EW, Zachariah P, Gorelik M, et al. Multisystem inflammatory syndrome related to COVID-19 in previously healthy children and adolescents in New York city. JAMA 2020;324(3):294–6.

92. Choi NH, Fremed M, Starc T, et al. MIS-C and cardiac conduction abnormalities. Pediatrics 2020; 146(6). https://doi.org/10.1542/peds.2020-009738.

93. Sperotto F, Friedman KG, Son MBF, et al. Cardiac manifestations in SARS-CoV-2-associated multisystem inflammatory syndrome in children: a comprehensive review and proposed clinical approach. Eur J Pediatr 2021;180(2):307–22.

94. Wu EY, Campbell MJ. Cardiac manifestations of multisystem inflammatory syndrome in children (MIS-C) following COVID-19. Curr Cardiol Rep 2021;23(11):168.

95. Verdoni L, Mazza A, Gervasoni A, et al. An outbreak of severe Kawasaki-like disease at the Italian epicentre of the SARS-CoV-2 epidemic: an observational cohort study. Lancet 2020; 395(10239):1771–8.

96. Whittaker E, Bamford A, Kenny J, et al. Clinical characteristics of 58 children with a pediatric inflammatory multisystem syndrome temporally associated with SARS-CoV-2. JAMA 2020;324(3): 259–69.

97. Yasuhara J, Watanabe K, Takagi H, et al. COVID-19 and multisystem inflammatory syndrome in children: a systematic review and meta-analysis. Pediatr Pulmonol 2021;56(5):837–48.

98. Hoste L, Van Paemel R, Haerynck F. Multisystem inflammatory syndrome in children related to COVID-19: a systematic review. Eur J Pediatr 2021;180(7): 2019–34.

99. McCormick DW, Richardson LC, Young PR, et al. Deaths in children and adolescents associated with COVID-19 and MIS-C in the United States.

Pediatrics 2021;148(5). https://doi.org/10.1542/peds.2021-052273.

100. Soriano JB, Murthy S, Marshall JC, et al. A clinical case definition of post-COVID-19 condition by a Delphi consensus. Lancet Infect Dis 2022;22(4): e102–7.

101. CDC. Post-COVID conditions: overview for healthcare providers. Available at: https://www.cdc.gov/coronavirus/2019-ncov/hcp/clinical-care/post-covid-conditions.html. Accessed 8 20, 2022.

102. Zimmermann P, Pittet LF, Curtis N. Long covid in children and adolescents. BMJ Jan 20 2022;376: o143.

103. Zimmermann P, Pittet LF, Curtis N. How common is long COVID in children and adolescents? Pediatr Infect Dis J 2021;40(12):e482–7.

104. Lopez-Leon S, Wegman-Ostrosky T, Ayuzo del Valle NC, et al. Long-COVID in children and adolescents: a systematic review and meta-analyses. Scientific Rep 2022;12(1):9950.

105. Kikkenborg Berg S, Palm P, Nygaard U, et al. Long COVID symptoms in SARS-CoV-2-positive children aged 0-14 years and matched controls in Denmark (LongCOVIDKidsDK): a national, cross-sectional study. Lancet Child Adolesc Health 2022;6(9): 614–23.

106. Funk AL, Kuppermann N, Florin TA, et al. Post-COVID-19 conditions among children 90 Days after SARS-CoV-2 infection. JAMA Netw Open 2022;5(7): e2223253. https://doi.org/10.1001/jamanetworkopen.2022.23253.

107. Antonelli M, Penfold RS, Merino J, et al. Risk factors and disease profile of post-vaccination SARS-CoV-2 infection in UK users of the COVID Symptom Study app: a prospective, community-based, nested, case-control study. Lancet Infect Dis 2022;22(1):43–55.

108. Kuodi P, Gorelik Y, Zayyad H, et al. Association between vaccination status and reported incidence of post-acute COVID-19 symptoms in Israel: a cross-sectional study of patients tested between March 2020 and November 2021. medRxiv 2022. https://doi.org/10.1101/2022.01.05.22268800.2022.01.05.22268800.

109. Antonelli M, Pujol JC, Spector TD, et al. Risk of long COVID associated with delta versus omicron variants of SARS-CoV-2. Lancet 2022;399(10343): 2263–4.

110. Coronavirus (COVID-19) Update: FDA Approves First COVID-19 Treatment for Young Children. 2022. https://www.fda.gov/news-events/press-announcements/coronavirus-covid-19-update-fda-approves-first-covid-19-treatment-young-children. [Accessed 20 August 2022].

111. Gottlieb RL, Vaca CE, Paredes R, et al. Early remdesivir to prevent progression to severe Covid-19 in outpatients. N Engl J Med 2022;386(4): 305–15.

112. Panel. C-TG. Coronavirus disease 2019 (COVID-19) treatment guidelines. National Institutes of Health. Available at: https://www.covid19treatmentguidelines.nih.gov/. Accessed August 20, 2022.

113. Spinner CD, Gottlieb RL, Criner GJ, et al. Effect of remdesivir vs standard care on clinical status at 11 Days in patients with moderate COVID-19: a randomized clinical trial. JAMA 2020;324(11):1048–57.

114. Beigel JH, Tomashek KM, Dodd LE, et al. Remdesivir for the treatment of covid-19 - final report. N Engl J Med 2020;383(19):1813–26.

115. Consortium WHOST. Remdesivir and three other drugs for hospitalised patients with COVID-19: final results of the WHO Solidarity randomised trial and updated meta-analyses. Lancet 2022;399(10339): 1941–53.

116. Ali K, Azher T, Baqi M, et al. Remdesivir for the treatment of patients in hospital with COVID-19 in Canada: a randomized controlled trial. CMAJ 2022;194(7):E242–51.

117. Ahmed A., Rojo P., Agwu A., et al. Remdesivir treatment for COVID-19 in hospitalized children: CARAVAN interim results. 2022. Available at: https://www.croiconference.org/abstract/remdesivir-treatment-for-covid-19- in-hospitalized-children-caravan-interim-results/. Accessed August 20, 2022.

118. Administration. FaD. Fact sheet for healthcare providers: emergency use authorization for Paxlovid.. Available at: https://www.fda.gov/media/155050/download. Accessed August 20, 2022.

119. Hammond J, Leister-Tebbe H, Gardner A, et al. Oral nirmatrelvir for high-risk, nonhospitalized adults with covid-19. N Engl J Med 2022;386(15): 1397–408.

120. Administration FaD. Fact sheet for healthcare providers: emergency use authorization for bebtelovimab. Available at: https://www.fda.gov/media/156152/download. Accessed August 20, 2022.

121. Group RC, Horby P, Lim WS, et al. Dexamethasone in hospitalized patients with covid-19. N Engl J Med 2021;384(8):693–704.

122. Kalil AC, Patterson TF, Mehta AK, et al. Baricitinib plus remdesivir for hospitalized adults with covid-19. N Engl J Med 2021;384(9):795–807.

123. Wolfe CR, Tomashek KM, Patterson TF, et al. Baricitinib versus dexamethasone for adults hospitalised with COVID-19 (ACTT-4): a randomised, double-blind, double placebo-controlled trial. Lancet Respir Med 2022. https://doi.org/10.1016/S2213-2600(22)00088-1.

124. Group RC. Baricitinib in patients admitted to hospital with COVID-19 (RECOVERY): a randomised,

controlled, open-label, platform trial and updated meta-analysis. Lancet 2022;400(10349):359–68.

125. Guimaraes PO, Quirk D, Furtado RH, et al. Tofacitinib in patients hospitalized with covid-19 pneumonia. N Engl J Med 2021;385(5):406–15.

126. Group RC. Tocilizumab in patients admitted to hospital with COVID-19 (RECOVERY): a randomised, controlled, open-label, platform trial. Lancet 2021; 397(10285):1637–45.

127. Investigators R-C, Gordon AC, Mouncey PR, et al. Interleukin-6 receptor antagonists in critically ill patients with covid-19. N Engl J Med Apr 22 2021; 384(16):1491–502.

128. WHO. Interim statement on COVID-19 vaccination for children. Available at: https://www.who.int/news/item/11-08-2022-interim-statement-on-covid-19-vaccination-for-children. Accessed 8 20, 2022.

129. Infectious Diseases CO. COVID-19 vaccines in infants, children, and adolescents. Pediatrics 2022. https://doi.org/10.1542/peds.2022-058700.

130. Fleming-Dutra KE, Wallace M, Moulia DL, et al. Interim recommendations of the advisory committee on immunization Practices for use of Moderna and pfizer-BioNTech COVID-19 vaccines in children aged 6 Months-5 Years - United States, june 2022. MMWR Morb Mortal Wkly Rep 2022; 71(26):859–68.

131. Young-Xu Y, Epstein L, Marconi VC, et al. Tixagevimab/cilgavimab for prevention of COVID-19 during the omicron surge: retrospective analysis of national VA electronic data. medRxiv 2022. https://doi.org/10.1101/2022.05.28.22275716. 2022.05.28.22275716.

132. Al Jurdi A, Morena L, Cote M, et al. Tixagevimab/cilgavimab pre-exposure prophylaxis is associated with lower breakthrough infection risk in vaccinated solid organ transplant recipients during the omicron wave. Am J Transplant 2022. https://doi.org/10.1111/ajt.17128.

133. Laboratory-confirmed COVID-19-associated hospitalizations. Centers for disease control and prevention. Available at: https://gis.cdc.gov/grasp/COVIDNet/COVID19_3.html. Accessed June 28, 2022.

134. The COVKID project women's institute for independent social enquiry. Available at: https://www.covkidproject.org. Accessed June 29, 2022.

Coronavirus Disease-2019 in Pregnancy

Jose Rojas-Suarez, MD, MSc[a],*, Jezid Miranda, MD, PhD[a,b]

KEYWORDS

- Acute respiratory distress syndrome • COVID-19 • Perinatal outcomes • Pregnancy • SARS-CoV-2

KEY POINTS

- Pregnant women are susceptible to coronavirus disease-2019 (COVID-19) and are at higher risk of complications than the general population.
- COVID-19 infection during pregnancy severely affects maternal health, increasing the risk of hospitalization, the requirement of mechanical ventilatory support, and maternal death.
- COVID-19 infection during pregnancy increases the risk of pregnancy complications such as preeclampsia and preterm birth.
- Despite the lack of evidence in obstetrics, pharmacologic and nonpharmacological therapies during pregnancy diminish severe complications and should be balanced against the potential risks.
- Vaccination during pregnancy is safe and reduces the risk of severe disease.

INTRODUCTION

Coronavirus disease 2019 (COVID-19) infection during pregnancy is associated with severe complications and adverse effects for the mother, fetus, and neonate.[1,2] Pregnancy constitutes a risk factor for hospitalization, intensive care admission, and death among COVID-19 women of reproductive age.[3] The physiologic adaptations in the respiratory system during pregnancy impose a significant challenge in managing pregnant women who develop acute respiratory distress syndrome (ARDS) in the context of COVID-19 infection.[4] In addition, the thromboembolic risk of pregnancy increases the likelihood of thrombosis, including pulmonary embolism.[5]

Even though this situation was identified during the pandemic, many pregnant women died without access to intensive care units (ICus).[6] COVID-19 infection might increase the risk of preterm delivery and stillbirth.[7] Conversely, inconsistent evidence suggests that vertical transmission is probable but infrequent.[8] Despite all pregnancy-related complications during the COVID-19 pandemic, many pregnant patients

decline to be vaccinated, assuming uncertainty regarding the safety and protection against current variants. This review summarizes the lessons learned in assessing, managing, and caring for pregnant patients with COVID-19 infection.

Epidemiology

The epidemiology of COVID-19, including its complications, should be demarcated to the historical moment (prevaccination or postvaccination), the geographic region, and the predominant COVID-19 variant, among others. Global maternal and fetal outcomes have worsened during the COVID-19 pandemic, increasing maternal deaths, stillbirth, ruptured ectopic pregnancies, and maternal depression in many regions. Some of these outcomes show a considerable disparity between low–middle-income (LMICs) and high-income countries (HICs). Comorbidities such as diabetes, hypertension, and asthma were more frequent in HICs. In contrast, others, such as hypothyroidism, anemia, and coinfections, were more prevalent in LMICs, and the overall risk of adverse pregnancy outcomes was higher in LMICs than in

a Intensive Care and Obstetric Research Group (GRICIO), Department of Obstetrics and Gynecology, Universidad de Cartagena, Colombia; b Department of Obstetrics and Gynecology, Maternal-Fetal Medicine Division, Centro Hospitalario Serena del Mar, Cartagena, Colombia
* Corresponding author.
E-mail address: jrojass@unicartagena.edu.co

Clin Chest Med 44 (2023) 373–384
https://doi.org/10.1016/j.ccm.2022.11.015
0272-5231/23/© 2022 Elsevier Inc. All rights reserved.

HICs, including abortion, stillbirths, and maternal death. Significant perinatal adverse events, such as neonatal deaths, pneumonia, and neonatal severe acute respiratory syndrome coronavirus 2 (SARS-CoV-2) infection, are generally reported in LMICs.[9]

Nevertheless, some lessons were learned after the worst period of the pandemic, highlighting an urgent need to prioritize safe, accessible, and equitable maternity care in response to this pandemic and future health crises.[7] COVID-19 affected antenatal care by decreasing the number of visits and unscheduled care and increasing virtual or remote antenatal care and hospitalizations. This suggests that reduced maternity health-care-seeking and health care providers during the COVID-19 pandemic influenced the pregnancy outcomes observed during the pandemic.[10] In LMICs, evidence describing telemedicine services did not show the expected benefit in the pregnant population by supplementing the existing protocols in antenatal care.[11]

CLINICAL RELEVANCE
Risk Factors for Severe Coronavirus Disease-2019 During Pregnancy

The evidence regarding COVID-19 and pregnancy has changed with the advance of the pandemic. The evidence suggests that some risk factors, including comorbidities and ethnicity, increase the likelihood of pregnant women being symptomatic.[12] Preexisting diabetes (not gestational diabetes) was associated with severe COVID-19 in pregnancy (odds ratio [OR]: 2.12; 95% confidence interval [CI]: 1.62 to 2.78).[13] In SARS-CoV-2 (+) pregnant women, Rh- status was associated with a lower risk of symptomatic COVID-19, with an increase in obstetric hemorrhage and preterm premature rupture of membranes in pregnant women with Rh+ and blood A group, respectively.[14] A systematic review and meta-analysis focused on the relationship between comorbidities and COVID-19 severity, including 13 studies and 154 deceased patients. The presence of at least one severe comorbidity showed a twofold increased risk of death. Overall, overweight (body mass index > 25 kg/m^2) and obesity doubled the risk of death, with no differences in gestational diabetes or asthma. ICU admission was related to fivefold increased risk of death, with no difference in respiratory support or mechanical ventilation.[15] Another study showed the main predictors of mortality (increase in the odds of maternal mortality (OR: 1.15, [95% CI: 1.05 to 1.26]) were the need for invasive mechanical ventilation and a more prolonged ICU stay.[16]

Pathophysiology of Coronavirus Disease-2019 Complications in Pregnancy

During the pandemic, pregnant women were at significant risk of presenting with more severe forms of COVID-19 infection and a high risk of pregnancy complications.[17] COVID-19 causes a severe systemic inflammatory response associated with vascular alterations that could be of particular interest considering the physiologic changes in the immune, respiratory, cardiovascular, coagulation, and renal systems during pregnancy.[18] Alterations of the respiratory system include mucosal edema, capillary engorgement of nasal and oropharyngeal mucosa, and laryngeal tissues. In addition, the diaphragm is displaced 4 cm upward, decreasing functional residual capacity by 10% to 25% at term. In the cardiovascular system, there is a reduction in systemic vascular resistance that allows the homeostatic control of pregnancy-related hemodynamic changes, an increase in cardiac output, an expanded blood volume, and a decrease in blood pressure. Based on these changes, despite the low level of evidence and some debate raised by the difficulties in achieving improvements in oxygenation during COVID-19, many experts and clinical societies propose an O_2 saturation (SpO_2) at $\geq$ 95%.[19]

SARS-CoV-2 causes severe alterations in the cardiovascular system, including the recruitment of inflammatory leukocytes in the vascular tissue, leading to tissue damage and cytokine release, followed by disseminated intravascular coagulation. To an extent, specific clinical responses of pregnant women to COVID-19 could be related to changes in the levels of ACE2 with reduced sensitivity to Ang II.[20] In terms of severity, thrombotic microangiopathy was invoked as one of the mechanisms in severe COVID-19 cases. The protease ADAMTS13 (A Disintegrin-like and Metalloprotease with thrombospondin type 1 motif no. 13) is a marker of microangiopathy responsible for controlling von Willebrand multimer size. Recent evidence shows an imbalance of the von Willebrand/ADAMTS13 axis in pregnant women with COVID-19, indicating that nulliparous women group O showed Willebrand/ADAMTS-13 ratios significantly lower than those in non-O. In this population, the Willebrand to ADAMTS13 ratio was associated with preterm delivery.[21]

Obstetric Complications Associated with Coronavirus Disease-2019 During Pregnancy

Infection in pregnant women was associated with a higher risk of adverse pregnancy outcomes, such as fetal growth restriction, premature rupture of membranes, fetal distress, preterm birth (delivery before 37 weeks of gestation), spontaneous abortion, and stillbirth.[2] SARS-CoV-2 during pregnancy was associated with a higher risk of developing preeclampsia.[22,23] **Table 1** describes accumulative evidence from a total of 706 pregnant women with COVID-19 in 18 countries, demonstrating that the risk of obstetric complications varies according to symptom status.[2] An observational cohort study from the United States involving 683,905 patients, including the pre- and postpandemic periods (2019 to 2021), showed that women with COVID-19 were more likely to experience both early and late preterm birth, preeclampsia, disseminated intravascular coagulopathy, pulmonary edema, the need for invasive mechanical ventilation and in-hospital mortality than women without COVID-19.[24]

In pregnant patients with COVID-19, the cesarean section rate was high, and iatrogenic preterm birth was reported to be as high as 25%.[25] A recent meta-analysis including 42 studies and 438,548 pregnant women reported that COVID-19 during pregnancy increased the risk of preeclampsia (OR: 2.11), preterm birth (OR: 1.82), and stillbirth (OR: 2.11).[26] Another meta-analysis including 790,754 pregnant women also described an increased risk of preeclampsia in patients infected with SARS-CoV-2.[23] A meta-analysis including 45 studies with a low-to-moderate risk of bias reported 1,843,665 pregnancies during the pandemic (2020) and 23,564,552 pregnancies during a variable pre-pandemic period (from 2002 to 2019, depending on the studies included). This meta-analysis did not find a difference in the odds of stillbirth between the pandemic and pre-pandemic periods, with an increase in mean birth weight during the pandemic compared with the pre-pandemic period and a reduction in unadjusted but not adjusted estimates of preterm birth.[16]

Fetal and Neonatal Disease

A link between fetal or neonatal disease and COVID-19 has not been well elucidated. During the pandemic, some data support that being pregnant with COVID-19 increases the risk of adverse pregnancy and birth outcomes and a low risk of congenital transmission.[27] Pregnant women who test positive for COVID-19 seem to be at a higher risk of lower birth weight and premature birth.[28] In a recent publication, the overall miscarriage rate in pregnant women with COVID-19 ranged between 15.3% (95% CI: 10.94 to 20.59) and 23.1% (95% CI: 13.17 to 34.95), a miscarriage rate within the normal population range.[29]

The vertical transmission of SARS-CoV-2 has been reported but remains highly debated.[30] A recent assessment of 177 pregnancies with a confirmed infection by reverse transcriptase-PCR using nasopharyngeal swabs within the first 24 to 48 hours of life and after 2 weeks of life showed that 5.1% of babies were SARS-CoV-2 positive in the neonatal period, with 1.7% considered intrauterine and 3.4% considered intrapartum or early postnatal transmission cases.[31] **Table 2** shows the rate of positivity of SARS-CoV-2 according to the type of biological sample. Thus, although rare, the intrauterine transmission of SARS-CoV-2 is possible, with early postnatal transmission occurring more frequently. SARS-CoV-2 has been isolated in the human placenta.[32] Many placentas showed histopathologic findings in pregnant women with COVID-19, suggesting placental hypoperfusion and inflammation (**Fig. 1**).[31,33] Angiotensin-converting enzyme 2 (ACE2) is the receptor of SARS-CoV-2, the placental mRNA expression of ACE2 is gestational age-dependent and plays a key role in pregnancy infection and complications.[34] Infected newborns reported in the literature remained asymptomatic or had mild symptoms resolved during follow-up.[35]

EVALUATION
Clinical Assessment and Disease Severity

Most pregnant women with COVID-19 present with mild-to-moderate symptoms (81% to 86% of cases) and are monitored as outpatients for 7 to 14 days after the onset of symptoms.[36] More than 70% of infected women were in their third trimester, with no evidence that supports an association between gestational age and COVID-19 mortality and morbidity.[37] However, SARS-CoV-2 was more severe in pregnant women than in the general population, with an increased risk of hospital admission, with 5% developing a severe form requiring ICU admission and approximately 35% requiring intubation, with a maternal mortality of close to 2.7%.[25] The most common symptoms were fever, cough, chest pain, dyspnea, and fatigue.[38]

Pregnant patients appear to present more commonly with more advanced COVID-19 chest tomography findings than the general adult population, but characteristic laboratory abnormalities are similar to the general population.[38] Early in 2020, the World Health Organization (WHO) proposed a guideline describing a clinical categorization of COVID-19 that has been used indistinctly for the obstetric population. This illness severity in COVID-19 defined patients as critical (criteria for ARDS, sepsis, septic shock, and the provision

Table 1
According to symptom status, the risk ratio for maternal, and perinatal outcomes among pregnant women with coronavirus disease-2019

	Risk Ratio (95% Confidence Interval)
Asymptomatic	
Preeclampsia	1.63 (1.01 to 2.63)
Preterm birth	0.99 (0.72 to 1.36)
Severe perinatal morbidity and mortality index	1.08 (0.69 to 1.69)
Severe neonatal morbidity index	1.42 (0.465 to 3.08)
Maternal morbidity and mortality index	1.24 (1.0 to 1.54)
Any symptoms	
Preeclampsia	2.00 (1.34 to 2.99)
Preterm birth	2.76 (1.77 to 4.30)
Severe perinatal morbidity and mortality index	2.79 (1.57 to 4.95)
Severe neonatal morbidity index	4.66 (1.93 to 11.3)
Maternal morbidity and mortality index	1.76 (1.49 to 2.08)

Maternal morbidity and mortality index includes at least one of the following complications during pregnancy: vaginal bleeding, pregnancy-induced hypertension, preeclampsia, eclampsia, HELLP, preterm labor, infections requiring antibiotics or maternal death, admission to intensive care unit, or referral for higher dependency care. *Severe neonatal morbidity index* includes at least one of the following morbidities: bronchopulmonary dysplasia, hypoxic-ischemic encephalopathy, sepsis, anemia requiring transfusion, patent ductus arteriosus, intraventricular hemorrhage, necrotizing enterocolitis, or retinopathy of prematurity. *The severe perinatal morbidity* and mortality index includes any morbidities listed in the SNMI, intrauterine or neonatal death, or neonatal intensive care unit stay >7 d.

(*Data from* Villar J, Ariff S, Gunier RB, et al. Maternal and Neonatal Morbidity and Mortality Among Pregnant Women With and Without COVID-19 Infection: The INTERCOVID Multinational Cohort Study [published correction appears in JAMA Pediatr. 2022 Jan 1;176(1):104]. JAMA Pediatr. 2021;175(8):817-826.)

of invasive or noninvasive mechanical ventilation or vasopressor therapy), severe (oxygen saturation < 90% on room air, signs of pneumonia, or severe respiratory distress) and nonsevere (in the absence of any severe or critical COVID-19).[39] International societies, including the Society for Maternal and Fetal Medicine (SMFM) and the Royal College of Obstetricians and Gynecologists (RCOG), proposed a disease severity classification based on oxygenation (**Box 1**). Almost half of all patients with COVID-19 admitted to the ICU developed persistent critical illness, requiring high resource utilization. Refractory hypoxemia remained significantly associated with mortality, yet evidence-based ARDS interventions, particularly prone positioning in the late second and third trimesters, were either not implemented or delayed, resulting in worse outcomes. Real-time service evaluation techniques offer opportunities to assess the level of care and improve the protocolized implementation of evidence-based ARDS interventions, which might be associated with improvements in survival.[40]

THERAPEUTIC OPTIONS
General Considerations

Clinical guidelines have made several recommendations for pregnancy during COVID-19: (1) hospitalization only for severe disease; (2) fetal growth scan after SARS-COV-2 infection; and (3) thromboprophylaxis with low molecular weight heparin (LMWH). In addition, a general agreement, supported by all current guidelines, is not to recommend cesarean section solely for maternal COVID-19 infection. A vaccine booster is recommended 6 months after the primary vaccination series. Inpatient management depends on disease severity. To assess clinical deterioration, the SMFM suggests a vital sign assessment every 4 to 8 hours for patients in the general ward and every 2 to 4 hours in cases of severe disease. Continuous monitoring (invasive or noninvasive) in critical illness is preferred as indicated or depending on hospital resources and policies. The inability to maintain oxygen saturation >94% with supplemental oxygen therapy, hemodynamic instability, or the presence of warning signs through any early warning systems (EWSs) should be indications for ICU consultation and transfer. Furthermore, some current and validated obstetric warning systems include SpO_2 as a crucial parameter to identify patients at risk of rapid deterioration.[41]

Pharmacologic Interventions

Six studies involving a total of 599 women reported pharmacologic treatment of COVID-19 in

Table 2
Rate of positivity for severe acute respiratory syndrome coronavirus 2 in maternal, fetal, and neonatal biological samples among pregnant women with coronavirus disease-2019

Sample Site	% (n/N)
Nasopharyngeal swab	2.88 (27/936)
Placenta	7.69 (2/26)
Cord blood	2.94 (1/34)
Amniotic fluid	0 (0/51)
Neonatal urine sample	0 (0/17)
Neonatal rectal swab	9.67(3/31)
IgM neonatal serology	3.66 (3/82)

Data from Kotlyar AM, Grechukhina O, Chen A, et al. Vertical transmission of coronavirus disease 2019: a systematic review and meta-analysis. Am J Obstet Gynecol. 2021;224(1):35-53.e3.

pregnancy that included antiviral therapy, systemic corticosteroids, antibiotics, and immunotherapy; however, the types and doses of the medications were not specified.[42] Antenatal corticosteroids may be used routinely for fetal lung maturation between 24 and 34 weeks. However, clinicians should make decisions in those < 24 or > 34 weeks of gestation on a case-by-case basis. Magnesium sulfate may be used cautiously for seizure prevention in the context of severe preeclampsia and fetal neuroprotection to reduce the risk of cerebral palsy associated with prematurity in those with hypoxia and renal compromise. Thromboprophylaxis in pregnant patients with COVID-19 should consider disease severity, the timing of delivery to disease onset, inpatient vs. outpatient status, underlying comorbidities, and contraindications to the use of anticoagulation.[43] To date, corticosteroids, particularly dexamethasone, are the most proven and recommended treatment for pregnant patients with COVID-19 who are mechanically ventilated or require supplemental oxygen.[44] Although no subgroup analysis was performed on pregnant women, the RCOG and the WHO stated that no harm is expected from steroid use. Concerns about pregnancy safety led to recommending prednisolone as the first choice instead of dexamethasone because prednisolone is extensively metabolized in the placenta, with minimal transfer to the fetus. Other

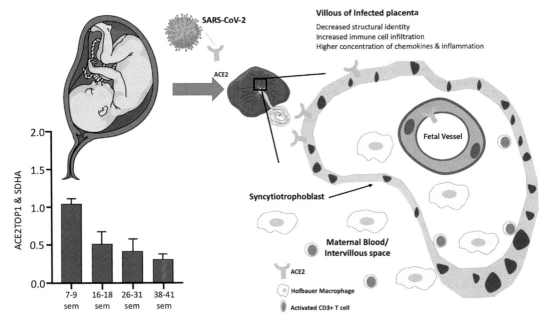

Fig. 1. Inflammatory responses in the placenta upon SARS-CoV-2 infection. Infected placentas show extensive infiltration of maternal immune cells. Angiotensin-converting enzyme 2 (ACE2) is the receptor of SARS-CoV-2 and plays a key role in pregnancy infection and complications. The placental mRNA expression of ACE2 is gestational age-dependent, increasing from the first- (7 to 9 weeks) through the third trimester (38 to 41 weeks). ACE2 is highly expressed in maternal-fetal interface cells, including stromal cells and perivascular cells of decidua, the cytotrophoblast, and syncytiotrophoblast in the placenta. In response to maternal-fetal infection, the syncytiotrophoblast shows increased chemokines and inflammatory markers expression.[33,34] ACE2, angiotensin-converting enzyme 2; SDHA, succinate-ubiquinone oxidoreductase; TOP1, topoisomerase 1. (*Adapted from* Argueta LB, Lacko LA, Bram Y, et al. Inflammatory responses in the placenta upon SARS-CoV-2 infection late in pregnancy. iScience. 2022;25(5):104223.)

> **Box 1**
> **COVID-19 classification based on maternal oxygenation**
>
> Asymptomatic:
>
> A positive test with no symptoms.
>
> Mild disease:
>
> A positive test, but not requiring oxygen and no evidence of sepsis.
>
> Moderate
>
> A positive test and symptoms of lower respiratory tract infection (dyspnea, abnormal blood gases, and persistent fever) but without oxygen desaturation ($SpO_2 < 94\%$ at room air) or requiring oxygen therapy to achieve this oxygen level.
>
> Severe:
>
> A positive test and tachypnea (respiratory rate >30 breaths per minute, $SpO_2 < 94\%$ at room air or a ratio of arterial partial pressure of oxygen to fraction of inspired oxygen < 300 mm Hg).
>
> Critical:
>
> A positive test and multiorgan dysfunction, septic shock, or need for respiratory support with high flow nasal cannula (HFNC), noninvasive or invasive mechanical ventilation (NIMV and IMV).
>
> *Adapted from* the Society for Maternal and Fetal Medicine (SMFM) and the Royal College of Obstetricians and Gynecologists (RCOG). Available at: https://www.smfm.org/. Accessed Sep 7 2022.

options are methylprednisolone or hydrocortisone for pregnant women.[45]

Antivirals with different mechanisms of action, such as protease inhibitors and nucleotide or nucleoside analogs, have been proposed for COVID-19 treatment.[46] Although the efficacy and safety profile of remdesivir among pregnant women remains inconclusive, a recent systematic review reporting nine case reports and case series showed clinical recovery after remdesivir treatments.[47] Remdesivir improved the clinical condition of pregnant patients with COVID-19, especially those with a better clinical status at baseline and who received treatment earlier in the course of the disease.[47,48] The current WHO guidelines updates the use of remdesivir for patients with nonsevere COVID-19: its use reduces hospital admission in the highest risk group, although with little or no impact on mortality.[49]

Adverse reactions and transaminase enzyme levels should be followed after remdesivir administration; the most common adverse event following remdesivir treatment is transaminitis.[47]

There are sufficient data on the role of tocilizumab, an interleukin-6 antagonist, in improving outcomes, including survival, in hospitalized patients with hypoxia with evidence of systemic inflammation. Tocilizumab improved survival and clinical outcomes in hospitalized COVID-19 patients with hypoxia and systemic inflammation.[50] Based on these results, the National Institute for Health and Care Excellence (NICE) guidance recommends using tocilizumab in hospitalized patients who have or had completed a course of steroids, an increase in C-reactive protein (CRP) > 75, the need for supplemental oxygen, or within 48 h of initiating mechanical ventilation. Data on the use of tocilizumab in pregnancy are scarce, but no adverse effects have been reported. The RCOG recommends offering tocilizumab to pregnant women when they fit the criteria. The decision should involve a multidisciplinary team (MDT) to analyze whether the benefits outweigh the risks.[51]

Although hydroxychloroquine and lopinavir/ritonavir are used during pregnancy and lactation within clinical trials, data from nonpregnant populations have not shown benefits. Although some studies describe the effects of hydroxychloroquine and antibiotics, this has now been shown not to be beneficial and is not recommended for either nonpregnant patients or pregnant women. Adverse events with treatment were three-fold higher than placebo, but very few serious adverse events were found.[52] Case reports suggest that convalescent plasma administered to pregnant women with severe COVID-19 benefits both the mother and the fetus. However, these studies suffer from relevant reporting bias.[53] Clinical trials to investigate the use of convalescent plasma for COVID-19 during pregnancy are lacking. More recent evidence showed no benefit, including in pregnant and nonpregnant populations.[54]

The use of convalescent plasma in patients who tested negative for anti-SARS-CoV-2 antibodies at baseline has not been associated with improved survival (RR 0.94, 95% CI 0.87 to 1.02). In patients with COVID-19, treatment with convalescent plasma, compared with control, was not associated with lower all-cause mortality or improved disease progression, irrespective of disease severity and baseline antibody status.[53] Immunomodulators (tacrolimus), interferon, and inhaled nitric oxide in pregnancy and lactation are not routinely recommended and need further evaluation.[55]

Nonpharmacological Interventions for Coronavirus Disease-2019 in Pregnancy

In the context of moderate to severe COVID-19 infection, the same treatment principles apply to pregnant women and nonpregnant patients regarding nonpharmacological interventions, such as oxygen supplementation or mechanical ventilation. However, invasive mechanical ventilation is arduous in pregnant patients. This is due to the increased demand for oxygen in pregnancy secondary to a higher metabolic rate and increased oxygen consumption. The gravid uterus contributes to ventilatory impairment, and achieving the required volumes during mechanical ventilation can be challenging.[56]

Prone positioning has been proven to help ventilate patients in the presence of ARDS. Although no trials include pregnant women, techniques describe how proning can be performed in this group of patients. For example, some authors describe how they place pillows in a specific way to put the pregnant woman in a comfortable position without compromising the pregnancy.[57] However, this should not be practiced in patients with a wound from a recent cesarean section (first 2 weeks) or when pregnancy is over 34 weeks pregnant; the heavily pregnant uterus can make this position more difficult. Furthermore, after 24 to 28 weeks, there is the risk of aortocaval compression when proning a pregnant woman.

Oxygen Therapy, High Flow Nasal Cannula, and Ventilatory Support

International guidelines recommend maintaining a $SpO_2 > 94\%$ in pregnancy. Another recommendation focuses on supplemental oxygen modalities, including a face mask or high-flow nasal cannula (HFNC). Using HFNC in patients with severe COVID-19 decreased the need for mechanical ventilation support and time for clinical recovery. Despite these benefits, pregnancy-specific or COVID-19-related interventions are poorly reported in the published literature. None of the randomized trials using HFNC reported outcomes in pregnant women or pregnancy was an exclusion criterion.[58] Comparative data for pregnant women for treatments proven effective in the general population lack clinically meaningful interpretation. Thus, despite a potential benefit, there is little evidence to support recommendations regarding using HFNC in obstetrics.

Eleven studies reported nonpharmacological interventions, of which mechanical ventilation was reported in six studies and oxygen administration in eight. In total, 1738 women were included in these studies; 240 were exposed to interventions, 28 patients had mechanical ventilation, and 212 had oxygen administration.[42] Prone positioning remains a well-proven intervention in ARDS and should be considered in pregnant women when indicated. We recognize that proning might not be effective in all cases. However, prone positioning is an option to improve oxygenation in patients with moderate to severe hypoxemia ($PaFiO_2 \leq 150$ mm Hg) before considering delivering a premature infant or maternal cannulation for extracorporeal membrane oxygenation (ECMO).[57] The use of ECMO in pregnancy has increased, and evidence supports its use, feasibility, and favorable outcomes. A recent publication, including six ECMO centers from three different continents and 60 cases over 10 years, describes a maternal survival rate of 87% with an acceptable neonatal outcome.[59] In summary, proven therapies from the nonpregnant critically ill COVID-19 patient population can be extrapolated to critically ill pregnant patients, resulting in good maternal ICU survival and limited extreme premature delivery. Furthermore, in very premature gestations (<32 weeks), the continuation of pregnancy during mechanical ventilation and prone positioning is feasible with good fetal monitoring (**Fig. 2**).[60]

Delivery and Anesthesia

Pregnancy-specific interventions, including delivery or anesthesia, were related to the severity of COVID-19. Scientific societies such as the Society for Obstetric Anesthesia and Perinatology (SOAP) and the SMFM issued recommendations for types of anesthesia for pregnant women with COVID-19. However, no trials have been conducted regarding the management or outcomes of such women. The liberal use of neuraxial labor analgesia may reduce the need for emergency general anesthesia.[61] A systematic review found an association between having a cesarean section and being admitted to the ICU or having COVID-19 pneumonia. The decision to proceed with a cesarean section may be prompted by the need to improve ventilation.[42] In the event of cesarean delivery, neuraxial anesthesia was performed over general anesthesia.[62]

PREVENTION
Vaccination in Pregnancy and Lactation

SARS-CoV-2 mRNA vaccines are the most important strategy for preventing maternal illness.[63] Vaccination prevented pregnant women from SARS-CoV-2 infection (OR: 0.50 [95% CI: 0.35 to 0.79]) and COVID-19-related hospitalization (OR: 0.50 [95% CI: 0.31 to 0.82]). Messenger RNA

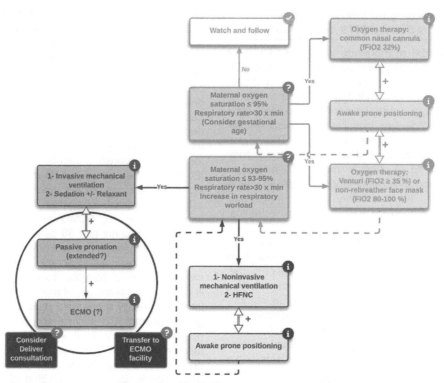

Fig. 2. Flowchart of management of severely critically ill pregnant women with COVID-19.

vaccines reduced the risk of infection in pregnant women (OR: 0.13 [95% CI: 0.03 to 0.57]).[64] Moreover, COVID-19 mRNA vaccination in pregnancy seems safe and is associated with a reduction in stillbirth.[65] However, excluding pregnant women from the initial COVID-19 vaccine trials resulted in a significant hesitancy to accept COVID-19 vaccination among pregnant women around the globe.[66] Worldwide analyses have reported an acceptance rate of 50% in pregnant women and 60% in breastfeeding women.[67] Safety concerns are the most common reason for the decline in COVID-19 vaccination during pregnancy.[68] There is evidence that administering a COVID-19 vaccine is safe and poses no additional risk to the breastfeeding woman or the breastfed baby.[63,69] After COVID-19 vaccination, pregnant patients develop a robust immune response, conferring protective immunity to newborns through breast milk and placental transfer and providing humoral immunity to the infant against COVID-19.[70–74]

In a population-based study including 24,288 singleton livebirths, the risk of preterm birth and small birth weight were similar between newborns prenatally exposed and unexposed to maternal vaccination.[75] Furthermore, the rate of congenital malformations in the exposed population was not higher than that in the unexposed population.[75] Therefore, professional associations and government health authorities should recommend COVID-19 vaccines to breastfeeding women, as the potential benefits of maternal vaccination outweigh the risks.[76] Vaccination campaigns are urgently needed to drive more confidence into the vaccine to help reduce the spread of the infection and the possible consequences during pregnancy.[67] However, pros and cons should be discussed extensively with both parents.[77]

SUMMARY

Although there is conflicting evidence, pregnant women were a potentially vulnerable population during the COVID-19 pandemic, with a significant risk of developing severe forms of COVID-19 and pregnancy complications. International guidelines recommend maintaining a SpO_2 >94% in pregnancy and supplemental oxygen delivery with a face mask or HFNC. Most COVID-19 pregnant women present with mild to moderate symptoms and can be monitored as outpatients for 7 to 14 days after the onset of symptoms. However, SARS-CoV-2 is more severe in pregnant women than in the general population, with an increased risk of hospital admission and severe forms requiring ICU admission, intubation, and mechanical ventilation. Finally, SARS-CoV-2 mRNA vaccines are the most important strategy for preventing maternal illness.

CLINICS CARE POINTS

- Coronavirus disease-2019 (COVID-19) infection during pregnancy is associated with severe complications and adverse effects for the mother, fetus, and neonate.
- Although there is conflicting evidence, pregnant women were a potentially vulnerable population during the COVID-19 pandemic, with a significant risk of presenting with severe COVID-19 and pregnancy complications. In addition, pregnancy is a risk factor for hospitalization, intensive care admission, and death among COVID-19 women of reproductive age.
- International societies have proposed a disease severity classification based on oxygen requirement and saturation. In addition, treatment recommendations do not differ significantly from the general population.
- SARS-CoV-2 mRNA vaccines are an essential strategy for preventing maternal illness and should be encouraged in all pregnant women.

DISCLOSURE

The authors have no relevant conflicts of interest.

REFERENCES

1. Metz TD, Clifton RG, Hughes BL, et al. Association of SARS-CoV-2 infection with serious maternal morbidity and mortality from obstetric complications. JAMA 2022;327:748–59.
2. Villar J, Ariff S, Gunier RB, et al. Maternal and neonatal morbidity and mortality among pregnant women with and without COVID-19 infection: the INTERCOVID multinational cohort study. JAMA Pediatr 2021;175:817–26.
3. Ellington S, Strid P, Tong VT, et al. Characteristics of women of reproductive age with laboratory-confirmed SARS-CoV-2 infection by pregnancy status — United States, january 22–june 7, 2020. MMWR Morb Mortal Wkly Rep 2020;69:769–75.
4. DeBolt CA, Bianco A, Limaye MA, et al. Pregnant women with severe or critical coronavirus disease 2019 have increased composite morbidity compared with nonpregnant matched controls. Am J Obstet Gynecol 2021;224:510.e1–12.
5. Servante J, Swallow G, Thornton JG, et al. Haemostatic and thrombo-embolic complications in pregnant women with COVID-19: a systematic review and critical analysis. BMC Pregnancy Childbirth 2021;21:108.
6. Maza-Arnedo F, Paternina-Caicedo A, Sosa CG, et al. Maternal mortality linked to COVID-19 in Latin America: results from a multi-country collaborative database of 447 deaths. Lancet Reg Heal Am 2022;12:100269.
7. Chmielewska B, Barratt I, Townsend R, et al. Effects of the COVID-19 pandemic on maternal and perinatal outcomes: a systematic review and meta-analysis. Lancet Glob Heal 2021;9:e759–72.
8. Hu X, Gao J, Luo X, et al. Severe acute respiratory syndrome coronavirus 2 (SARS-CoV-2) vertical transmission in neonates Born to mothers with coronavirus disease 2019 (COVID-19) pneumonia. Obstet Gynecol 2020;136:65–7.
9. Gajbhiye RK, Sawant MS, Kuppusamy P, et al. Differential impact of COVID-19 in pregnant women from high-income countries and low- to middle-income countries: a systematic review and meta-analysis. Int J Gynecol Obstet 2021;155:48–56.
10. Townsend R, Chmielewska B, Barratt I, et al. Global changes in maternity care provision during the COVID-19 pandemic: a systematic review and meta-analysis. EClinicalMedicine 2021;37:100947.
11. Goyal LD, Garg P, Verma M, et al. Effect of restrictions imposed due to COVID-19 pandemic on the antenatal care and pregnancy outcomes: a prospective observational study from rural North India. BMJ Open 2022;12:e059701.
12. Khan DSA, Hamid LR, Ali A, et al. Differences in pregnancy and perinatal outcomes among symptomatic versus asymptomatic COVID-19-infected pregnant women: a systematic review and meta-analysis. BMC Pregnancy Childbirth 2021;21:801.
13. Allotey J, Stallings E, Bonet M, et al. Clinical manifestations, risk factors, and maternal and perinatal outcomes of coronavirus disease 2019 in pregnancy: living systematic review and meta-analysis. BMJ 2020;370:m3320.
14. Sainz Bueno JA, Cerrillos González L, Abascal-Saiz A, et al. Association of ABO and Rh blood groups with obstetric outcomes in SARS-CoV-2 infected pregnancies: a prospective study with a multivariate analysis. Eur J Obstet Gynecol Reprod Biol 2021;264:41–8.
15. La Verde M, Riemma G, Torella M, et al. Maternal death related to COVID-19: a systematic review and meta-analysis focused on maternal comorbidities and clinical characteristics. Int J Gynecol Obstet 2021;154:212–9.
16. Yang J, D'Souza R, Kharrat A, et al. Coronavirus disease 2019 pandemic and pregnancy and neonatal outcomes in general population: a living systematic review and meta-analysis (updated Aug 14, 2021). Acta Obstet Gynecol Scand 2022;101:7–24.

17. Leung C, de Paiva KM. Is pregnancy a risk factor for in-hospital mortality in reproductive-aged women with SARS-CoV-2 infection? A nationwide retrospective observational cohort study. Int J Gynecol Obstet 2022;157:121–9.

18. Ayala-Ramírez P, González M, Escudero C, et al. Severe acute respiratory syndrome coronavirus 2 infection in pregnancy. A non-systematic review of clinical presentation, potential effects of physiological adaptations in pregnancy, and placental vascular alterations. Front Physiol 2022;13:785274.

19. Society for Maternal-Fetal Medicine. Society for maternal-fetal medicine management considerations for pregnant patients with COVID-19 developed with guidance from torre halscott, MD, MS; jason vaught, MD; and the SMFM COVID-19 task force. 2021. https://s3.amazonaws.com/cdn.smfm.org/media/2734/SMFM_COVID_Management_of_COVID_pos_preg_patients_2-2-21_(final).pdf. [Accessed 30 November 2021].

20. Liu H, Wang LL, Zhao SJ, et al. Why are pregnant women susceptible to COVID-19? An immunological viewpoint. J Reprod Immunol 2020;139:103122.

21. Yang J, D'Souza R, Kharrat A, et al. COVID-19 pandemic and population-level pregnancy and neonatal outcomes: a living systematic review and meta-analysis. Acta Obstet Gynecol Scand 2021; 100:1756–70.

22. Conde-Agudelo A, Romero R. SARS-CoV-2 infection during pregnancy and risk of preeclampsia: a systematic review and meta-analysis. Am J Obstet Gynecol 2022;226:68–89. e3.

23. Papageorghiou AT, Deruelle P, Gunier RB, et al. Preeclampsia and COVID-19: results from the INTERCOVID prospective longitudinal study. Am J Obstet Gynecol 2021;225:289.e1–17.

24. Litman EA, Yin Y, Nelson SJ, et al. Adverse perinatal outcomes in a large United States birth cohort during the COVID-19 pandemic. Am J Obstet Gynecol MFM 2022;4:100577.

25. Han Y, Ma H, Suo M, et al. Clinical manifestation, outcomes in pregnant women with COVID-19 and the possibility of vertical transmission: a systematic review of the current data. J Perinat Med 2020;48:912–24.

26. Wei SQ, Bilodeau-Bertrand M, Liu S, et al. The impact of COVID-19 on pregnancy outcomes: a systematic review and meta-analysis. CMAJ 2021; 193(16):E540–8.

27. Ciapponi A, Bardach A, Comandé D, et al. COVID-19 and pregnancy: an umbrella review of clinical presentation, vertical transmission, and maternal and perinatal outcomes. PLoS One 2021;16:e0253974.

28. Marchand G, Patil AS, Masoud AT, et al. Systematic review and meta-analysis of COVID-19 maternal and neonatal clinical features and pregnancy outcomes up to June 3, 2021. AJOG Glob Rep 2022;2:100049.

29. Cavalcante MB, de Melo Bezerra Cavalcante CT, Cavalcante ANM, et al. COVID-19 and miscarriage: from immunopathological mechanisms to actual clinical evidence. J Reprod Immunol 2021;148:103382.

30. Fenizia C, Biasin M, Cetin I, et al. Analysis of SARS-CoV-2 vertical transmission during pregnancy. Nat Commun 2020;11:5128.

31. Di Girolamo R, Khalil A, Alameddine S, et al. Placental histopathology after SARS-CoV-2 infection in pregnancy: a systematic review and meta-analysis. Am J Obstet Gynecol MFM 2021;3:100468.

32. Vivanti AJ, Vauloup-Fellous C, Prevot S, et al. Transplacental transmission of SARS-CoV-2 infection. Nat Commun 2020;11:3572.

33. Argueta LB, Lacko LA, Bram Y, et al. Inflammatory responses in the placenta upon SARS-CoV-2 infection late in pregnancy. iScience 2022;25:104223.

34. Bloise E, Zhang J, Nakpu J, et al. Expression of severe acute respiratory syndrome coronavirus 2 cell entry genes, angiotensin-converting enzyme 2 and transmembrane protease serine 2, in the placenta across gestation and at the maternal-fetal interface in pregnancies complicated by preterm. Am J Obstet Gynecol 2021;224(3):298.e1–8.

35. Vigil-Vázquez S, Carrasco-García I, Hernanz-Lobo A, et al. Impact of gestational COVID-19 on neonatal outcomes: is vertical infection possible? Pediatr Infect Dis J 2022;41:466–72.

36. Li N, Han L, Peng M, et al. Maternal and neonatal outcomes of pregnant women with coronavirus disease 2019 (COVID-19) pneumonia: a case-control study. Clin Infect Dis 2020;71:2035–41.

37. Leung C, Simões-E-Silva AC, Oliveira EA. Is in-hospital COVID-19 mortality and morbidity associated with gestational age? Ultrasound Obstet Gynecol 2022;60(2):234–42.

38. Oshay RR, Chen MYC, Fields BKK, et al. COVID-19 in pregnancy: a systematic review of chest CT findings and associated clinical features in 427 patients. Clin Imaging 2021;75:75–82.

39. Organization WH. Clinical management of COVID-19: interim guidance, 2020. Geneve, Switzerland: World Health Organization; 2020.

40. Patel BV, Haar S, Handslip R, et al. Natural history, trajectory, and management of mechanically ventilated COVID-19 patients in the United Kingdom. Intensive Care Med 2021;47:549–65.

41. Singh S, McGlennan A, England A, et al. A validation study of the CEMACH recommended modified early obstetric warning system (MEOWS). Anaesthesia 2012;67:12–8.

42. Giesbers S, Goh E, Kew T, et al. Treatment of COVID-19 in pregnant women: a systematic review

and meta-analysis. Eur J Obstet Gynecol Reprod Biol 2021;267:120–8.

43. Society for Maternal-Fetal Medicine. Society for Maternal-Fetal Medicine Management Considerations for Pregnant Patients With COVID-19 Developed with guidance from Torre Halscott, MD, MS; Jason Vaught, MD; and the SMFM COVID-19 Task Force. 2021.

44. Group RC. Dexamethasone in hospitalized patients with covid-19. N Engl J Med 2021;384:693–704.

45. RCOG. Coronavirus (COVID-19), infection in pregnancy. 2022. https://www.rcog.org.uk/guidance/coronavirus-covid-19-pregnancy-and-women-s-health/coronavirus-covid-19-infection-in-pregnancy/. [Accessed 27 December 2021].

46. Nasrallah S, Nguyen AQ, Hitchings L, et al. Pharmacological treatment in pregnant women with moderate symptoms of coronavirus disease 2019 (COVID-19) pneumonia. J Matern Neonatal Med 2021; 35(25):1–8.

47. Budi DS, Pratama NR, Wafa IA, et al. Remdesivir for pregnancy: a systematic review of antiviral therapy for COVID-19. Heliyon 2022;8(1). https://doi.org/10.1016/j.heliyon.2022.e08835.

48. Burwick RM, Yawetz S, Stephenson KE, et al. Compassionate use of remdesivir in pregnant women with severe coronavirus disease 2019. Clin Infect Dis Off Publ Infect Dis Soc Am 2021;73: e3996–4004.

49. WHO. Therapeutics and COVID-19: living guideline. https://www.who.int/publications/i/item/WHO-2019-nCoV-therapeutics-2022.3. [Accessed 17 February 2022].

50. Abani O, Abbas A, Abbas F, et al. Tocilizumab in patients admitted to hospital with COVID-19 (RECOVERY): a randomised, controlled, open-label, platform trial. Lancet 2021;397(10285):1637–45.

51. Royal College of Obstetricians and Gynaecologists. Coronavirus (COVID-19), infection in pregnancy. 2022. https://www.rcog.org.uk/guidance/coronavirus-covid-19-pregnancy-and-women-s-health/coronavirus-covid-19-infection-in-pregnancy/. [Accessed 27 December 2021].

52. Singh B, Ryan H, Kredo T, et al. Chloroquine or hydroxychloroquine for prevention and treatment of COVID-19. Cochrane Database Syst Rev 2021; 2(2):CD013587.

53. Franchini M, Prefumo F, Grisolia G, et al. Convalescent plasma for pregnant women with covid-19: a systematic literature review. Viruses 2021;13:1194.

54. Qian Z, Zhang Z, Ma H, et al. The efficiency of convalescent plasma in COVID-19 patients: a systematic review and meta-analysis of randomized controlled clinical trials. Front Immunol 2022;13: 964398.

55. D'Souza R, Ashraf R, Rowe H, et al. Pregnancy and COVID-19: pharmacologic considerations. Ultrasound Obstet Gynecol 2021;57:195–203.

56. Lapinsky SE. Management of acute respiratory failure in pregnancy. Semin Respir Crit Care Med 2017;38:201–7.

57. Cojocaru L, Turan OM, Levine A, et al. Proning modus operandi in pregnancies complicated by acute respiratory distress syndrome secondary to COVID-19. J Matern Neonatal Med 2022;35(25): 9043–52.

58. Ospina-Tascón GA, Calderón-Tapia LE, García AF, et al. Effect of high-flow oxygen therapy vs conventional oxygen therapy on invasive mechanical ventilation and clinical recovery in patients with severe COVID-19: a randomized clinical trial. JAMA 2021; 326:2161–71.

59. Malfertheiner SF, Brodie D, Burrell A, et al. Extracorporeal membrane oxygenation during pregnancy and peripartal. An international retrospective multicenter study. Perfusion 2022. https://doi.org/10.1177/02676591221090668.

60. van Genderen ME, van Uitert E, Duvekot JJ, et al. Management and outcome of critically ill pregnant women with COVID-19. Intensive Care Med 2022; 48(5):613–5.

61. Bhatia K. Obstetric analgesia and anaesthesia in SARS-CoV-2-positive parturients across 10 maternity units in the north-west of England: a retrospective cohort study. Anaesthesia 2022;77:389–97.

62. Keita H, James A, Bouvet L, et al. Clinical, obstetrical and anaesthesia outcomes in pregnant women during the first COVID-19 surge in France: a prospective multicentre observational cohort study. Anaesthesia, Crit Care Pain Med 2021;40:100937.

63. Goldshtein I, Nevo D, Steinberg DM, et al. Association between BNT162b2 vaccination and incidence of SARS-CoV-2 infection in pregnant women. JAMA 2021;326:728–35.

64. Ma Y, Deng J, Liu Q, et al. Effectiveness and safety of COVID-19 vaccine among pregnant women in real-world studies: a systematic review and meta-analysis. Vaccines 2022;10(2):246.

65. Prasad S, Kalafat E, Blakeway H, et al. Systematic review and meta-analysis of the effectiveness and perinatal outcomes of COVID-19 vaccination in pregnancy. Nat Commun 2022;13:2414.

66. Samannodi M. COVID-19 vaccine acceptability among women who are pregnant or planning for pregnancy in Saudi Arabia: a cross-sectional study. Patient Prefer Adherence 2021;15:2609–18.

67. Carbone L, Di Girolamo R, Mappa I, et al. Worldwide beliefs among pregnant women on SARS-CoV-2 vaccine: a systematic review. Eur J Obstet Gynecol Reprod Biol 2022;268:144–64.

68. Kuciel N, Mazurek J, Hap K, et al. COVID-19 vaccine acceptance in pregnant and lactating women

and mothers of young children in Poland. Int J Womens Health 2022;14:415–24.

69. Kachikis A, Englund JA, Singleton M, et al. Short-term reactions among pregnant and lactating individuals in the first wave of the COVID-19 vaccine rollout. JAMA Netw Open 2021;4(8):e2121310.

70. Gray KJ, Bordt EA, Atyeo C, et al. Coronavirus disease 2019 vaccine response in pregnant and lactating women: a cohort study. Am J Obstet Gynecol 2021;225:303.e1–17.

71. Collier A-RY, McMahan K, Yu J, et al. Immunogenicity of COVID-19 mRNA vaccines in pregnant and lactating women. JAMA 2021;325:2370–80.

72. Shimabukuro TT, Kim SY, Myers TR, et al. Preliminary findings of mRNA covid-19 vaccine safety in pregnant persons. N Engl J Med 2021;384(24):2273–82.

73. Falsaperla R, Leone G, Familiari M, et al. COVID-19 vaccination in pregnant and lactating women: a systematic review. Expert Rev Vaccin 2021;20:1619–28.

74. Pratama NR, Wafa IA, Budi DS, et al. mRNA Covid-19 vaccines in pregnancy: a systematic review. PLoS One 2022;17:e0261350.

75. Goldshtein I, Steinberg DM, Kuint J, et al. Association of BNT162b2 COVID-19 vaccination during pregnancy with neonatal and early infant outcomes. JAMA Pediatr 2022;176:470–7.

76. Muyldermans J, De Weerdt L, De Brabandere L, et al. The effects of COVID-19 vaccination on lactating women: a systematic review of the literature. Front Immunol 2022;13:852928.

77. De Rose DU, Salvatori G, Dotta A, et al. SARS-CoV-2 vaccines during pregnancy and breastfeeding: a systematic review of maternal and neonatal outcomes. Viruses 2022;14:539.

COVID-19 in Patients with Chronic Lung Disease

Jessica Fae Calver[a], Laura Fabbri, MD[b], James May, MBBS, MRCP[c],
R. Gisli Jenkins, MD, PhD, FRCP, FERS[b],*

KEYWORDS

- Chronic lung disease • Asthma • COPD • Cystic fibrosis • Interstitial lung disease
- Pulmonary arterial hypertension • COVID-19 susceptibility • Vaccination

KEY POINTS

- Severe acute respiratory syndrome coronavirus 2 infection targets the respiratory epithelium.
- Patients with chronic lung disease (CLD) are at risk of more severe coronavirus disease 2019 (COVID-19).
- Patients with CLD should continue with standard therapy, although patients receiving immunosuppression, particularly rituximab, are at higher risk of infection and severe disease.
- Patients with CLD do not seem at higher risk of adverse vaccine reactions and therefore should be offered vaccination, which reduces the chance of severe COVID-19.

Severe acute respiratory syndrome coronavirus 2 (SARS-CoV-2) is a novel coronavirus that leads to an acute respiratory tract infection, and for the first couple of years of the pandemic, it lead to acute lung injury in a substantial proportion of people. The combination of improved therapy, vaccination, and mutant strains with a lower trophism for alveolar epithelium seem to have reduced the number of people overall with severe respiratory complications of severe coronavirus disease 2019 (COVID-19). However, patients with a preexisting chronic lung disease (CLD) may have an increased risk of acquiring SARS-CoV-2 infection and also have an increased risk of COVID-19 following with poor outcomes.[1–3] It is therefore crucial to understand the interaction between SARS-CoV-2 and the respiratory tract, especially in patients with compromised pulmonary physiology, to understand the pathogenesis of severe COVID-19 and complications such as "long COVID."

MECHANISMS OF SEVERE ACUTE RESPIRATORY SYNDROME CORONAVIRUS 2 INFECTION IN THE LUNG

Severe COVID-19 has been associated with SARS-CoV-2 infection of the lower respiratory tract with the primary site of infection being type II alveolar epithelial cells (AT2) in the distal lung.[4] Early in February 2020, it was reported that the major mechanism for SARS-CoV-2 viral entry into cells was through angiotensin-converting enzyme 2 (ACE2) expressed on the cell surface.[5] Yet, single-cell RNA-sequencing and protein atlas assessment of ACE2 determined low ACE2 gene expression and rare ACE2 protein expression in the airway epithelium and alveoli of control and CLD groups.[4,6] The low level of ACE2 expression at the major site of infection within the lungs suggests that it is likely that alternative non-ACE2–mediated mechanisms of cell infection exist in the lung and that these might be responsible for the

[a] University of Nottingham, Medical School, Nottingham NG7 2UH, United Kingdom; [b] National Heart and Lung Institute, Imperial College London, Guy Scadding Building, Cale Street, London SW3 6LY, United Kingdom; [c] Guy's and St Thomas' NHS Trust, Westminster Bridge SE1 7EH, United Kingdom
* Corresponding author.
E-mail address: Gisli.jenkins@imperial.ac.uk

Clin Chest Med 44 (2023) 385–393
https://doi.org/10.1016/j.ccm.2022.11.013

worse outcomes of patients with CLD. The virus has been shown to use several coreceptors including CD147/Basigin/BSG; NRP1 (Neuropilin-1); GRP78 (78 kDa glucose-regulated protein)/HSPA5 (Heat Shock Protein Family A (Hsp70) Member 5); and proteases Transmembrane serine protease 2 (TMPRSS2), Cathepsin L/CTSL (cathepsin L), FURIN (Furin), and ADAM17 (A disintegrin and metalloprotease 17) to facilitate infection.[1,4,7-13] Difference in these coreceptors explain the different pathogenicity of the newer Omicron variants[14]; however, the overall differences in SARS-CoV-2 entry factors are minimal in CLD, suggesting that viral entry alone does not explain the variation in disease severity observed between patients with and without CLD.[4] More recently, it has been hypothesized that in addition to increased susceptibility to infection, CLD patients have altered expression profiles of antiviral and immune response genes, altering their alveolar microenvironment and ability to fight infection. Having impaired innate immunity reduces the antiviral defense, which may promote host permissiveness and an increase in viral replication. As a result, they may be predisposed to severe lung injury.[4]

Although CLD has been cited as a risk factor for severe COVID-19, the different types of CLD have distinct pathologic mechanisms and treatment modalities. Subsequently, the molecular characteristics influencing SARS-CoV-2 severity differ between the groups.

ASTHMA

Asthma is an inflammatory condition of the airways occurring in all age groups but is more common in younger patients and is commonly associated with allergic diseases such as rhinosinusitis. Exacerbations of asthma are frequently caused by viral infections including rhinovirus and influenza and may be life-threatening. Asthma patients have impaired type-I interferon (IFN-I) responses, yet the risk of severe COVID-19 differs between the 2 main asthma endotypes: type-2 (allergic and eosinophilic) versus non-type-2 (neutrophilic and paucigranulocytic).[15]

In type-2 asthma, the proinflammatory cytokines interleukin (IL)-4, IL-5, and IL-13 are secreted to drive a Th2-type immune response, which perhaps modulates SARS-CoV-2 infectivity with IL-13 shown to downregulate ACE2 expression by airway epithelial cells (AECs).[16-18] In addition, type-2 cytokines and IgE cross-linking have previously been shown to suppress toll-like receptor (TLR) expression, possibly preventing an IFN-driven upregulation of ACE2.[19,20] Yet IL-13 increases TMPRSS2 expression, although a low frequency of dual ACE2+/ TMPRSS2+ expressing cells are present for viral entry.[18] It has been suggested that the preventative inhaled corticosteroid (ICS), ciclesonide, may even have inhibitory effects on viral replication by binding to the SARS-CoV-2 viral endonuclease NSP15.[21,22] In a randomized trial, patients treated with ciclesonide had reduced hospital attendance, although symptom duration was not reduced.[23] Additional protective factors in type-2 asthma patients include eosinophilia contributing to antiviral immunity and preexisting ICS usage for the long-term management of asthma.[24] Preexisting eosinophilia (>150 cells/μL) was protective against hospital admission, and the development of eosinophilia during admission was protective against mortality.[25] Consequently, concerns are raised regarding the use of biologic agents that directly interfere with Th2 inflammation and eosinophil function, yet their use is lifesaving in those with the worst forms of asthma. Reassuringly, a large cohort study did not find higher prevalence or worse outcomes in asthma patients on biologic therapy.[26]

By comparison, it has been suggested that individuals with non-type-2 asthma have an increased risk of severe COVID-19. In non-type-2 asthma, there is a greater involvement of Th1 and Th17 responses, predominantly through the cytokines IL-1β, IL-8, IL-6, and IL-17, many of which play a central role in the "cytokine storm."[15] Non-type-2 cytokines have been associated with an increased expression of ACE2 in epithelial cells, which may increase SARS-CoV-2 infection and similarly these individuals have low eosinophil levels, which usually have a protective role in viral infection.[27] Adding to this, IL-17 induces neutrophil migration during asthma onset, and these neutrophil levels (%) have been shown to significantly associate with FURIN gene expression in sputum.[28]

The different responses of eosinophilic and neutrophilic phenotypes may be the cause of conflicting data from studies of asthmatic patient. Early large-scale studies concluded that there was a higher incidence of COVID-19 in patients with asthma that there was a higher risk of severe COVID-19 (although asthma was not an independent risk factor) and that asthma treatment including biologic therapy did not influence disease course.[29,30] However, a more recent meta-analysis found that the risk of contracting COVID-19 was lower in patients with asthma versus nonasthmatics, and importantly, there were no significant differences in hospitalization, intensive care admission, or mechanical ventilation requirements.[31] Although once intubated, asthma patients are more likely to require longer periods of mechanical ventilation, which has been identified as an independent risk factor.[32]

Few cases of asthma exacerbation after COVID-19 vaccination have been reported.[33] However, the overall benefit of vaccination against SARS-CoV-2 outweighs the extremely low overall risk of an allergic reaction should not discourage the vaccination.

CHRONIC OBSTRUCTIVE PULMONARY DISEASE

Chronic obstructive pulmonary disease (COPD) is a common respiratory disease characterized by airway inflammation and alveolar destruction.[34] Expiratory airflow limitation with an FEV1/FVC ratio of less than 0.7 is diagnostic and the condition is associated with former smoking, current smoking, or noxious fume exposure. Pharmacotherapy includes bronchodilators and in certain cases ICS.[35] Acute exacerbations of COPD are characterized by worsening symptoms relative to the stable state, which frequently cause hospitalization and lung function deterioration in this patient group. An exacerbation is commonly triggered by infection, particularly viruses.[36] Subsequently, the emergence of SARS-CoV-2 raised concerns about the deleterious influence COVID-19 may have on the "clinically extremely vulnerable" patients with COPD with an increased risk of mortality.[37–39] Patients with COPD are at higher risk of hospitalization and have 4-fold higher risk of developing severe COVID-19.[38,40]

Patients with COPD have dampened IFN-I responses, which may consequently increase the risk of SARS-CoV-2 infection in the airway epithelium.[41] Recent evidence has implicated a reduction in the expression of the pattern recognition receptors (PRRs) retinoic acid-inducible gene I-like receptors and melanoma differentiation-associated protein 5.[41] These PRRs are a part of the innate immunity defense and recognize pathogen-associated molecular patterns and/or damage-associated molecular patterns to induce an antiviral IFN-I response. In addition, the expression of the type-I interferon IFN-β and its transcription factor IRF-7 are also decreased in patients with COPD.[41,42] In contrast, TLR2 and TLR4 expressions are increased in patients with COPD, which may be driving inflammation and an IFN-driven upregulation of the interferon-stimulated gene ACE2.[42–44] Alongside the dysregulation of these immune factors, TMPRSS2 protein expression is upregulated in COPD lung homogenates and NRP1 expression slightly upregulated in COPD macrophages.[4,45] Whether ACE2, CD147, and FURIN are upregulated in COPD to facilitate viral entry remains to be determined.[4,6,45–49]

To date, the overall prevalence of COVID-19 does not seem to be increased in patients with COPD. The impact of smoking on COVID-19 outcomes remains a topic of debate, although never smokers are likely to have better outcomes than current or former smokers.[39] There are several factors that may increase the risk of severe disease with poor outcomes in patients with COPD. Impaired lung function including air flow limitation, hyperinflation with poor inspiratory reserve, reduced gas transfer and impaired host defense blunt the ability to compensate for the vast pathologic condition, which affects the lungs in COVID-19 pneumonitis (inflammatory infiltrates, interstitial edema progressing to ARDS, and thromboembolism/in situ thrombosis).[50,51]

Similar to asthma, patients with COPD have continued with their established management therapies and have not adjusted, withdrawn, or escalated treatment during the COVID-19 pandemic. No harm has been reported with inhaled bronchodilator therapy although ICS is a more contentious issue. It has been demonstrated by in vivo and in vitro studies that ICS attenuate ACE2 receptor expression, yet a large cohort of patients with COPD receiving ICS were reported to be at increased risk of death from COVID-19 compared with those on Long Acting Beta Agonist and Long Acting Muscarinic antagonist (LABA/LAMA) therapy.[52,53] However, there was likely significant unmeasured confounding from disease severity, given that most patients on ICS tend to experience frequent exacerbations and/or have more severe airflow obstruction. The consensus is that inhaled treatment should be continued unaltered in stable patients.[54]

Initially, concerns were raised regarding the management of COPD acute exacerbations with oral corticosteroids. Early in the pandemic, there was significant anxiety over their use, especially given previous data from the Middle East respiratory syndrome coronavirus (MERS-CoV) pandemic.[55] This has now been superseded by the findings of the RECOVERY trial, which demonstrated a mortality benefit of dexamethasone for all patients requiring supplemental oxygen therapy; this is now accepted standard of care for severe COVID-19.[56] Surprisingly, there has been a 50% reduction in hospital admission from COPD exacerbations in prepandemic versus pandemic times. This is likely reflective of patients isolating from the general public resulting in reduced viral transmission (not limited to SARS-CoV-2). Although these observations may guide important public health strategy, significant depression and anxiety associated with social isolation is likely to result.[57] Currently, there is neither evidence of an adverse effect of COVID-19 vaccines in patients with COPD nor evidence of diminished efficacy.

BRONCHIECTASIS

Bronchiectasis is a condition of abnormally dilated airways and impaired mucociliary clearance. There are various causes including genetic (cystic fibrosis [CF] and primary ciliary dyskinesia), post-infectious (bacterial pneumonia, whooping cough, and tuberculosis), autoimmune (rheumatoid arthritis and inflammatory bowel disease), and immune dysfunction. The architectural distortion of the airways causes chronic sputum production and increased susceptibility to pulmonary infection. In comparison with some other forms of CLD, patients with bronchiectasis have a higher risk of contracting COVID-19, more severe disease, and poorer outcomes.[58] This may relate to the structural pulmonary abnormalities and impaired host defense response causing a greater risk of infection and respiratory failure. Corticosteroid treatments (inhaled or oral) are less commonly used in the chronic management of bronchiectasis or exacerbation management compared with asthma and COPD. Similar to patients with COPD and CF, studies demonstrate a significant decrease in the frequency of reported exacerbations during the COVID-19 pandemic.[59]

CYSTIC FIBROSIS

CF is an autosomal recessive disease affecting the lungs, digestive system, sweat glands, and reproductive tract. The primary abnormality is in chloride and sodium transport across secretory epithelia causing thickened viscous secretions in the bronchi, biliary tract, pancreas, intestines, and reproductive system. Although the disease is systemic, progressive lung disease continues to be the major cause of morbidity and mortality for most patients.[60] The thick airway secretions cause chronic airway obstruction, which gets progressively colonized by pathogenic bacteria. Once infection is established, neutrophils are unable to control the bacteria and release elastase, which overwhelms the antiproteases of the lung and contributes to tissue destruction.[61] In addition, large amounts of DNA and cytosol matrix proteins are released by degranulating neutrophils, contributing to the increased viscosity of the airway mucus. Chronic infection and an ineffective inflammatory response seem to be the major stimulus for an exuberant, which subsequently results in bronchiectasis.[62,63]

Although the sputum levels of IL-6 are lower in patients with CF, which may protect against severe COVID-19, CF patients are still categorized as a high-risk group.[64] ACE2 messenger RNA (mRNA) level is elevated in CF AECs when compared with non-CF cells but TMPRSS2 mRNA level is decreased.[65] CF cells also display elevated FURIN activity, which has been shown to increase TGF-β1 production.[66] Cystic fibrosis transmembrane conductance regulator (CFTR) modulators administered for CF treatment are thought to be protective against severe COVID-19.[67]

To date, the literature suggests that CF individuals seem to be contracting SARS-CoV-2 viral infection at a lower rate compared with the general population. Lower rates of SARS-CoV-2 infection in CF individuals are likely explained by the increased awareness of infection, prevention, and control practices including frequent hand hygiene, mask wearing, and continued social distancing. Although the hospitalization rates are higher in CF than in the general population, individuals with CF seem to have better outcomes than initially anticipated, when compared with other respiratory viral infections. There are no specific concerns regarding the safety of mRNA vaccines in patients with CF. A small cohort study showed that CF patients mounted sufficient antibody responses after immunization irrelevant of CFTR genotype, related comorbidities, or treatment type.[68]

INTERSTITIAL LUNG DISEASE

The term interstitial lung disease (ILD) encompasses a group of respiratory diseases affecting the alveolar parenchyma, with inflammation and/or fibrosis affecting the alveolar interstitium. These alterations cause increased morbidity and mortality. ILDs can have a known etiology such as occupational exposure to mold, metals, chemical substances or drugs, and autoimmune diseases. However, a large number of ILDs have no known cause with idiopathic pulmonary fibrosis (IPF) being the most well studied.[69]

ILD patients have an increased frequency of COVID-19 infection compared with the general population; however, COVID-19 susceptibility differs among the ILD subtypes. The incidence of COVID-19 is higher in patients with IPF; however, patients with sarcoidosis and chronic hypersensitivity pneumonitis do not show increased susceptibility to the disease.[70–73] In addition to increased susceptibility, patients with ILD have more severe disease than those without ILD. After COVID-19 infection, they require more oxygen therapy, intensive care admission, and mechanical ventilation.[73]

In IPF, there is an increase in ACE2 protein expression, specifically in the small airways.[4] There are also significantly lower plasma levels of soluble ACE2 in patients with pulmonary fibrosis, which normally acts as a decoy protein to neutralize SARS-CoV-2 infectivity.[45] This regional increase in ACE2+ cells in the distal lung alongside an upregulation of the epithelial-restricted αvβ6 integrin in AT2 cells, may explain the increased severity in IPF patients despite overall low ACE2 expression levels.[4] The integrin αvβ6 is critical in the pathogenesis of IPF and is upregulated in the fibrotic regions of an IPF lung.[74] The Arg-Gly-Asp (RGD)-binding integrin was suggested as a coreceptor for SARS-CoV-2 infectivity as unlike any other coronavirus, the SARS-CoV-2 spike protein has acquired an RGD motif.[75] The SARS-CoV-2 spike protein S1 subunit can bind to αvβ6, and its overexpression has been shown to augment ACE2-dependent SARS-CoV-2 pseudoviral entry into epithelial cells. The αvβ6 integrin also mediates TGF-β1 activation in human epithelial cells, and this enhanced TGF-β1 signaling can suppress antiviral IFN-I signaling activity by alveolar macrophages.[74,76–78] This may explain the increased severity in patients with IPF despite overall low-ACE2 expression levels. A positive correlation between NRP1 and FURIN expression also exists in IPF AT2 cells, which may facilitate viral entry.[4] The MUC5B promoter rs35705950 T allele is a genetic risk factor for IPF development and has additionally been associated with COVID-19 but seems to be protective against severe disease, perhaps because MUC5B forms part of the innate immune response.[79] The 2 antifibrotic therapies approved for IPF treatment, nintedanib and pirfenidone, may also protect against severe COVID-19 by attenuating profibrotic pathways and IL-6 cytokine levels.[4] Yet short telomere length is a risk factor for both familial and sporadic IPF and has been shown to be associated with increased COVID-19 infection and disease severity.[80]

Studies have suggested that COVID-19 vaccines may be less effective in immunocompromised patients, who are at increased risk of severe COVID-19.[81] Particularly, those with autoimmune diseases and associated ILDs may fail to mount the desired antibody response with mRNA vaccinations.[82] The lower responses correlated with coexistent ongoing treatments, particularly glucocorticoids, mycophenolate mofetil and rituximab.[83] Similarly, patients with IPF did not mount expected antispike antibody responses to 2 doses of SARS-CoV-2 mRNA, irrespective of current antifibrotic treatment.[84] Anecdotally, acute exacerbation of IPF has been reported after vaccine administration in people with ILD-related autoimmune diseases and IPF. These episodes might suggest that the immune response induced by the vaccine may activate a pathobiological

cascades leading to the acute exacerbation in susceptible patients. Still, vaccine-associated exacerbation should be considered a rare event occurring in a small minority of vaccinated patients with IPF.[83,85,86] These cases do however raise an important question, which can only be answered by larger, prospective studies comparing the rate of ILD exacerbations between vaccinated and unvaccinated groups.

PULMONARY ARTERIAL HYPERTENSION

Pulmonary arterial hypertension (PAH) is a vasculopathy characterized by remodeling and thickening of the pulmonary arteries with increased vascular resistance and right heart dysfunction. Early in the COVID-19 pandemic, there was a suggestion that patients with PAH may be protected from severe COVID-19.[87] Successively, large cohort studies showed that cumulative incidence was similar to the general population; however, outcomes were worse with half of patients requiring hospitalization and a 12% rate of mortality.[88]

A possible pathogenic mechanism explaining these findings is the reduction of ACE2 in patients with PAH.[89] This downregulation leads to higher circulating levels of angiotensin II with worsened ensuing lung.[90] PAH-specific therapies, including the endothelin receptor antagonists and phosphodiesterase type 5 inhibitors, are also very likely to be important. Endothelin I stabilizes ACE2 expression, which may not only enhance viral binding and replication but also protect against high expression of angiotensin II. Similarly, some of these agents may have anti-inflammatory and antithrombotic properties. However, most importantly their vasodilatory effect may worsen V:Q mismatch by enhancing blood flow to poor ventilated areas of lung and worsening hypoxemia.[91]

It is recommended that established PAH therapy is continued unchanged in the face of infection with COVID-19. However, this patient group may display a more challenging management approach regarding oxygen and ventilatory support. Positive-pressure ventilation (including high flow nasal oxygen, continuous positive airway pressure, and bilevel positive airway pressure) is often used to manage severe hypoxemia, as a bridge or to delay intubation. However, increased airway pressure from these modalities may decrease venous return to the right ventricle and worsen the already struggling cardiopulmonary hemodynamic, making these patients unstable. Similarly, invasive ventilation requires general anesthesia to manage an anticipated reduction in vascular tone and worsening right heart failure. In these situations, patients may require vasopressor support, which presents its own challenges.[92] No evidence of contraindication of COVID-19 vaccines in patients with pulmonary hypertension has been reported nor is there evidence of diminished vaccine efficacy in this group of patients.

SUMMARY

In summary, the presence of some preexisting CLD may increase the risk of contracting COVID-19, which frequently leads to worse outcomes including increased disease severity and mortality. However, the baseline health status and comorbidities also influence the evolution of COVID-19, and these need to be evaluated in the context of CLD. No evidence currently supports the change of chronic therapy, nor is there convincing evidence of an increased risk of adverse reaction to COVID-19 vaccination thus vaccine uptake should be encouraged. There continues to be a considerable health burden of COVID-19 in patients with CLD, and health-care policy should prioritize the use of antiviral therapies in these vulnerable patients.

CLINICS CARE POINTS

- Patients with Chronic Lung Disease are at increased risk of severe COVID-19 and its complications.
- Patients with Chronic Lung Disease should be prioritised for anti-viral therapy.
- Patients with Chronic Lung Disease are not at increased risk of adverse reactions to COVID-19 vaccines and should be encouraged to have vaccination.

DISCLOSURE

RGJ: Astra Zeneca; Biogen; Galecto; GlaxoSmithKline; Nordic Biosciences RedX; Pliant; Bristol Myers Squibb; Chiesi; Cohbar; Daewoong; Veracyte; Resolution Therapeutics; Boehringer Ingelheim; Chiesi; Roche; PatientMPower; Galapagos; Vicore; NuMedii; Action for Pulmonary Fibrosis.

ACKNOWLEDGEMENTS

UKRI Covid-19 Rapid Response - (EP/V051490/1) The UK Interstitial Lung Disease Long-COVID19 study (UKILD-Long COVID): understanding the burden of Interstitial Lung Disease in Long COVID.

REFERENCES

1. Halpin DMG, Faner R, Sibila O, et al. Do chronic respiratory diseases or their treatment affect the risk of SARS-CoV-2 infection? Lancet Respir Med 2020; 8(5):436–8.
2. George PM, Wells AU, Jenkins RG. Pulmonary fibrosis and COVID-19: the potential role for antifibrotic therapy. Lancet Respir Med 2020;8(8): 807–15.
3. Williamson EJ, Walker AJ, Bhaskaran K, et al. Factors associated with COVID-19-related death using OpenSAFELY. Nature 2020;584(7821):430–6.
4. Bui LT, Winters NI, Chung MI, et al. Chronic lung diseases are associated with gene expression programs favoring SARS-CoV-2 entry and severity. Nat Commun 2021;12(1):4314.
5. Zhou P, Yang XL, Wang XG, et al. A pneumonia outbreak associated with a new coronavirus of probable bat origin. Nature 2020;579(7798):270–3.
6. Aguiar JA, Tremblay BJ, Mansfield MJ, et al. Gene expression and in situ protein profiling of candidate SARS-CoV-2 receptors in human airway epithelial cells and lung tissue. Eur Respir J 2020;56(3): 2001123.
7. Cantuti-Castelvetri L, Ojha R, Pedro LD, et al. Neuropilin-1 facilitates SARS-CoV-2 cell entry and infectivity. Science 2020;370(6518):856–60.
8. Carlos AJ, Ha DP, Yeh DW, et al. The chaperone GRP78 is a host auxiliary factor for SARS-CoV-2 and GRP78 depleting antibody blocks viral entry and infection. J Biol Chem 2021;296:100759.
9. Hoffmann M, Kleine-Weber H, Schroeder S, et al. SARS-CoV-2 cell entry Depends on ACE2 and TMPRSS2 and is Blocked by a clinically Proven protease inhibitor. Cell 2020;181(2):271–80. e278.
10. Ibrahim IM, Abdelmalek DH, Elshahat ME, et al. COVID-19 spike-host cell receptor GRP78 binding site prediction. J Infect 2020;80(5):554–62.
11. Ou X, Liu Y, Lei X, et al. Characterization of spike glycoprotein of SARS-CoV-2 on virus entry and its immune cross-reactivity with SARS-CoV. Nat Commun 2020;11(1):1620.
12. Wang K, Chen W, Zhang Z, et al. CD147-spike protein is a novel route for SARS-CoV-2 infection to host cells. Signal Transduct Target Ther 2020; 5(1):283.
13. Zhao MM, Yang WL, Yang FY, et al. Cathepsin L plays a key role in SARS-CoV-2 infection in humans and humanized mice and is a promising target for new drug development. Signal Transduct Target Ther 2021;6(1):134.
14. Zhang Y-N, Zhang Z-R, Zhang H-Q, et al. Different pathogenesis of SARS-CoV-2 Omicron variant in wild-type laboratory mice and hamsters. Signal Transduction Targeted Ther 2022;7(1):62.

15. Lombardi C, Gani F, Berti A, et al. Asthma and COVID-19: a dangerous liaison? Asthma Res Pract 2021;7(1):9.

16. Jackson DJ, Busse WW, Bacharier LB, et al. Association of respiratory allergy, asthma, and expression of the SARS-CoV-2 receptor ACE2. J Allergy Clin Immunol 2020;146(1):203–206 e203.

17. Kimura H, Francisco D, Conway M, et al. Type 2 inflammation modulates ACE2 and TMPRSS2 in airway epithelial cells. J Allergy Clin Immunol 2020; 146(1):80–88 e88.

18. Sajuthi SP, DeFord P, Li Y, et al. Type 2 and interferon inflammation regulate SARS-CoV-2 entry factor expression in the airway epithelium. Nat Commun 2020;11(1):5139.

19. Contoli M, Ito K, Padovani A, et al. Th2 cytokines impair innate immune responses to rhinovirus in respiratory epithelial cells. Allergy 2015;70(8):910–20.

20. Gill MA, Bajwa G, George TA, et al. Counterregulation between the FcepsilonRI pathway and antiviral responses in human plasmacytoid dendritic cells. J Immunol 2010;184(11):5999–6006.

21. Kimura H, Kurusu H, Sada M, et al. Molecular pharmacology of ciclesonide against SARS-CoV-2. J Allergy Clin Immunol 2020;146(2):330–1.

22. Matsuyama S, Kawase M, Nao N, et al. The inhaled steroid ciclesonide blocks SARS-CoV-2 RNA replication by targeting the viral replication-transcription complex in cultured cells. J Virol 2020;95(1):e01648–720.

23. Clemency BM, Varughese R, Gonzalez-Rojas Y, et al. Efficacy of inhaled ciclesonide for outpatient treatment of adolescents and adults with symptomatic COVID-19: a randomized clinical trial. JAMA Intern Med 2022;182(1):42–9.

24. Padayachee Y, Faiez TS, Singanayagam A, et al. Asthma and viruses: a focus on rhinoviruses and SARS-CoV-2. J Allergy Clin Immunol 2021;147(5): 1648–51.

25. Ferastraoaru D, Hudes G, Jerschow E, et al. Eosinophilia in asthma patients is protective against severe COVID-19 illness. J Allergy Clin Immunol Pract 2021;9(3):1152–62. e1153.

26. Matucci A, Caminati M, Vivarelli E, et al. COVID-19 in severe asthmatic patients during ongoing treatment with biologicals targeting type 2 inflammation: results from a multicenter Italian survey. Allergy 2021;76(3):871–4.

27. Camiolo M, Gauthier M, Kaminski N, et al. Expression of SARS-CoV-2 receptor ACE2 and coincident host response signature varies by asthma inflammatory phenotype. J Allergy Clin Immunol 2020;146(2): 315–324 e317.

28. Kermani NZ, Song WJ, Badi Y, et al. Sputum ACE2, TMPRSS2 and FURIN gene expression in severe neutrophilic asthma. Respir Res 2021;22(1):10.

29. Choi YJ, Park JY, Lee HS, et al. Effect of asthma and asthma medication on the prognosis of patients with COVID-19. Eur Respir J 2021;57(3):2002226.

30. Izquierdo JL, Almonacid C, Gonzalez Y, et al. The impact of COVID-19 on patients with asthma. Eur Respir J 2021;57(3):2003142.

31. Sunjaya AP, Allida SM, Di Tanna GL, et al. Asthma and COVID-19 risk: a systematic review and meta-analysis. Eur Respir J 2022;59(3):2101209.

32. Mahdavinia M, Foster KJ, Jauregui E, et al. Asthma prolongs intubation in COVID-19. J Allergy Clin Immunol Pract 2020;8(7):2388–91.

33. Colaneri M, De Filippo M, Licari A, et al. COVID vaccination and asthma exacerbation: might there be a link? Int J Infect Dis 2021;112:243–6.

34. Adeloye D, Song P, Zhu Y, et al. Global, regional, and national prevalence of, and risk factors for, chronic obstructive pulmonary disease (COPD) in 2019: a systematic review and modelling analysis. Lancet Respir Med 2022;10(5):447–58.

35. Gupta N, Malhotra N, Ish P. GOLD 2021 guidelines for COPD- what's new and why. Adv Respir Med 2021;89(3):344–6.

36. Wedzicha JA, Singh R, Mackay AJ. Acute COPD exacerbations. Clin Chest Med 2014;35(1):157–63.

37. Gerayeli FV, Milne S, Cheung C, et al. COPD and the risk of poor outcomes in COVID-19: a systematic review and meta-analysis. EClinicalMedicine 2021;33: 100789.

38. Lacedonia D, Scioscia G, Santomasi C, et al. Impact of smoking, COPD and comorbidities on the mortality of COVID-19 patients. Sci Rep 2021;11(1):19251.

39. Patanavanich R, Glantz SA. Smoking is associated with COVID-19 progression: a meta-analysis. Nicotine Tob Res 2020;22(9):1653–6.

40. Zhao Q, Meng M, Kumar R, et al. The impact of COPD and smoking history on the severity of COVID-19: a systemic review and meta-analysis. J Med Virol 2020;92(10):1915–21.

41. Garcia-Valero J, Olloquequi J, Montes JF, et al. Deficient pulmonary IFN-beta expression in COPD patients. PLoS One 2019;14(6):e0217803.

42. Guo-Parke H, Linden D, Weldon S, et al. Deciphering respiratory-virus-associated interferon signaling in COPD airway epithelium. Medicina (Kaunas) 2022;58(1):121.

43. Hansbro PM, Haw TJ, Starkey MR, et al. Toll-like receptors in COPD. Eur Respir J 2017;49(5):1700739.

44. Ziegler CGK, Allon SJ, Nyquist SK, et al. SARS-CoV-2 receptor ACE2 is an interferon-stimulated gene in human airway epithelial cells and is Detected in specific cell subsets across tissues. Cell 2020;181(5): 1016–1035 e1019.

45. Fliesser E, Birnhuber A, Marsh LM, et al. Dysbalance of ACE2 levels - a possible cause for severe COVID-19 outcome in COPD. J Pathol Clin Res 2021;7(5): 446–58.

46. Saheb Sharif-Askari N, Saheb Sharif-Askari F, Alabed M, et al. Airways expression of SARS-CoV-2 receptor, ACE2, and TMPRSS2 is lower in children than adults and increases with smoking and COPD. Mol Ther Methods Clin Dev 2020;18:1–6.

47. Maremanda KP, Sundar IK, Li D, et al. Age-dependent assessment of genes involved in cellular senescence, telomere, and mitochondrial pathways in human lung tissue of smokers, COPD, and IPF: associations with SARS-CoV-2 COVID-19 ACE2-TMPRSS2-furin-DPP4 Axis. Front Pharmacol 2020; 11:584637.

48. Radzikowska U, Ding M, Tan G, et al. Distribution of ACE2, CD147, CD26, and other SARS-CoV-2 associated molecules in tissues and immune cells in health and in asthma, COPD, obesity, hypertension, and COVID-19 risk factors. Allergy 2020;75(11): 2829–45.

49. Aloufi N, Traboulsi H, Ding J, et al. Angiotensin-converting enzyme 2 expression in COPD and IPF fibroblasts: the forgotten cell in COVID-19. Am J Physiol Lung Cell Mol Physiol 2021;320(1):L152–7.

50. Hu W, Dong M, Xiong M, et al. Clinical courses and outcomes of patients with chronic obstructive pulmonary disease during the COVID-19 epidemic in Hubei, China. Int J Chron Obstruct Pulmon Dis 2020;15:2237–48.

51. Thomas M, Price OJ, Hull JH. Pulmonary function and COVID-19. Curr Opin Physiol 2021;21:29–35.

52. Finney LJ, Glanville N, Farne H, et al. Inhaled corticosteroids downregulate the SARS-CoV-2 receptor ACE2 in COPD through suppression of type I interferon. J Allergy Clin Immunol 2021;147(2):510–9. e515.

53. Schultze A, Walker AJ, MacKenna B, et al. Risk of COVID-19-related death among patients with chronic obstructive pulmonary disease or asthma prescribed inhaled corticosteroids: an observational cohort study using the OpenSAFELY platform. Lancet Respir Med 2020;8(11):1106–20.

54. Halpin DMG, Singh D, Hadfield RM. Inhaled corticosteroids and COVID-19: a systematic review and clinical perspective. Eur Respir J 2020;55(5): 2001009.

55. Arabi YM, Mandourah Y, Al-Hameed F, et al. Corticosteroid therapy for critically ill patients with Middle East respiratory syndrome. Am J Respir Crit Care Med 2018;197(6):757–67.

56. Group RC, Horby P, Lim WS, et al. Dexamethasone in hospitalized patients with covid-19. N Engl J Med 2021;384(8):693–704.

57. Alqahtani JS, Oyelade T, Aldhahir AM, et al. Reduction in hospitalised COPD exacerbations during COVID-19: a systematic review and meta-analysis. PLoS One 2021;16(8):e0255659.

58. Choi H, Lee H, Lee SK, et al. Impact of bronchiectasis on susceptibility to and severity of COVID-19: a nationwide cohort study. Ther Adv Respir Dis 2021;15. 1753466621995043.

59. Crichton ML, Shoemark A, Chalmers JD. The impact of the COVID-19 pandemic on exacerbations and symptoms in bronchiectasis: a prospective study. Am J Respir Crit Care Med 2021;204(7):857–9.

60. Guggino WB. Cystic fibrosis and the salt controversy. Cell 1999;96(5):607–10.

61. Griese M, Kappler M, Gaggar A, et al. Inhibition of airway proteases in cystic fibrosis lung disease. Eur Respir J 2008;32(3):783–95.

62. DiMango E, Ratner AJ, Bryan R, et al. Activation of NF-kappaB by adherent Pseudomonas aeruginosa in normal and cystic fibrosis respiratory epithelial cells. J Clin Invest 1998;101(11):2598–605.

63. Heeckeren A, Walenga R, Konstan MW, et al. Excessive inflammatory response of cystic fibrosis mice to bronchopulmonary infection with Pseudomonas aeruginosa. J Clin Invest 1997;100(11):2810–5.

64. Marcinkiewicz J, Mazurek H, Majka G, et al. Are patients with lung cystic fibrosis at increased risk of severe and fatal COVID-19? Interleukin 6 as a predictor of COVID-19 outcomes. Pol Arch Intern Med 2020;130(10):919–20.

65. Stanton BA, Hampton TH, Ashare A. SARS-CoV-2 (COVID-19) and cystic fibrosis. Am J Physiol Lung Cell Mol Physiol 2020;319(3):L408–15.

66. Ornatowski W, Poschet JF, Perkett E, et al. Elevated furin levels in human cystic fibrosis cells result in hypersusceptibility to exotoxin A-induced cytotoxicity. J Clin Invest 2007;117(11):3489–97.

67. Peckham D, McDermott MF, Savic S, et al. COVID-19 meets Cystic Fibrosis: for better or worse? Genes Immun 2020;21(4):260–2.

68. Michos A, Filippatos F, Tatsi EB, et al. Immunogenicity of the COVID-19 BNT162b2 vaccine in adolescents and young adults with cystic fibrosis. J Cyst Fibros 2022;21(3):e184–7.

69. American thoracic S, European respiratory S. American thoracic society/European respiratory society international multidisciplinary consensus classification of the idiopathic interstitial pneumonias. This joint statement of the American thoracic society (ATS), and the European respiratory society (ERS) was adopted by the ATS board of directors, june 2001 and by the ERS executive committee, june 2001. Am J Respir Crit Care Med 2002;165(2):277–304.

70. Baughman RP, Lower EE, Buchanan M, et al. Risk and outcome of COVID-19 infection in sarcoidosis patients: results of a self-reporting questionnaire. Sarcoidosis Vasc Diffuse Lung Dis 2020;37(4): e2020009.

71. George LJ, Philip AM, John KJ, et al. A review of the presentation and outcome of sarcoidosis in coronavirus disease 2019. J Clin Transl Res 2021;7(5): 657–65.

72. Kahlmann V, Manansala M, Moor CC, et al. COVID-19 infection in patients with sarcoidosis: susceptibility and clinical outcomes. Curr Opin Pulm Med 2021; 27(5):463–71.

73. Lee H, Choi H, Yang B, et al. Interstitial lung disease increases susceptibility to and severity of COVID-19. Eur Respir J 2021;58(6):2004125.

74. Munger JS, Huang X, Kawakatsu H, et al. A mechanism for regulating pulmonary inflammation and fibrosis: the integrin αvβ6 binds and activates latent TGF β1. Cell 1999;96(3):319–28.

75. Sigrist CJ, Bridge A, Le Mercier P. A potential role for integrins in host cell entry by SARS-CoV-2. Antivir Res 2020;177:104759.

76. Jenkins RG, Su X, Su G, et al. Ligation of protease-activated receptor 1 enhances alpha(v)beta6 integrin-dependent TGF-beta activation and promotes acute lung injury. J Clin Invest 2006;116(6): 1606–14.

77. Meliopoulos VA, Van de Velde LA, Van de Velde NC, et al. An epithelial integrin regulates the amplitude of protective lung interferon responses against multiple respiratory pathogens. Plos Pathog 2016;12(8): e1005804.

78. Xu MY, Porte J, Knox AJ, et al. Lysophosphatidic acid induces alphavbeta6 integrin-mediated TGF-beta activation via the LPA2 receptor and the small G protein G alpha(q). Am J Pathol 2009;174(4): 1264–79.

79. van Moorsel CHM, van der Vis JJ, Duckworth A, et al. The MUC5B promoter Polymorphism associates with severe COVID-19 in the European population. Front Med (Lausanne) 2021;8:668024.

80. Drake TM, Docherty AB, Harrison EM, et al. Outcome of Hospitalization for COVID-19 in patients with interstitial lung disease. An international multicenter study. Am J Respir Crit Care Med 2020; 202(12):1656–65.

81. Galmiche S, Luong Nguyen LB, Tartour E, et al. Immunological and clinical efficacy of COVID-19 vaccines in immunocompromised populations: a systematic review. Clin Microbiol Infect 2022;28(2): 163–77.

82. Furer V, Eviatar T, Zisman D, et al. Immunogenicity and safety of the BNT162b2 mRNA COVID-19 vaccine in adult patients with autoimmune inflammatory rheumatic diseases and in the general population: a multicentre study. Ann Rheum Dis 2021; 80(10):1330–8.

83. Ferri C, Ursini F, Gragnani L, et al. Impaired immunogenicity to COVID-19 vaccines in autoimmune systemic diseases. High prevalence of non-response in different patients' subgroups. J Autoimmun 2021;125:102744.

84. Karampitsakos T, Papaioannou O, Dimeas I, et al. Reduced immunogenicity of the mRNA vaccine BNT162b2 in patients with idiopathic pulmonary fibrosis. ERJ Open Res 2022;8(2):00082–2022.

85. Sgalla G, Magri T, Lerede M, et al. COVID-19 vaccine in patients with exacerbation of idiopathic pulmonary fibrosis. Am J Respir Crit Care Med 2022; 206(2):219–21.

86. Ehteshami-Afshar S, Raj R. COVID-19 mRNA vaccines and ILD exacerbation: causation or just a temporal association? Am J Respir Crit Care Med 2022; 206(7):919.

87. Horn EM, Chakinala M, Oudiz R, et al. Could pulmonary arterial hypertension patients be at a lower risk from severe COVID-19? Pulm Circ 2020;10(2). 2045894020922799.

88. Lee JD, Burger CD, Delossantos GB, et al. A survey-based estimate of COVID-19 incidence and outcomes among patients with pulmonary arterial hypertension or chronic thromboembolic pulmonary hypertension and impact on the Process of care. Ann Am Thorac Soc 2020;17(12):1576–82.

89. Hemnes AR, Rathinasabapathy A, Austin EA, et al. A potential therapeutic role for angiotensin-converting enzyme 2 in human pulmonary arterial hypertension. Eur Respir J 2018;51(6):1702638.

90. Kuba K, Imai Y, Penninger JM. Angiotensin-converting enzyme 2 in lung diseases. Curr Opin Pharmacol 2006;6(3):271–6.

91. Farha S, Heresi GA. COVID-19 and pulmonary arterial hypertension: early data and many questions. Ann Am Thorac Soc 2020;17(12):1528–30.

92. Sahay S, Farber HW. Management of hospitalized patients with pulmonary arterial hypertension and COVID-19 infection. Pulm Circ 2020;10(3). 2045894020933480.

Coronavirus Disease-2019 in the Immunocompromised Host

Christopher D. Bertini Jr, MD[a], Fareed Khawaja, MD[b],
Ajay Sheshadri, MD, MS[c],*

KEYWORDS

- COVID-19 • SARS-CoV-2 • Immunocompromised host • Pneumonia • Hematologic malignancy
- Immunosuppression

KEY POINTS

- Immunocompromise refers to a host's inability to combat infections from a variety of partial or total immune defects and can occur in the setting of diseases such as hematologic malignancies, immunosuppression use, primary immunodeficiency syndromes, and human immunodeficiency virus infection.
- Hospitalization risk, intensive care unit admission, and mortality are substantially higher after severe acute respiratory syndrome coronavirus 2 pneumonia in immunocompromised hosts.
- Immunocompromised hosts are underrepresented in clinical trials of vaccines and other treatments, and therefore efficacy data are often inferred or based upon small studies.
- Vaccines and treatments are often effective in immunocompromised hosts, but persistent viral replication due to impaired immunity can hinder the efficacy of these interventions.

INTRODUCTION

Severe acute respiratory syndrome coronavirus 2 (SARS-CoV-2) is a respiratory virus that originated in Wuhan, China in 2019. Since that time, SARS-CoV-2 has been responsible for over 6 million deaths from coronavirus disease-2019 (COVID-19).[1] Respiratory viral infections, in general, place an outsized burden on immunocompromised hosts, and increase the mortality.[2] Therefore, there was significant concern from the outset of the pandemic that SARS-CoV-2 infection would similarly impact immunocompromised patients disproportionately. This review focuses on the specific impact of COVID-19 on immunocompromised patients.

The term "immunocompromise" describes patients who have an impaired or absent immune system, limiting a host's ability to combat pathogens. Immunodeficiencies are classified as either primary or secondary. Primary immunodeficiencies (PIDs) are intrinsic to the immune system. Examples include congenital conditions such as severe combined immunodeficiency (SCID), caused by various mutations which can impact many immune cell lineages, and common variable immune deficiency (CVID), which is caused by a diverse array of genetic conditions that result in varying degrees of hypogammaglobulinemia.[3] Secondary immunodeficiencies refer to those acquired through conditions that depress the immune system. These include

The authors have nothing to disclose.
[a] Department of Internal Medicine, UTHealth Houston McGovern Medical School, 6431 Fannin, MSB 1.150, Houston, TX 77030, USA; [b] Department of Infectious Diseases, Infection Control, and Employee Health, The University of Texas MD Anderson Cancer Center, 1515 Holcombe Boulevard, Unit 1469, Houston, TX 77030, USA; [c] Department of Pulmonary Medicine, The University of Texas MD Anderson Cancer Center, 1400 Pressler Street Unit 1462, Houston, TX 77030, USA
* Corresponding author.
E-mail address: asheshadri@mdanderson.org
Twitter: @ajaysheshadri (A.S.)

Clin Chest Med 44 (2023) 395–406
https://doi.org/10.1016/j.ccm.2022.11.012

hematological malignances, solid and hematopoietic transplantation, infection with the human immunodeficiency virus (HIV), chronic immunosuppressive medication use, and others. In these cases, the period of immunocompromise may be limited in duration; for example, a patient with leukemia may no longer be immunocompromised once their disease is in remission and leukocyte counts recover, or a patient receiving biologic immunosuppressive therapy may no longer be immunocompromised once therapy has completed and enough time has lapsed to allow for immune recovery. On the contrary, comorbidities that may impact immune function, such as diabetes, do not necessarily connote an immunocompromised state, but are worthy of consideration because they are often independently associated with poor outcomes after COVID-19.[4,5] **Table 1** shows examples of high-risk groups who we consider to be immunocompromised and their attendant immune deficits.

Immunocompromised hosts are at considerable risk for a variety of infections. For example, bacterial pneumonia has been estimated to account for 30% of intensive care unit (ICU) admissions in patients with cancer.[6] In another study of severe influenza pneumonia, 12.5% of patients admitted

to the ICU were immunocompromised, indicative of a higher propensity toward critical illness after infection.[7] Indeed, mortality was over twofold higher among immunocompromised patients with influenza pneumonia. Other respiratory viruses also affect the immunocompromised; a recent retrospective cohort study of 1643 hematopoietic cell transplant (HCT) patients found increased mortality in allogeneic recipients infected with human rhinovirus (HRV) and adenovirus lower respiratory infections.[2] Finally, human herpesvirus-6 (HHV-6) and cytomegalovirus (CMV) have long been associated with increased mortality amongst HCT recipients.[8]

Considering that over 500 million cases of COVID-19 have been reported worldwide since the pandemic began, it is likely that several million immunocompromised hosts were infected, extrapolating from the estimate that 2.7% of the American adult population are immunocompromised.[9] Research within this specific vulnerable population has not been commensurate to the substantial body of literature for COVID-19 in general. This review will summarize the current scientific literature that discusses the impact of COVID-19 on immunocompromised hosts. We will discuss mechanisms for COVID-19's affinity for the

Table 1
Examples of immunocompromised conditions and possible mechanisms of immunocompromise

Immunocompromised Condition	Mechanism of Immunocompromise	Immune Deficits
Hematologic malignancies	Marrow infiltration and cytotoxic chemotherapy	Lymphopenia Neutropenia Impaired cellular immunity Impaired humoral immunity
Hematopoietic cell transplantation	Corticosteroid use, immunosuppressive medications (eg, tacrolimus, sirolimus, and ibrutinib)	Lymphopenia Neutropenia Impaired cellular immunity Impaired humoral immunity
Solid organ transplant (kidney, lung, and heart)	Corticosteroid use, immunosuppressive medications (eg, tacrolimus, sirolimus, and cyclosporine)	Impaired cellular immunity Impaired humoral immunity
Human immunodeficiency virus (HIV)	Apoptosis of T cells	Lymphopenia Impaired cellular immunity Impaired humoral immunity
Autoimmune rheumatology diseases requiring immunosuppressive drug therapy	Use of immunosuppressive agents (eg, methotrexate, TNF-alpha inhibitors, and specific interleukin inhibitors)	Lymphopenia Impaired cellular immunity Impaired humoral immunity Impaired innate immunity
Primary immunodeficiency syndromes	Hereditary agammaglobulinemia, defective phagocytosis, and impaired leukopoiesis	Lymphopenia Neutropenia Impaired cellular immunity Impaired humoral immunity Impaired innate immunity

immunocompromised, compare clinical data between immunocompromised and immunocompetent hosts, and examine the evidence supporting treatment strategies within immunocompromised hosts who develop COVID-19.

MECHANISMS OF IMMUNOCOMPROMISE

The innate immune response is driven by cells such as neutrophils, macrophages, and natural killer cells. The innate immune response is evolutionarily ancient and is often the first defense against many pathogens, including SARS-CoV-2. Impaired innate immunity may be correlated with COVID-19 severity. For example, in a study of 84 COVID-19 patients, of whom 44 were critically ill, the presence of immature neutrophils, defined by low CD13 expression and characterized by diminished antimicrobial and phagocytic activity, was associated with a critical illness.[10] Similar findings were seen in monocytes, and the diminished functional capacity of monocytes was correlated with increased risk for septic shock rate and mortality. Impaired type 1 interferon responses measured in the peripheral blood were also associated with severe illness in 50 patients with COVID-19 of variable severity.[11] On the contrary, more exuberant type 1 interferon responses that occur later in the course of infection have been associated with a worsening of lung injury, indicating that these innate immune responses may have salutary or harmful roles depending upon when they occur within the course of disease.[12] Of note, these studies were conducted in immunocompetent hosts and were performed during an acute infection, and although the findings indicate that innate immune impairments are associated with higher COVID-19 severity, these findings require validation in immunocompromised hosts who are evaluated before the onset of disease.

Cellular, or cell-mediated, immunity, typically refers to host response involving T cells, though notably many innate immune cells also have a direct cell-mediated anti-pathogen response. In many immunocompromised hosts, cellular immunity can be impaired and lead to worsened outcomes after COVID-19. In a study comparing over 1400 immunocompetent COVID-19 patients to 166 immunocompromised patients, lymphopenia was associated with threefold mortality increase in the latter.[13] The immunocompromised cohort consisted of patients with autoimmune rheumatologic diseases (ARD) (39.2%) as well as patients with hematologic malignancies (21.1%), solid malignances (19.3%), and solid organ transplant (SOT) recipients (18.1%). Specifically, CD8 cells may have an important role in determining outcomes after COVID-19. In a prospective cohort study of 106 patients with cancer, lower peripheral blood CD8 T-cell counts were correlated with a higher COVID-19 viral load and associated with higher mortality.[14] However, hematologic patients with cancer with preserved CD8 counts had low viral loads and decreased mortality, even among patients with impaired humoral immunity. Of note, 23% of patients with hematologic malignancy had no detectable anti-SARS-CoV-2 T-cell responses. In another cohort of 79 COVID-19 patients, 36 immunocompromised hosts had significantly fewer CD3+ T -cells and CD3+/CD4+ T cells compared with 20 patients above age 60 and 23 patients with diabetes.[15] T cells from immunocompromised patients produced less interferon-gamma compared with elderly patients, but there was no difference in interferon production between diabetic and immunocompromised patients. However, this study included patients with renal disease and cirrhosis as part of its definition of immunocompromised hosts. Further detailing the role CD8 cells play, a retrospective case-control study of 174 COVID-19 hospitalized patients in Spain showed that patients admitted to the ICU had lower CD8 counts compared with patients admitted to the general wards.[16] CD4 counts did not vary between ICU and non-ICU admitted patients. However, in general, the classification of immunocompromise should precede the infection, and in this study, most of the patients did not have a disease that would indicate immunocompromise.

In addition to impaired cellular immunity, immunocompromised hosts may have diminished humoral immunity, defined by an impaired ability to produce pathogen-specific antibodies against COVID-19 and other pathogens. For example, a study of 103 patients with cancer showed that delayed viral clearance was associated with loss of antibody production, despite adequate T cell response to infection.[17] Prolonged viremia was driven by B-cell depletion, potentially indicating that the resolution of infection depends upon adequate humoral immunity. In a study of lymphoma patients, B-cell-depleting therapies, such as rituximab, were associated with higher rates of hospital readmission and persistent SARS-CoV-2 positivity.[18] This diminished humoral response may increase the risk in for adverse outcomes; a study of 111 patients with lymphoma admitted to French hospitals for the treatment of COVID-19 found that anti-CD20 therapies increased the risk of mortality by over two-fold.[19] With regards to the development of humoral immunity after infection, Wunsch and colleagues[15] found in a cohort of 70 patients with SARS-CoV-

2 infection IgG ELISA antibody responses measured after infection that 16 patients lacked antibodies. Of these 16 patients, 11 were immunocompromised. This lack of humoral immunity can in rare instances lead to immune escape by SARS-CoV-2 variants.

Long-term shedding of COVID-19 in immunocompromised patients has been well described in transplant recipients and patients with cancer with B cell depletion.[20–24] Many of these cases describe changes in viral spike protein despite repeated treatment with antivirals. For example, one renal transplant patient with COVID-19, over a 145-day course of infection, SARS-CoV-2 viral spike proteins showed increased resistance to neutralizing antibodies.[20] These mutations have been shown to mimic variants from Brazil and the United Kingdom, though no clear link between long-term shedding and the evolution of COVID-19 variants have been identified.[20] In addition to the potential for mutations in the spike protein, resistance to antiviral agents may also arise in patients with long-term shedding[24]; this was most recently described in a cancer patient with B cell depletion.[24] These examples cite the risk long-term shedding of COVID-19 poses in immunocompromised patients and the need for effective prevention and treatment methods.

Clinical Outcomes After Coronavirus Disease-2019 Infection in Immunocompromised Hosts

Immunocompromised patients generally develop more severe illness after SARS-CoV-2 infection than immunocompetent patients. However, the studies discussed here need to be interpreted in the context of which variants dominated during the time of study and the availability of vaccines and effective therapies. We will discuss COVID-19 disease severity in the immunocompromised and considerations amongst different types of immunocompromised patients.

Immunocompromised patients may have a higher ICU admission rate and longer hospital lengths of stay. A Turkish retrospective case-control study reported a 22% ICU admission rate among 156 immunocompromised patients compared with 9% ICU admission rate among 312 nonimmunocompromised patients between April 2020 and October 2020.[25] Length of stay was longer in the immunocompromised cohort as well. The immunocompromised cohort included people living with HIV (PLWH), cancer, rheumatologic disease, and those who were on immunosuppressive medications. Immunocompromised patients may also have higher mortality rates compared with those in the immunocompetent.

For example, a separate Korean retrospective cohort study of 871 immunocompromised patients and 5564 nonimmunocompromised patients found that immunocompromised patients had a mortality of 9.6%, over four times higher than the 2.3% mortality rate observed in immunocompetent patients.[26] Immunocompromised patients included those with HIV/AIDs, malignancy, SOT, and immunosuppressive medication use. Smaller cohort studies have also shown a mortality rate three to four times higher in immunocompromised patients.[25]

Immunocompromised patients who are mechanically ventilated often present with more severe acute respiratory distress syndrome (ARDS). For example, a retrospective cohort of 1594 patients with COVID-19, of whom 166 were immunocompromised, found that the mean Sap02/Fi02 ratio was 251 in immunocompromised patients, compared with 276 in immunocompetent patients.[13] Mild ARDS (Sap02/FiO2 >235 mm Hg) occurred in 42.3% of the immunocompetent grouped, compared with 33.7% of the immunocompromised group, and moderate ARDS (Sap02/FiO2 >160 mm Hg) occurred in 25.6% of the immunocompetent group compared with 33.1% of the immunocompromised group. No significant difference was observed in the rate of severe ARDS (Sap02/FiO2 <100 mm Hg) between the two groups. Immunocompromised patients had higher mortality, and among immunocompromised patients, older age, the presence of ARDS, and severe lymphopenia were predictors of mortality. These studies show the shift to a higher disease severity among COVID-19 patients.

Hematologic malignancy

Patients with hematologic malignancy have been shown to have high rates of hospitalization for COVID-19. For example, a European multicenter analysis of 3801 patients with hematologic malignancies who developed COVID-19 reported a hospitalization rate of 74%.[27] Other studies have also reported high hospitalization rates; for example, Mato and colleagues[28] reported a 25% admission rate among 174 patients with chronic lymphocytic leukemia (CLL). ICU admission rate has high as 18% have been observed, with a median length of stays as long as 15 days.[27] Mortality is often high in hematologic patients with cancer. For example, in 174 patients with CLL, 33% of patients died during the analysis.[28] Similarly, a study of 3801 patients with hematologic malignancies showed a mortality rate of 31%, with the highest found in patients with AML or myelodysplastic syndrome (~40%).[27] Smaller cohort studies have confirmed a case fatality rate of about 40%

among patients with hematologic malignancy. Lastly, patients with hematologic malignancies often require vasopressor support and renal replacement; in a cohort of patients with CLL, 27% required vasopressor support and 11% required hemodialysis.[28] Reassuringly, survival in patients with CLL may be improving with newer variants.[29]

Solid malignancy

Several studies have shown that solid malignancy COVID-19 patients have a high hospitalization rate. A French retrospective cohort study of 212 solid tumor patients with cancer, of whom about 75% were undergoing active treatment of cancer, found a similar 70% rate of hospitalization, but a lower rate of ICU admission (12%).[30] Half of this cohort had undergone chemotherapy in the first 3 months, and overall mortality was 30%.

Furthermore, Dai and colleagues[31] showed an ICU admission rate of 20% for 105 hospitalized patients with cancer, compared with 8% in 536 non-patients with cancer, and ICU survivors with cancer had a mean 27-day length of stay compared with 17 in ICU survivors without cancer. The cancer cohort in this study included patients with lung, breast, thyroid, blood, cervical and esophageal cancer. In addition, death occurred in 11% of the cancer cohort compared with 4% in the noncancer cohort. Of all the cancers, hematologic and lung cancers had the highest mortality rates at 33% and 18%, respectively. This suggests that though patients with lung cancer usually do not meet the definition of immunocompromise, their risk of death is substantially higher than in non-patients with cancer. Though it is not clear how lung cancer increases mortality in patients with COVID-19, it is possible that this is either due to the extent of preexisting lung disease or a direct effect from smoking.[32] Further work is necessary to understand the mechanisms driving increased in mortality in lung patients with cancer with COVID-19.

In general, patients with hematologic and lung cancers or metastatic cancers had more severe COVID-19 illness. To wit, Dai and colleagues[31] found that 10% of patients with cancer required mechanical ventilation, compared with less than 1% of non-patients with cancer. The authors also found that patients with cancer had higher rates of renal replacement therapy and extracorporeal membrane oxygenation compared with non-patients with cancer, in addition to symptoms such as fever or chest pain.

Risk factors that have been reported to correlate with disease severity in immunocompetent patients have been validated in patients with cancer.[33] For example, a Chinese comparative study showed that old age, d-dimer, elevated tumor necrosis factor (TNF) alpha and N terminal pro-brain natriuretic peptide (pro-BNP) may be correlated worsening hypoxemia in solid and hematological patients with cancer admitted with COVID 19.[34] Furthermore, in an analysis of 218 solid and hematologic patients with cancer, D-dimer levels were twice as high in patients with cancer who died; serum lactate and lactate dehydrogenase were also higher among decedents.[35] Furthermore, CRP and ferritin have been shown to be higher in immunocompromised patients compared with immunocompetent patients.[25] This suggests that serum biomarkers which correlate with disease severity in non-patients with cancer are also applicable to patients with cancer.

Hematopoietic cell transplantation

A study of 382 HCT recipients in Europe during the first few months of the pandemic showed a mortality of 22% in allogeneic transplant recipients and 28% in autologous transplant recipients; children had a mortality of 7%, lower than adults but exponentially higher than the mortality observed in children who were not HCT recipients.[36,37] Older age and more severe immunodeficiency were associated with a higher chance for death. Furthermore, an observational cohort study of 86 HCT recipients in Brazil showed that 70% required hospitalization and 14% required ICU admission.[38] Mortality in this cohort was 30%, with a 34% mortality rate among the 62 adult patients compared with 21% in the 24 pediatric patients. In general, large studies of HCT recipients who are infected with SARS-CoV-2 are lacking.

Solid organ transplant

SOT recipients also have poorer outcomes after COVID-19. In over 17,000 patients with SOT, of whom 1682 developed COVID-19, COVID-19 increased the rate of death by nearly ten-fold, and SOT recipients hospitalized with COVID-19 were about 2.5 times more likely to die than those hospitalized with non-SARS-CoV-2 pneumonia.[39] In-hospital mortality among those who developed COVID-19 was 17%, and 21% required ICU admission. SOT recipients with COVID-19 had an increased length of stay (LOS) compared with SOT patients with non-COVID-19 pneumonia (6 vs. 4 days). Similar to the general population, certain comorbidities increase hospitalization risk in SOT recipients. For example, a case-control series of 47 SOT recipients found that chronic kidney disease (CKD), type 2 diabetes mellitus (T2DM), and hypertension (HTN) were more prevalent in the hospitalized patients compared with the non-hospitalized control group.[40]

In 49 advanced heart failure (HF) patients admitted for COVID-19, heart transplant (HTx) patients had worse mortality compared with left ventricular assist device (LVAD) and HF patients.[41] Specifically, mortality for the HTx group was 18.9% compared with 12.5% for LVAD and 11.5% for HF, respectively. Similarly, HTx patients, who are often on immunosuppressive medications, have been shown to have higher ICU LOS compared with HF patients. Kidney transplant recipients (KTx) show similar vulnerability to COVID-19. An international registry of 9845 KTx recipients reported that 144 patients required hospitalization.[42] The mortality rate was 32%; 29% were intubated and 52% developed acute kidney injury. Lymphopenia, elevated lactate dehydrogenase and elevated procalcitonin were all correlated with increased mortality. Outcomes may be more severe among lung transplant (LTx) recipients, as a French cohort analysis of 35 LTx patients with COVID-19 reported a hospitalization rate of 88.6%.[43] 42% were admitted to the ICU, and 52% required mechanical ventilation. 14% of the 35 LTx patients died after COVID-19.

People living with human immunodeficiency virus

COVID-19 may more severely affect PLWH who have uncontrolled HIV as compared with their well-controlled counterparts. For example, in an Italian study of 69 PLWH, 38 hospitalized patients had an average nadir CD4 count of 167 compared 399 in those who were not hospitalized.[44] However, the hospitalization rate remains high even among PLWH on antiretroviral therapy (ART). In a large Spanish cohort of 77,590 PLWH on ART, 63% of the 236 PLWH diagnosed with COVID-19 required hospitalization.[45] Of those 151 hospitalized patients, the ICU admission rate was about 9% and the mortality rate was 11%. Of the 15 PLWH admitted to the ICU, the mortality rate was 33%. The median LOS for 116 patients who survived to hospital discharge was 7 days. Similar to the general population and other immunocompromised patients, age and number of comorbidities were highly correlated with hospitalization, ICU admission, and death rates.

Autoimmune rheumatologic disease

Patients with rheumatologic illness are also at high risk for severe complications from COVID-19. For example, a cohort of 58,052 Danish patients with inflammatory rheumatologic diseases had a 50% higher probability of admission compared with the general Danish population of 4.5 million.[46]

The risk was 30% higher for patients with rheumatoid arthritis and over 80% higher for patients with vasculitis. However, the use of immunosuppressive agents (TNF-alpha inhibitors and steroids) surprisingly did not impact admission rate. Hospitalized patients with rheumatoid arthritis, particularly those with lung or cardiovascular disease, may have the more severe infection than hospitalized patients without ARD. In a case-control study comparing 2,379 patients with ARD to those without, ARD increased the risk of hospitalization by 14%, ICU admission by 32%, acute kidney injury by 81%, and venous thromboembolism by 74%, but did not increase the risk for mechanical ventilation or death.[47] Severe outcomes were more common for patients on glucocorticoids, but not DMARDs (disease-modifying antirheumatic drugs). In a study of 52 patients with systemic ARD, of whom 75% were on immunosuppressive therapy and 31% on biologic therapies, the requirement for mechanical ventilation was threefold higher in patients with rheumatologic disease compared with matched controls. However, mortality was indistinguishable between the two groups. Similar to other patients, a greater number of comorbidities increases the likelihood of severe COVID-19 in patients with ARD. For example, in patients with inflammatory bowel disease with two or more comorbidities, such as heart disease, diabetes, and kidney disease, severe COVID-19 was more common than in patients with one or zero comorbidities.[48]

Primary immunodeficiency

Little data exist for patients who have non-HIV immunodeficiency. In an Italian case series of seven patients with PIDs, six were hospitalized, and three were admitted the ICU.[49] Of the hospitalized patients at time of publication, 1 patient died in hospital, three were discharged and two were still being treated. The length of stay ranged between 3 days to 25 days.

TREATMENT

In general, there is a paucity of randomized controlled trial data examining the efficacy of anti-SARS-CoV-2 treatments in immunocompromised hosts. For example, in a recent randomized controlled trial of high-risk individuals who developed COVID-19 and were randomized to nirmatrelivir/ritonavir or placebo, fewer than 30 patients met any criteria for immunocompromise as we outline above.[50] Most data comes from observational or case-control studies. In this section, we will discuss studies that show the efficacy of antiviral, monoclonal antibodies, and convalescent plasma to treat, preempt, or prevent COVID-19 in immunocompromised patients.

Little data exist regarding antiviral therapy and its efficacy specifically in the immunocompromised. One challenge with the use of antiviral therapy is that the kinetics of viral replication necessitate prompt therapy to ensure an adequate outcome[51]; there is no clear evidence that replication is more rapid in immunocompromised hosts, despite the possibility due to impaired innate and cellular immunity. In one series of 31 ARD patients treated with nirmatrelivir/ritonavir (29) and molnupiravir during the first 5 days of COVID-19 diagnosis, no patients were hospitalized, but most (94%) were fully vaccinated,[52] and no comparator arm was studied. Little efficacy data is available for remdesivir in immunocompromised hosts; a case study suggested that remdesivir can reduce viral load in immunocompromised patients with persistent infections.[53] A recent randomized, double-blind, placebo-controlled trial found that a 3-day course of remdesivir in non-hospitalized patients with COVID-19 with high-risk conditions reduced the risk for hospitalization or death by 87%; however, only 4% of patients were immunocompromised.[54] Given the possibility of prolonged viral replication, multiple courses or longer courses of remdesivir may be necessary in immunocompromised hosts, but prospective studies comparing these strategies to usual care are necessary. In general, the evidence for the efficacy of antiviral therapy in immunocompromised hosts is lacking, but antiviral therapies are reasonable to use given the high probability of adverse outcomes in immunocompromised hosts.

It is unclear as to whether anti-inflammatory drugs are as effective in immunocompromised COVID-19 patients as in the general population. For example, a multicenter cohort study of 80 KTx patients showed that the mortality rate among patients treated with the interleukin-6 inhibitor tocilizumab was around 33%,[55,56] whereas the overall mortality rate for KTx patients with COVID-19 has been estimated to be around 24%. However, it is likely there is a selection bias as sicker patients tend to be treated with monoclonal antibodies, and prospective studies with appropriate controls are lacking. Similarly, studies regarding the use of the interleukin-6 inhibitor sarilumab have also excluded patients on immunosuppressive medications. The Infectious Disease Society of America (IDSA) does not promote nor discourage the use of tocilizumab and sarilumab in immunocompromised due to lack of available evidence.[57] Janus Kinase Inhibitors such as

baricitinib have not been well studied in the immunocompromised. Both the RECOVERY trial and COV-BARRIER trial showed that baricitinib reduced risk of death in COVID-19 patients; however, only RECOVERY included immunocompromised patients, whereas COV-BARRIER excluded them.[58,59] The IDSA points out that data supporting the use of Janus kinase inhibitors in immunocompromised hosts is lacking.

COVID-19 convalescent plasma (CCP) has been used in immunocompetent patients with variable evidence for efficacy. Although this may be useful in immunocompromised patients who cannot generate a humoral response, high-quality randomized, placebo-controlled trials have shown no benefit.[60] Lower quality studies have suggested efficacy under some circumstances. For example, in a propensity score-matched analysis of 112 patients with hematologic malignancies, most of whom received other nonplasma therapies, the use of convalescent plasma decreased mortality by 63% among patients who were exposed to anti-CD20 antibodies in the subgroup of patients with B-cell neoplasms.[61] Transfusion reactions were rare. A Swedish cohort of 28 immunocompromised COVID-19 patients showed that 46% had clinical improvement by at least one score one WHO scale on week after convalescent plasma administration.[62] No comparator arm was studied. The United States Food and Drug Administration Emergency Use Authorization authorizes CCP use in patients with immunosuppressive conditions, but data is limited and caution is necessary when extrapolating data from immunocompetent hosts.[57]

VACCINATION

Vaccinations are effective for reducing mortality in immunocompromised patients. For example, a retrospective British study examining vaccine efficacy in SOT patients including 39260 double vaccinated patients, 1141 single vaccinated patients and 3080 unvaccinated patients showed a 20% reduction in risk of death in vaccinated patients.[63] However, vaccination may not effectively decrease risk of positive SARS-CoV-2 test, as the risk-adjusted infection incidence rate was 1.29. Moreover, although two doses of ChAdOx1-S vaccines reduced the risk of death, similar efficacy was not observed with BNT162b2.

However, vaccines may be less effective for the immunocompromised compared with the immunocompetent. For example, one comparison prospective study detailing humoral immune response between 54 immunocompetent patients and 57 immunocompromised patients showed that some immunocompromised patients, namely patients with PIDs and rheumatologic disease, show declining immunity to COVID-19 as time progresses after two administrations of BNT162b2 vaccine.[64] Among the immunocompetent patients, PLWH and CKD patients, all had detectable antibodies at 2 weeks and 3 months post vaccination. The mean CD4 count for the PLWH was 254. However, subgroup analysis showed that 50% of the rheumatologic patients and 94.5% of the (PID) group had antibodies at two weeks. An inferior response to SARS-CoV-2 vaccination in immunocompromised patients has been shown in other studies. For example, an Austrian prospective cohort studied antibody response to COVID-19 vaccination in 15 healthy controls compared this to 74 patients previously treated with rituximab.[65] All healthy patients developed antibodies, but only 39% of the rituximab group developed antibodies to spike proteins following vaccination.

Lastly, COVID-19 hospitalization following vaccination, commonly referred to as "breakthrough cases," are more frequent in the immunocompromised. For example, an American study of 45 vaccine breakthrough COVID-hospitalizations reported that 44% were immunocompromised, and an Israeli cohort of 152 hospitalized fully vaccinated patients reported that 40% were immunocompromised.[66,67] Of the 60 immunocompromised fully vaccinated patients in the Israeli cohort, 18 had a poor outcome, which was defined as either requiring mechanical ventilation or death. Knowing that the prevalence of immunocompromise in the United States is around 2%, it follows that breakthrough infection seems to occur much more frequently among immunocompromised patients. Two studies prove this point more definitively. In a study of 6,860 cases of breakthrough COVID-19 after vaccination, patients with hematologic malignancies had over a four-fold higher risk for breakthrough infection,[68] with the highest rates seen in patients with leukemia or myeloma. Proteasome inhibitors and other immunomodulators significantly increased the risk for breakthrough infection. Similarly, in a study of over 45,000 patients with cancer, primarily with solid tumors, the overall incidence of breakthrough COVID-19 was 13.6%.[69] Mortality rate may be higher after breakthrough infection in immunocompromised patients. A cohort study of 54 fully vaccinated hematologic and solid tumor patients with cancer who developed breakthrough COVID-19 reported a 65% hospitalization rate, 19% ICU admission rate and 13% mortality rate,[70] not markedly different from adverse event rates among unvaccinated patients with cancer.

Pre-Exposure Prophylaxis

A preexposure prophylaxis strategy may be effective to mitigate COVID-19 severity in the immunocompromised. The PROVENT trial is a 2:1 randomized double-blind placebo-controlled study of 5197 patients investigating the use of tixagevimab and cilgavimab, a cocktail of two monoclonal antibodies that bind to non-overlapping sites from the SARS-CoV-2 spike protein, in preventing symptomatic COVID-19 in the at-risk patients, such as those with chronic obstructive pulmonary disease, immunocompromise, or elderly. Results show that the medication has a 77% risk reduction compared with placebo and 83% reduction at 6 months analysis.[71] As a result, the Infectious Diseases Society of America guidelines and US Food and Drug Administration agree about its use for the immunocompromised to provide further protection. However, only 7.4% of the cohort had any cancer, only 3.3% were receiving immunosuppressive therapies, and only 0.5% had a PID; therefore, these results are not necessarily indicative of efficacy in all immunocompromised hosts. Nevertheless, the use of tixagevimab and cilgavimab is reasonable given the frequent lack of humoral response to vaccination in immunocompromised hosts.

Post-Acute Sequelae of Coronavirus Disease-2019

Post-acute Sequelae of COVID-19 (PASC) refer to a range of ongoing health problems that people experience usually in the weeks and months following SARS-CoV-2 pneumonia,.[72] PASC refers to symptoms that are not explained by an alternative diagnosis, including fatigue, shortness of breath, anosmia, chest pain, diarrhea, and fever.[73,74] In immunocompromised patients, persistent respiratory symptoms and fatigue may be the most common.[74] These symptoms can persist for an extended period of time and, in some cases, may persist indefinitely.

PASC presents unique challenges to immunocompromised patients. A study of 1557 COVID-19 survivors with cancer showed that 15% reported PASC symptoms at a median of 44 days after COVID-19 diagnosis, suggesting a higher incidence than in the general population.[74] The study also reported a higher hospitalization rate and mortality rate due to PASC, but this must be interpreted in the context of other factors related to cancer, such as the discontinuation of cancer treatment which was independently associated with mortality. Lastly, the analysis revealed a few characteristics that were more frequent in the 234 patients with PASC as compared with the 1323 patients without

PASC. Compared with patients without COVID-19 sequalae, a larger portion of the PASC group was male (54.5% vs 47.2%), over the age 65 (55.1% vs 48.1%), and had two or more comorbidities (48.4% vs 36.4%).[74]

One possibility for why immunocompromised patients may experience PASC is the possibility of delayed viral clearance. Some reports have shown that immunocompromised patients may display persistent viral infection well after initial COVID-19 diagnosis. For example, in addition to prior examples, one follicular lymphoma patient showed an increase in SARS-CoV-2 viral load 54 days after symptoms onset, whereas another patient receiving showed persistent RT-PCR (reverse transcription polymerase chain reaction) positivity 238 days following SARS-Cov-2 diagnosis.[53,75] A recent report suggested that the presence of spike proteins could be associated with PASC; in a recent study of 37 PASC patients, 84% had evidence of circulating spike protein, as compared with 0 in 26 recovered COVID-19 patients.[76] Whether the circulating spike protein represents active SARS-CoV-2 replication or simply viral remnants is unclear. Further work is needed to understand PASC in patients with or without immunocompromise.

SUMMARY

COVID-19 often results in more severe infections in immunocompromised patients. Hospitalization rate, disease severity, and mortality rates are generally higher for the immunocompromised, especially those with hematologic malignancies, SOT recipients, and patients with ARD. Treatment strategies for these patients are similar to those in the immunocompetent, but high-quality data are lacking. Vaccinations are recommended but less effective in immunocompromised patients. As the pandemic continues, the vulnerability of immunocompromised patients should garner the attention of the medical and scientific communities. Studies focusing on immunocompromised patients will help illuminate the best strategies to mitigate harms in these high-risk patients.

CLINICS CARE POINTS

- Immunocompromised patients have often develop severe SARS-CoV-2 pneumonia, and the threshold to escalate the level of care should be low given the possibility for rapid deterioration.

- Despite the possibility of inferior rates of response to vaccination, vaccinatiion is recommended in most immunocompromsied patients.
- Though most antiviral and anti-inflammatory agents have not been specifically tested in immunocompromised hosts, these should be initiated early given the possibility for clinical worsening without prompt intervention.

REFERENCES

1. WHO. WHO Coronavirus disease (COVID-19) dashboard In:2022. Available at: https://covid19.who.int/
2. Kim Y, Waghmare A, Xie H, et al. Respiratory viruses in hematopoietic cell transplant candidates: impact of preexisting lower tract disease on outcomes. Blood Adv 2022;6:5307–16.
3. Raje N, Dinakar C. Overview of immunodeficiency disorders. Immunol Allergy Clin N Am 2015;35(4):599–623.
4. Chinen J, Shearer WT. Secondary immunodeficiencies, including HIV infection. J Allergy Clin Immunol 2010;125(2):S195–203.
5. Mahamat-Saleh Y, Fiolet T, Rebeaud ME, et al. Diabetes, hypertension, body mass index, smoking and COVID-19-related mortality: a systematic review and meta-analysis of observational studies. BMJ Open 2021;11(10):e052777.
6. Azoulay E, Pickkers P, Soares M, et al. Acute hypoxemic respiratory failure in immunocompromised patients: the Efraim multinational prospective cohort study. Intensive Care Med 2017;43(12):1808–19.
7. Garnacho-Montero J, Leon-Moya C, Gutierrez-Pizarraya A, et al. Clinical characteristics, evolution, and treatment-related risk factors for mortality among immunosuppressed patients with influenza A (H1N1) virus admitted to the intensive care unit. J Crit Care 2018;48:172–7.
8. Seo S, Renaud C, Kuypers JM, et al. Idiopathic pneumonia syndrome after hematopoietic cell transplantation: evidence of occult infectious etiologies. Blood 2015;125(24):3789–97.
9. Harpaz R, Dahl RM, Dooling KL. Prevalence of immunosuppression among US adults, 2013. JAMA 2016;316(23):2547.
10. Peyneau M, Granger V, Wicky P-H, et al. Innate immune deficiencies are associated with severity and poor prognosis in patients with COVID-19. Scientific Rep 2022;12(1):638.
11. Hadjadj J, Yatim N, Barnabei L, et al. Impaired type I interferon activity and inflammatory responses in severe COVID-19 patients. Science 2020;369(6504):718–24.
12. Lee JS, Park S, Jeong HW, et al. Immunophenotyping of COVID-19 and influenza highlights the role of

type I interferons in development of severe COVID-19. Sci Immunol 2020;5(49):eabd1554.

13. Martínez-Urbistondo M, Gutiérrez-Rojas A, Andrés A, et al. Severe lymphopenia as a predictor of COVID-19 mortality in immunosuppressed patients. J Clin Med 2021;10(16):3595.

14. Bange E, Han N, Wileyto EP, et al. CD8 T cells compensate for impaired humoral immunity in COVID-19 patients with hematologic cancer. In: Research Square; 2021.

15. Wünsch K, Anastasiou OE, Alt M, et al. COVID-19 in elderly, immunocompromised or diabetic patients—from immune monitoring to clinical management in the hospital. Viruses 2022;14(4):746.

16. Urra JM, Cabrera CM, Porras L, et al. Selective CD8 cell reduction by SARS-CoV-2 is associated with a worse prognosis and systemic inflammation in COVID-19 patients. Clin Immunol 2020;217(108486): 108486.

17. Lyudovyk O, Kim JY, Qualls D, et al. Impaired humoral immunity is associated with prolonged COVID-19 despite robust CD8 T cell responses. Cancer Cell 2022;40(7):738–753 e735.

18. Lee CY, Shah MK, Hoyos D, et al. Prolonged SARS-CoV-2 infection in patients with lymphoid malignancies. Cancer Discov 2022;12(1):62–73.

19. Dulery R, Lamure S, Delord M, et al. Prolonged in-hospital stay and higher mortality after Covid-19 among patients with non-Hodgkin lymphoma treated with B-cell depleting immunotherapy. Am J Hematol 2021;96(8):934–44.

20. Weigang S, Fuchs J, Zimmer G, et al. Within-host evolution of SARS-CoV-2 in an immunosuppressed COVID-19 patient as a source of immune escape variants. Nat Commun 2021;12(1):6405.

21. Choi B, Choudhary MC, Regan J, et al. Persistence and evolution of SARS-CoV-2 in an immuno-compromised host. N Engl J Med 2020;383(23): 2291–3.

22. Han A, Rodriguez TE, Beck ET, et al. Persistent SARS-CoV-2 infectivity greater than 50 days in a case series of allogeneic peripheral blood stem cell transplant recipients. Curr Probl Cancer Case Rep 2021;3:100057.

23. Baang JH, Smith C, Mirabelli C, et al. Prolonged severe acute respiratory syndrome coronavirus 2 replication in an immunocompromised patient. J Infect Dis 2021;223(1):23–7.

24. Gandhi S, Klein J, Robertson AJ, et al. De novo emergence of a remdesivir resistance mutation during treatment of persistent SARS-CoV-2 infection in an immunocompromised patient: a case report. Nat Commun 2022;13(1):1547.

25. Oztürk S, Kant A, Comoglu S, et al. Investigation of the clinical course and severity of covid-19 infection in immunocompromised patients. Acta Med Mediterranea 2021;37:2593–7.

26. Baek MS, Lee M-T, Kim W-Y, et al. COVID-19-related outcomes in immunocompromised patients: a nationwide study in Korea. PLOS ONE 2021; 16(10):e0257641.

27. Pagano L, Salmanton-García J, Marchesi F, et al. COVID-19 infection in adult patients with hematological malignancies: a European Hematology Association Survey (EPICOVIDEHA). J Hematol Oncol 2021; 14(1):1–168.

28. Mato AR, Roeker LE, Lamanna N, et al. Outcomes of COVID-19 in patients with CLL: a multicenter international experience. Blood 2020;136(10):1134–43.

29. Roeker LE, Eyre TA, Thompson MC, et al. COVID-19 in patients with CLL: improved survival outcomes and update on management strategies. Blood 2021;138(18):1768–73.

30. Martin S, Kaeuffer C, Leyendecker P, et al. COVID-19 in patients with cancer: a retrospective study of 212 cases from a French SARS-CoV-2 cluster during the first wave of the COVID-19 pandemic. The Oncologist 2021;26(9):e1656–9.

31. Dai M, Liu D, Liu M, et al. Patients with cancer appear more vulnerable to SARS-CoV-2: a multicenter study during the COVID-19 outbreak. Cancer Discov 2020;10(6):783–91.

32. Luo J, Rizvi H, Preeshagul IR, et al. COVID-19 in patients with lung cancer. Ann Oncol 2020;31(10): 1386–96.

33. Yao Y, Cao J, Wang Q, et al. D-dimer as a biomarker for disease severity and mortality in COVID-19 patients: a case control study. J Intensive Care 2020; 8(1).

34. Tian J, Yuan X, Xiao J, et al. Clinical characteristics and risk factors associated with COVID-19 disease severity in patients with cancer in Wuhan, China: a multicentre, retrospective, cohort study. Lancet Oncol 2020;21(7):893–903.

35. Mehta V, Goel S, Kabarriti R, et al. Case fatality rate of patients with cancer with COVID-19 in a New York hospital system. Cancer Discov 2020;10(7):935–41.

36. Ljungman P, De La Camara R, Mikulska M, et al. COVID-19 and stem cell transplantation; results from an EBMT and GETH multicenter prospective survey. Leukemia 2021;35(10):2885–94.

37. Smith C, Odd D, Harwood R, et al. Deaths in Children and Young People in England following SARS-CoV-2 infection during the first pandemic year: a national study using linked mandatory child death reporting data. Laurel Hollow, NY: Cold Spring Harbor Laboratory; 2021.

38. Karataş A, Malkan ÜY, Velet M, et al. The clinical course of COVID-19 in hematopoietic stem cell transplantation (HSCT) recipients. Turkish J Med Sci 2021;51(4):1647–52.

39. Jering KS, McGrath MM, Mc Causland FR, et al. Excess mortality in solid organ transplant recipients

hospitalized with COVID-19: a large-scale comparison of SOT recipients hospitalized with or without COVID-19. Clin Transplant 2022;36(1):e14492.

40. Chaudhry ZS, Williams JD, Vahia A, et al. Clinical characteristics and outcomes of COVID-19 in solid organ transplant recipients: a cohort study. Am J Transplant 2020;20(11):3051–60.

41. Cunningham LC, George S, Nelson D, et al. Outcomes of COVID-19 in an advanced heart failure practice: a single center study. J Heart Lung Transplant 2022;41(4):S176.

42. Cravedi P, Mothi SS, Azzi Y, et al. COVID-19 and kidney transplantation: results from the TANGO international transplant consortium. Am J Transplant 2020;20(11):3140–8.

43. Messika J, Eloy P, Roux A, et al. COVID-19 in lung transplant recipients. Transplantation 2021;105(1):177–86.

44. Di Biagio A, Ricci E, Calza L, et al. Factors associated with hospital admission for COVID-19 in HIV patients. AIDS 2020;34(13):1983–5.

45. Del Amo J, Polo R, Moreno S, et al. Incidence and severity of COVID-19 in HIV-positive persons receiving antiretroviral therapy : a cohort study. Ann Intern Med 2020;173(7):536–41.

46. Cordtz R, Lindhardsen J, Soussi BG, et al. Incidence and severeness of COVID-19 hospitalization in patients with inflammatory rheumatic disease: a nationwide cohort study from Denmark. Rheumatology 2021;60(SI):SI59–67.

47. D'Silva KM, Serling-Boyd N, Wallwork R, et al. Clinical characteristics and outcomes of patients with coronavirus disease 2019 (COVID-19) and rheumatic disease: a comparative cohort study from a US 'hot spot. Ann Rheum Dis 2020;79(9):1156–62.

48. Brenner EJ, Ungaro RC, Gearry RB, et al. Corticosteroids, but not TNF antagonists, are associated with adverse COVID-19 outcomes in patients with inflammatory bowel diseases: results from an international registry. Gastroenterology 2020;159(2):481–91.e483.

49. Quinti I, Lougaris V, Milito C, et al. A possible role for B cells in COVID-19? Lesson from patients with agammaglobulinemia. J Allergy Clin Immunol 2020;146(1):211–3.e214.

50. Hammond J, Leister-Tebbe H, Gardner A, et al. Oral nirmatrelvir for high-risk, nonhospitalized adults with covid-19. N Engl J Med 2022;386(15):1397–408.

51. Neant N, Lingas G, Le Hingrat Q, et al. Modeling SARS-CoV-2 viral kinetics and association with mortality in hospitalized patients from the French COVID cohort. Proc Natl Acad Sci U S A 2021;118(8):1.

52. Fragoulis GE, Koutsianas C, Fragiadaki K, et al. Oral antiviral treatment in patients with systemic rheumatic disease at risk for development of severe COVID-19: a case series. Ann Rheum Dis 2022;81(10):1477–9. annrheumdis-202.

53. Camprubí D, Gaya A, Marcos MA, et al. Persistent replication of SARS-CoV-2 in a severely immunocompromised patient treated with several courses of remdesivir. Int J Infect Dis 2021;104:379–81.

54. Gottlieb RL, Vaca CE, Paredes R, et al. Early remdesivir to prevent progression to severe covid-19 in outpatients. N Engl J Med 2022;386(4):305–15.

55. Pérez-Sáez MJ, Blasco M, Redondo-Pachón D, et al. Use of tocilizumab in kidney transplant recipients with COVID-19. Am J Transplant 2020;20(11):3182–90.

56. Hilbrands LB, Duivenvoorden R, Vart P, et al. COVID-19-related mortality in kidney transplant and dialysis patients: results of the ERACODA collaboration. Nephrol Dial Transplant 2020;35(11):1973–83.

57. Adarsh Bhimraj RLM, Amy Hirsch Shumaker, Valery Lavergne, LindseyBaden, Vincent Chi-Chung Cheng, Kathryn M. Edwards,Rajesh Gandhi,Jason Gallagher,William J. Muller, John C. O'Horo, Shmuel Shoham, M. Hassan Murad, Reem A.Mustafa, Shahnaz Sultan, Yngve Falck-Ytter3. Infectious Diseases Society of America Guidelines on the Treatment and Management of Patients with COVID-19. 2022. Version 10.1.1 Available at: http://www.idsociety.org/COVID19guidelines.

58. Kalil AC, Patterson TF, Mehta AK, et al. Baricitinib plus remdesivir for hospitalized adults with covid-19. N Engl J Med 2021;384(9):795–807.

59. Marconi VC, Ramanan AV, De Bono S, et al. Efficacy and safety of baricitinib in patients with COVID-19 infection: results from the randomised, double-blind, placebo-controlled, parallel-group COV-BARRIER phase 3 trial. Laurel Hollow, NY: Cold Spring Harbor Laboratory; 2021.

60. Ortigoza MB, Yoon H, Goldfeld KS, et al. Efficacy and safety of COVID-19 convalescent plasma in hospitalized patients: a randomized clinical trial. JAMA Intern Med 2022;182(2):115–26.

61. Hueso T, Godron A-S, Lanoy E, et al. Convalescent plasma improves overall survival in patients with B-cell lymphoid malignancy and COVID-19: a longitudinal cohort and propensity score analysis. Leukemia 2022;36(4):1025–34.

62. Ljungquist O, Lundgren M, Iliachenko E, et al. Convalescent plasma treatment in severely immunosuppressed patients hospitalized with COVID-19: an observational study of 28 cases. Infect Dis 2022;54(4):283–91.

63. Callaghan CJ, Mumford L, Curtis RMK, et al. Real-world effectiveness of the pfizer-BioNTech BNT162b2 and oxford-AstraZeneca ChAdOx1-S vaccines against SARS-CoV-2 in solid organ and islet transplant recipients. Transplantation 2022;106(3):436–46.

64. Oyaert M, De Scheerder MA, Van Herrewege S, et al. Evaluation of humoral and cellular responses

in SARS-CoV-2 mRNA vaccinated immunocompromised patients. Front Immunol 2022;13:858399.

65. Mrak D, Tobudic S, Koblischke M, et al. SARS-CoV-2 vaccination in rituximab-treated patients: B cells promote humoral immune responses in the presence of T-cell-mediated immunity. Ann Rheum Dis 2021;80(10):1345–50.

66. Tenforde MW, Patel MM, Ginde AA, et al. Effectiveness of SARS-CoV-2 mRNA vaccines for preventing covid-19 hospitalizations in the United States. Clin Infect Dis 2022;74(9):1515–24.

67. Brosh-Nissimov T, Orenbuch-Harroch E, Chowers M, et al. BNT162b2 vaccine breakthrough: clinical characteristics of 152 fully vaccinated hospitalized COVID-19 patients in Israel. Clin Microbiol Infect 2021;27(11):1652–7.

68. Song Q, Bates B, Shao YR, et al. Risk and outcome of breakthrough COVID-19 infections in vaccinated patients with cancer: real-world evidence from the national COVID cohort collaborative. J Clin Oncol 2022;40(13):1414–27.

69. Wang W, Kaelber DC, Xu R, et al. Breakthrough SARS-CoV-2 infections, hospitalizations, and mortality in vaccinated patients with cancer in the US between december 2020 and november 2021. JAMA Oncol 2022;8(7):1027–34.

70. Schmidt AL, Labaki C, Hsu CY, et al. COVID-19 vaccination and breakthrough infections in patients with cancer. Ann Oncol 2022;33(3):340–6.

71. Levin MJ, Ustianowski A, De Wit S, et al. LB5. PROVENT: phase 3 study of efficacy and safety of AZD7442 (Tixagevimab/Cilgavimab) for pre-exposure prophylaxis of COVID-19 in adults. Open Forum Infect Dis 2021; 8(Supplement_1):S810.

72. Center for Disease Control and Prevention. Long COVID or Post-COVID Conditions. In:2022. Available at: https//www.cdc.gov/coronavirus/2019-ncov/long-term-effects/index.html

73. Soriano JB, Murthy S, Marshall JC, et al. A clinical case definition of post-COVID-19 condition by a Delphi consensus. Lancet Infect Dis 2022;22(4): e102–7.

74. Pinato DJ, Tabernero J, Bower M, et al. Prevalence and impact of COVID-19 sequelae on treatment and survival of patients with cancer who recovered from SARS-CoV-2 infection: evidence from the OnCovid retrospective, multicentre registry study. Lancet Oncol 2021;22(12):1669–80.

75. Taramasso L, Sepulcri C, Mikulska M, et al. Duration of isolation and precautions in immunocompromised patients with COVID-19. J Hosp Infect 2021;111: 202–4.

76. Swank Z, Senussi Y, Alter G, et al. Persistent circulating SARS-CoV-2 spike is associated with postacute COVID-19 sequelae. Laurel Hollow, NY: Cold Spring Harbor Laboratory; 2022.

The Impact of Coronavirus Disease 2019 on Viral, Bacterial, and Fungal Respiratory Infections

Ashley Losier, MD[a,1,*], Gayatri Gupta, DO[a,1], Mario Caldararo, MD, MS[b,1], Charles S. Dela Cruz, MD, PhD[a,1]

KEYWORDS

- Coinfections • COVID-19 • Influenza • Respiratory syncytial virus • Social distancing
- Bacterial pneumonia

KEY POINTS

- The COVID-19 pandemic impacted the trends of other common respiratory viral illnesses between 2020 and 2022.
- Implementation of social distancing, mask wearing, and other behavioral interventions for COVID impacted levels of respiratory virus spread.
- Coinfection with other respiratory viruses can occur with COVID-19 infections, with influenza and RSV being among the most common.
- Coinfection with bacterial pneumonia can occur with COVID-19 infections, including community-acquired pneumonia and hospital-acquired pneumonia.
- Ventilator-associated pneumonia is a common nosocomial infection associated with COVID-19 infections and increased mortality.

INTRODUCTION

Since the emergence of the coronavirus disease 2019 (COVID-19) pandemic in Wuhan, China, in December 2019, there has been a significant focus placed on its transmission, pathogenesis, treatment, and prevention.[1] Although COVID-19 continues to have a global impact, concerns about other respiratory infections, including those caused by viruses and bacteria, remain.

The COVID-19 pandemic has shed unique light on the epidemiologic trends of common community-acquired respiratory viruses and the impacts of nonpharmacologic practices including social distancing and mask wearing. In addition, coinfections of COVID-19 with other respiratory viruses and bacterial organisms, along with nosocomial and opportunistic fungal infections, have been observed with variable outcomes.

This article highlights epidemiologic trends of common respiratory viruses during the COVID-19 pandemic and coinfections with common respiratory viruses and other infectious agents.

EPIDEMIOLOGIC TRENDS OF COMMON RESPIRATORY VIRUSES DURING THE SEVERE ACUTE RESPIRATORY SYNDROME CORONAVIRUS 2 PANDEMIC

Although there has been a primary focus on the severe acute respiratory syndrome coronavirus 2 (SARS-CoV-2) respiratory virus since the COVID-19

[a] Department of Internal Medicine, Section of Pulmonary and Critical Care Medicine, Yale University School of Medicine, New Haven, CT 06511, USA; [b] Veteran's Affairs Connecticut Healthcare System, West Haven, CT 06516, USA

[1] Present address. PO Box 208057, New Haven, CT 06520-8057.

* Corresponding author. Mario Caldararo is now at Saint Peter's Univesity Hospital, New Brunswick, NJ 08901.
E-mail address: Ashley.losier@yale.edu

Clin Chest Med 44 (2023) 407–423
https://doi.org/10.1016/j.ccm.2022.11.018

pandemic emerged in 2019, concern for other common community-acquired respiratory viruses remains. Community-acquired respiratory viruses include influenza, respiratory syncytial virus (RSV), paramyxoviruses, rhinovirus, and adenovirus, among others; all may have varied clinical presentations/severities depending on host factors. In the absence of laboratory testing, it may be difficult to distinguish between various respiratory viruses. Often respiratory viruses cause upper respiratory tract infections all with similar symptoms of fever, chills, myalgias, cough, and shortness of breath. However, several respiratory viruses including influenza may lead to lower respiratory tract infections with pneumonia, hypoxemic respiratory failure, and superimposed infections. Given the wide range of symptom severity, including those with asymptomatic infections, respiratory viral illnesses may be underestimated because many patients do not undergo diagnostic testing for non-COVID infections. Thus, the authors provide an overview of the epidemiologic trends in respiratory viruses during the SARS-CoV-2 pandemic and discuss recent updates and the impact of the pandemic on influenza, RSV, and other respiratory viruses.

Influenza Virus

Influenza is seasonal in North America occurring frequently in the winter but can occur year-round in tropical countries. The emergence of the H3N2 strain occurred in 1968 near Hong Kong, and since that time the origin of several antigenically diverse strains of seasonal influenza a (H3N2) has been attributed to the densely populous East, South, and Southeast Asia regions. Seasonal influenza epidemics are influenced by antigenic drift or small mutations in hemagglutinin and neuraminidase proteins, which produce closely related viruses. Antigenic shift occurs less frequently and is an abrupt change in the influenza virus that can cause pandemics due to lack of immunity in the general population to this genetic shift. Annual epidemics can result in up to 650,000 deaths worldwide according to the World Health Organization (WHO), and the last influenza pandemic was in 2009 to 2010, caused by the H1N1 virus with 284,000 deaths in more than 214 countries.[2,3] Surveillance done by WHO FluNet and Centers for Disease Control and Prevention ([CDC] FluView) include the most robust data on influenza; however, because influenza is not a reportable disease in the United States, these are compiled estimates (**Fig. 1**).

Indeed, studies early in the pandemic demonstrated that changes in population behavior were associated with both reduced transmission of SARS-CoV-2 and decreased influenza transmission.[4,5] In the United States, between September 2020 and May 2021, there was a marked reported reduction in reported influenza cases: the CDC reported that only 1899 (0.2%) of 1,081,671 clinical samples tested positive for influenza virus; influenza B comprised most of the reported cases at 62.5%.[6] In contrast to the 2020 to 2021 season, the CDC reported more than 250,000 positive influenza specimens of 1,491,430 total specimens in the 2019 to 2020 season[7] with a similar global trend.[8,9] Prediction models after the light 2020 to 2021 season anticipated a heavier compensatory season in 2021 to 2022 due to decreased immunity.[10]

Respiratory Syncytial Virus

RSV contributed substantially to the respiratory viral disease burden before the pandemic. RSV is common in the pediatric population where it causes significant mortality in children younger than 2 years due to bronchiolitis and pneumonia, although there are increasing data demonstrating significant burden in elderly, chronically ill, or immunocompromised adults.[11,12] Influenza is typically associated with more deaths than RSV in all age groups except for children younger than 1 year.[13] The CDC collects information on RSV in the United States using the National Respiratory and Enteric Virus Surveillance System (NREVSS).[14] According to the CDC, RSV contributes to 58,000 hospitalizations among children younger than 5 years and 14,000 deaths among adults older than 65 years annually.[15] RSV follows a similar seasonal trend to influenza in the United States,[16] starting in early December and peaking in February in the United States.[14] Longer infection seasons have been associated with more northern latitude.[17] Infection can be seen outside a seasonal trend in tropical countries and also when infection mitigation measures disrupt seasonal patterns as noted earlier. RSV activity can correlate with rainfall and humidity in tropical regions, as in Australia during 2020 when widespread spring RSV outbreaks extended into summer.[18] In addition, in the United States and France, RSV was reported later and extended into the spring and summer months.[14,19]

Similar to influenza, epidemiologic trends demonstrate a reduction in RSV cases across various countries from March 2020[20–23] that was also attributed to social distancing and nonpharmacologic interventions. Despite lifting social distancing restrictions in April 2020, no RSV cases were detected in western Australia until august

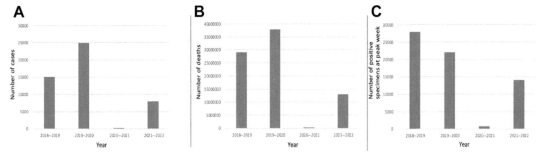

Fig. 1. Comparison of influenza seasons in the United States with compilation of data from WHO FluNet and CDC FluView between 2018 and 2022[4–8] including (A) total number of cases, (B) total number of deaths, and (C) total number of positive specimens at peak week.

2020, inferring that increased hygienic measures, such as hand washing, may have sustained prevention of viral transmission.[24] Another hypothesis for reduction in RSV was viral interference from SARS-CoV-2 because interferon-stimulated immunity by one virus reduces infectivity of additional viruses. In 2021 as pandemic measures were relaxed, the reemergence of RSV was noted in various regions even out of the usual seasonal trends in both northern and southern hemispheres where outbreaks began later than seasonally expected.[14,19] Another hypothesis for the reemergence of RSV was that fewer viral infections in 2020 led to lower concentrations of antibodies in pregnant women, subsequently impacting acquired immunity of infants.[25] Indeed, lack of immunity coupled with the resumption of normal societal activities is likely responsible for the surge of RSV cases in children that is overwhelming pediatric facilities in the fall of 2022.[26]

EPIDEMIOLOGIC TRENDS OF OTHER RESPIRATORY VIRUSES

Throughout the SARS-CoV-2 pandemic there remained concerns for other respiratory viruses including paramyxoviruses, respiratory adenovirus, seasonal coronavirus, and rhinovirus, among others. The NREVSS database showed that the epidemiology of non-RSV paramyxoviruses (including human metapneumovirus and parainfluenza virus) and respiratory adenovirus varied during the pandemic.[14]

The common seasonal coronavirus (the strains 229E, NL63, OC43, and HKU1) had a persistent role during the SARS-CoV-2 pandemic and was often found in cocirculation with SARS-CoV-2.[14] The data on the diagnosis of seasonal coronavirus may have been limited because it is often not part of the diagnostic panels. Seasonal coronavirus follows a trend of peaking during winter months, which may suggest that factors including low

temperature and low sunlight favor survival, and remains more common in the pediatric and adolescent populations.[27,28]

Rhinovirus is another commonly observed virus that is also noted to have persistence during the COVID-19 pandemic in various regions including the United Kingdom and Singapore.[29,30] Rhinovirus reductions were only seen after lockdown, and levels rebounded earlier than other respiratory viruses, which suggests that social distancing practices were more effective at suppressing other respiratory viruses.[30] The hypothesis surrounding the early reemergence of rhinovirus infections included its viral structure as a small, hydrophilic, nonenveloped virus with propensity for contact and droplet transmission.[29]

These various viruses have demonstrated some regional differences during the COVID-19 pandemic, but overall many regions exhibited similar trends of decreased annual seasonal respiratory viruses in 2020 to 2021 with reemergence in the 2021 to 2022 season.[31,32]

IMPACT OF SOCIAL DISTANCING AND VACCINATION ON THE SPREAD OF COMMON RESPIRATORY VIRAL INFECTIONS DURING THE CORONAVIRUS DISEASE 2019 PANDEMIC

Several interventions have influenced epidemiologic trends of respiratory infections since the pandemic began, including social distancing and implementation of nonpharmacologic measures such as wearing masks, eye protection, and strict hand hygiene practices.

Even before the COVID-19 pandemic, interventions to limit contact and droplet-related spread were studied. A systematic review of social distancing measures including crowd avoidance, workplace/school closures, lockdowns, isolation of infected persons, quarantining of exposed persons, and contract tracing had some benefit against influenza spread.[33–36] Transmission of viruses was noted to be lower when physical distance was greater than 1 m, and protection was increased as distance increased.[37] Hand hygiene has long been a key infection prevention method and has been associated with reduction in respiratory viral illnesses.[38] Chan and colleagues[39] observed an 88.9% decrease in the prototypical community-acquired pneumonia (CAP) syndrome with pneumococcal pneumonia from pandemic years 2020 to 2021 when compared with the 5 years before the pandemic, hypothesizing that public health policies (eg, universal masking and social distancing) may have been the primary drivers of such a decrease. A reduction in bronchiectasis exacerbations was noted during the first 12 months of the COVID-19 pandemic upon implementation of social distancing measures.[40]

In addition, the implementation of mask wearing resulted in a large reduction in risk of COVID-19 infection. The use of respirator masks (like N95 masks) was associated with stronger protection when compared with the use of disposable surgical masks.[37] An N95 respirator mask has efficient airborne filtration with a tight-fitting design allowing for a seal around the nose and mouth. In contrast, surgical masks are loose fitting and less efficiently filter airborne particles.

Apart from masks, eye protection provided an added layer for infection prevention. In a study of frontline emergency room workers, mandatory eye protection in conjunction with universal masking was effective at reducing COVID-19; additional reviews have suggested that use of eye protection may help prevent eye inoculation, which could lead to respiratory infections.[41,42]

SEVERE ACUTE RESPIRATORY SYNDROME CORONAVIRUS 2 AND VIRAL COINFECTIONS
Severe Acute Respiratory Syndrome Coronavirus 2 and Influenza

It can be expected that SARS-CoV-2 will become endemic and cocirculate with influenza, and therefore their similarities and differences should be reviewed. Before SARS-CoV-2, influenza was one of the largest public health challenges, resulting in approximately half a million deaths annually.[43] Several studies have compared both viruses given their similarity of symptoms and propensity to each cause severe illness (table 1).

Clinical presentation may be similar for both influenza and SARS-CoV-2; however, symptoms that tend to be more unique to SARS-CoV-2 include loss of taste and smell as a symptom. Additional variants of SARS-CoV-2, including the omicron variant, have been associated with less severe symptoms when compared with alpha and delta variants, and many individuals are asymptomatic and may be unaware of their infection. A large study demonstrated that patients with SARS-CoV-2 more frequently had conditions including obesity, diabetes, hypertension, and dyslipidemia when compared with patients with influenza, indicating the importance of metabolic syndrome as a risk factor for SARS-CoV-2 infection. Those with influenza more frequently had heart failure, chronic respiratory disease, and cirrhosis. This comparative study also demonstrated that patients hospitalized with SARS-CoV-2 infection more frequently developed acute respiratory failure, pulmonary embolism, septic shock, or hemorrhagic stroke than patients with influenza, although they were noted to have a lower incidence of myocardial infarction or atrial fibrillation. In-hospital mortality was higher in patients with SARS-CoV-2 than in patients with influenza,[62] and patients with SARS-CoV-2 more frequently have abnormal chest radiology and longer duration of stay during hospitalizations.[63]

Apart from the clinical presentations, the treatment and prevention for SARS-CoV-2 and influenza also differ. SARS-CoV-2 therapeutics include novel antiviral therapies such as remdesivir and vaccinations, which are currently the mainstay of outpatient therapy and prevention of SARS-CoV-2. For influenza, interferons and neuraminidase inhibitors play roles in the prophylaxis and treatment. Interferon types 1 and type 3 function to inhibit viral replication,[64] and neuraminidase inhibitors assist in preventing virions from being released from the surface of infected cells and are effective for both prophylaxis and treatment.[65] Antiviral medications for influenza are approved for use within the United States and have a mechanism of action based via neuraminidase inhibition and can lessen symptoms and shorten duration of illness. Annual influenza vaccination is recommended for everyone aged six months and older (**Table 2**), whereas CDC recommendations for SARS-CoV-2 vaccines include initial series and boosters. The efficacy for influenza vaccines varies by season and aids to reduce severity of illness.[66,67] There has been evidence that has also suggested that flu vaccination has the potential to reduce mortality of SARS-CoV-2 with lower risk of death at 60 days in patients who had received flu vaccinations.[68]

In cases of severe disease with refractory hypoxemia in both SARS-CoV-2 and influenza, extracorporeal membrane oxygenation can be considered as a salvage therapy.[72] When comparing symptoms after acute illness of SARS-CoV-2 and influenza infections, postacute sequalae of COVID ([PASC] or long COVID) has

Table 1
Comparison of characteristics of severe acute respiratory syndrome coronavirus 2, influenza, and respiratory syncytial virus

	SARS-CoV-2	Influenza	RSV
Viral structure	Single-stranded, positive-sense RNA	Negative-sense, single-stranded RNA with surface glycoproteins integral in determining influenza type	Filamentous enveloped, negative-sense, single-stranded RNA
Zoonotic infection	Bats	Avian and swine	Animal models of RSV infections in rodents and nonhumans primates
Virulence	Median r_0 2.79	Median r_0 1.28	Median r_0 1.2–.2.1
Population at risk	• Hypertension • Diabetes • Smoking history • Age: elderly • Male sex • Pregnancy • Obesity • History of heart disease • History of lung disease	• History of chronic disease • Neuromuscular disorders • Morbid obesity • Pregnancy • Age: elderly and young children	• Age: children and elderly • History of heart disease • History of lung disease
Time until postexposure presentation	3–7 d	2–5 d	4–6 d
Clinical symptoms	• Fever • Headache • Dyspnea • Cough • Myalgias • Fatigue • Anosmia and loss of taste May be asymptomatic	• Fever • Nasal congestion • Sore throat • Myalgias • Fatigue • Nausea?, vomiting • Abdominal pain • Diarrhea	• Fever • Poor appetite • Rhinorrhea • Cough • Dyspnea • Wheezing
Duration of symptoms	Depends on severity of illness	Typically resolves by day 8	Typically resolves by 3–7 d
Complications	Post-COVID syndrome and severe cases can lead to ARDS	Severe cases can lead to ARDS	Severe cases can lead to bronchiolitis and pneumonia (especially in pediatric cases)

Abbreviation: ARDS, acute respiratory distress syndrome.
Data regarding SARS-CoV-2 from Refs.[44–53]; data regarding influenza from Refs.[54–58]; data regarding RSV from Refs.[59–61]

been associated with symptoms of prolonged dyspnea, fatigue/malaise, chest/throat pain, headache, abdominal symptoms, myalgias, cognitive symptoms, and anxiety/depression.[73]

Systematic reviews report variable rates of coinfection, one stating rates of influenza infection were 0.8% in patients with confirmed SARS-CoV-2 with fever, cough, and shortness of breath being most common clinical manifestations.[74] Analyses also demonstrate higher coinfection rates in pediatrics compared with adults.[75] In one small pediatric study, nearly half of SARS-CoV-2 infected children had coinfection with other common respiratory pathogens.[76] Although there is no clear consensus on the implications of coinfection, one study suggests there is a potential for

Table 2
Influenza and severe acute respiratory syndrome coronavirus 2 vaccine comparison

	Influenza Vaccine	SARS-CoV-2 Vaccine		
Type	Inactivated, quadrivalent vaccine (live attenuated or recombinant vaccines also available)	mRNA vaccine		DNA viral vector
Mechanism	Surface glycoproteins hemagglutinin	RNA leads to generation of spike protein found on coronavirus and creation of antibodies against it		Modified virus is a vector carrying for COVID spike protein to trigger immune response
Brands	Not applicable	Pfizer-BioNTech	Moderna	Johnson & Johnson's Janssen (J&J)
Frequency of dosing	Annual	2 injections 21 d apart + booster	2 injections 28 d apart + booster	1 dose + booster
% Effectiveness	40–60	90	95	66
Population recommended for	6 mo and older	6 mo and older	6 mo and older	> 18 years old

Vaccine mechanisms reviewed from Refs.[69–71]

added harm with viral coinfection, because post-translational changes in angiotensin-converting enzyme-2 by influenza A may increase vulnerability to lung injury and acute respiratory distress syndrome (ARDS) during coinfections.[77] Although potential targets for therapy are under investigation,[78] no single medication is known to treat both SARS-CoV-2 and influenza simultaneously, although supportive care can be given for both. Similar to influenza infections, as many as one-fifth of patients with SARS-CoV-2 are found to have coinfection or superinfection with other pathogens, which increases mortality, and these coinfections and superinfections are discussed further in this article. Influenza is also associated with bacterial superinfection, specifically *Staphylococcus aureus* and *Streptococcus pneumoniae*.[79]

In the future, coinfection of SARS-CoV-2 and influenza virus will likely continue to occur because influenza epidemics may happen concurrently with the ongoing SARS-CoV-2 pandemic. WHO now recommends countries to prepare for the cocirculation of influenza and SARS-CoV-2 viruses with surveillance, monitoring, and vaccination programs for both SARS-CoV-2 and influenza.

Severe Acute Respiratory Syndrome Coronavirus 2 and Respiratory Syncytial Virus

Similar to influenza, we can expect that SARS-CoV-2 and RSV will start to cocirculate globally.

Both RSV and SARS-CoV-2 can present with typical viral symptoms including fever, chills, myalgias, rhinorrhea, cough, and sore throat. Apart from cold-type symptoms (see **Table 2**) RSV can also lead to serious conditions such as bronchiolitis and predominantly affects pediatric and elderly patient populations.

Treatment of RSV is largely supportive and includes antipyretics and hydration. However, severe cases of bronchiolitis or pneumonia may require hospitalization and respiratory support. For prophylaxis against RSV, the medication palivizumab can be given to select pediatric patient populations who are at high risk of serious complications including lower respiratory tract infections from RSV and has been shown to reduce hospitalizations.[80] Ribavarin is approved for severe RSV disease, but its effectiveness is unclear and not well studied, including in patients who are immunocompromised. At this time, there are limited effective antiviral medications targeted to RSV infections; however, there are ongoing trials to evaluate new antivirals and vaccines for RSV, including during pregnancy.[81]

RSV is among the most common coinfections in patients with SARS-CoV-2 pneumonia.[82] Viral coinfection of RSV and SARS-CoV-2 may be associated with prolonged hospitalization, need for higher level of care, complicated lower respiratory infections,[83] and elevated procalcitonin levels[84];

however, its contribution to increased mortality remains unclear.[85–88]

Severe Acute Respiratory Syndrome Coronavirus 2 and Epstein-Barr Virus

SARS-CoV-2 has also demonstrated interaction with other viruses, although data for these viruses is based on smaller studies and case reports. Immune dysregulation from SARS-CoV-2 may potentiate other viral infections, particularly those with an asymptomatic course with potential to reactivate.

Epstein-Barr virus (EBV) can cause a wide range of diseases, from infectious mononucleosis in younger adults to various cancers or lymphoproliferative disorders, or it may be asymptomatic. Co-infection with both viruses demonstrated increased inflammation and consequently increased steroid use.[89] Indeed, both SARS-CoV-2 and EBV can infect epithelial cells of the respiratory tract or cause liver function abnormalities, thus elevated liver function tests in coinfection can be expected, especially in setting of EBV reactivation.[90] One study demonstrated up to 25% reactivation rate of EBV in patients with SARS-CoV-2, particularly in older and female persons, and suggested an associated increased mortality.[91] This enhanced inflammation from EBV viral reactivation is thought to play a significant role in the development of PASC symptoms,[92] possibly due to alternations in mitochondrial function and senescence.[93]

Severe Acute Respiratory Syndrome Coronavirus 2 and Cytomegalovirus

There are case reports of SARS-CoV-2 and cytomegalovirus (CMV), which have been associated with various clinical presentations including the development of CMV pneumonitis and presentations of gastrointestinal symptoms.[94] CMV seropositivity is associated with increased risk of hospitalization with SARS-CoV-2 infection[15] and increased severe bacterial infections.[95] Furthermore, there has been suggestion to consider secondary infection with CMV in the differential of transaminitis for those with SARS-CoV-2 and EBV infections, because reactivation of CMV has also been described,[96] although EBV is most consistently shown among opportunistic viruses.[97]

Additional considerations for viral reactivation include the alterations of the immune system associated with SARS-CoV-2 vaccination, which have been associated with sequelae of viral reactivation in CMV and varicella zoster virus.[98–102]

Severe Acute Respiratory Syndrome Coronavirus 2 and Other Respiratory Viruses

Although viral coinfections remains relatively rare, case reports have described coinfections of SARS-CoV-2 with human metapneumovirus,[103] human parainfluenza virus,[104] and adenovirus,[105] among others. Case reports of SARS-CoV-2 and coinfection with adenovirus have suggested a more severe hospital course than when with isolated infections.[106] It should be noted that studies reviewed here are not specific to patients who undergo transplant, although transplant recipients are already at increased risk of reactivation of certain viruses due to immunosuppression.

SEVERE ACUTE RESPIRATORY SYNDROME CORONAVIRUS 2, BACTERIAL COINFECTIONS, AND SUPERINFECTIONS

Bacterial coinfection and superinfection during severe viral illness has been a prominent issue documented as early as the 1918 influenza pandemic. Autopsies showed that virtually all influenza deaths were complicated, and perhaps caused by bacterial pneumonia coinfection; *Streptococcus pneumoniae* was a particularly significant pathogen with high mortality.[107]

The reasons for bacterial involvement in viral disease are unclear and can occur through several mechanisms (**Fig. 2**). Dysbiosis of the pulmonary microbiome during invasive mechanical ventilation has been demonstrated and hypothesized to be due to a combination of antibiotic use, translocation of gastrointestinal flora, dysfunction of pulmonary mucosal immunity, and impaired microbial clearance.[108] Viruses also impair host defenses resulting in increased susceptibility to bacterial infection, namely, by compromising the integrity of the respiratory epithelium, which allows for better adherence and invasion of bacteria.[109] In addition, there is preliminary evidence in extrapulmonary infection models that viruses alter host cytokine expression potentially "distracting" the immune system away from a bacterial pathogen leading to worsening of bacterial infection.[110] Because it pertains to SARS-CoV-2 specifically, some evidence also points toward an early immunoparalysis driven by virally infected monocytes and macrophages.[111]

The diagnosis of contemporaneous and secondary bacterial infections during SARS-CoV-2 infections has implications for patient outcomes, antibiotic stewardship, and health care costs.

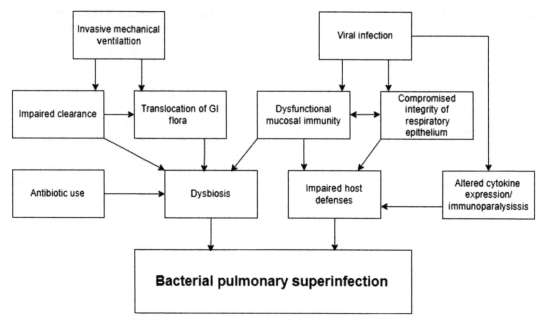

Fig. 2. The complex interplay of factors predisposing to bacterial pulmonary superinfection. GI, gastrointestinal.

SEVERE ACUTE RESPIRATORY SYNDROME CORONAVIRUS 2 AND COMMUNITY-ACQUIRED PNEUMONIA

Definition

CAP is defined in clinical terms as the presence of symptoms attributable to pneumonia (eg, dyspnea, cough) plus radiographic confirmation.[112]

Epidemiology

A multicenter study done by the CDC in 2015 showed that among approximately 2300 patients presenting with CAP, a bacterial cause was only identified 17% of the time.[113] Patients presenting with SARS-CoV-2 have bacterial coinfection even less frequently. Lehmann and colleagues[114] found bacterial coinfection to occur in 7 of 321 SARS-CoV-2 presentations, with 4 cases of S pneumoniae, 2 cases of S aureus, and 1 case of Proteus mirabilis. This finding was further confirmed when an additional study showed that community-acquired bacterial coinfection occurred in only 59 of 1705 SARS-CoV-2 admissions.

The contrast between higher rates of coinfection during the influenza pandemic and the lower rate of bacterial CAP as a coinfection in SARS-CoV-2 is potentially explained by differing public health landscapes. Amin-Choudhury and colleagues[115] confirmed that public health policies, such as social distancing practices, can lead to of decreased rates of pneumococcal CAP in the setting of coinfection; however, they noted that when coinfection happened it was associated with a 7-fold increase in 28-day mortality.[39]

Diagnosis

Discerning a patient presenting from the community with solitary COVID-19 pneumonia versus one with a bacterial coinfection remains difficult. Unfortunately, procalcitonin level drawn at admission is neither sensitive nor specific for this purpose.[116] Radiographically, there are some findings that are more "typical" for COVID-19 than for bacterial pneumonia. In COVID-19, computed tomography (CT) of the chest shows bilateral, multilobar ground-glass opacities (GGOS) in a peripheral and subpleural distribution and focal areas of consolidation may be found within areas of GGOS.[117] In the second week of illness the GGOS may continue to expand and evolve to contain areas of irregular linear opacities signaling the transformation into an organizing pneumonia.[117]

In contrast, bacterial pneumonia may more frequently have centrilobular nodules and bronchial wall thickening with mucoid impactions, as well as the characteristic lobar consolidation.[116]

Treatment

Treatment of suspected bacterial CAP coinfection should be according to published Infectious Diseases Society of America (IDSA)/American Thoracic Society (ATS) CAP guidelines.[112] Targeted diagnostics should include sputum culture and blood culture for severe disease or if treatment is targeting *Pseudomonas aeruginosa* or methicillin-resistant *S aureus*. Although guidelines only recommend pneumococcal urinary antigen testing for severe cases, it should likely be done whenever coinfection with SARS-CoV-2 is being considered given the higher odds of severe disease developing. Current IDSA guidelines for management of COVID-19 do not recommend for or against antibiotics for CAP, but do describe mostly negative effects of indiscriminate antibiotic use at the time of admission such as resistant superinfection.[118]

CORONAVIRUS DISEASE 2019 AND VENTILATOR-ASSOCIATED PNEUMONIA
Definition

Hospital-acquired pneumonia (HAP) is specified as a pneumonia not incubating at the time of hospital admission and occurring 48 hours or more after admission. Ventilator-associated pneumonia (VAP) is defined as a pneumonia developing greater than 48 hours after endotracheal intubation.[119] Diagnosis of HAP or VAP is based on finding a new lung infiltrate plus clinical evidence that the infiltrate is of an infectious origin (new fever, purulent sputum, leukocytosis, and decline in oxygenation).

Epidemiology

There are considerably more data regarding VAP infections in the setting of COVID-19 when compared with CAP. Mechanically ventilated patients with COVID-19 are at higher risk for VAP than mechanically ventilated patients without COVID-19, with a virtually universal agreement among large studies using strict definitions and microbiological confirmation.[120] Furthermore, autopsy studies of patients who died of severe COVID-19 show that at least 32% had a bacterial superinfection.[121]

VAP was found to be the cause of more than 50% of hospital-acquired infections with *P aeruginosa* and *Klebsiella pneumoniae* being the most common isolated organisms.[122] In a retrospective study observing 192 patients intubated for COVID-19 with early bronchoalveolar lavage (BAL) occurring before intubation in most cases, 11.6% had a superinfection meeting diagnostic criteria for HAP before intubation, with at least one episode of VAP occurring in 44.4% of patients. The average time to diagnosis was 10.8 days postintubation.[123] In a study of more than 70,000 patients in the medical intensive care unit (ICU) divided into groups of prepandemic, pandemic without COVID-19 infection, and pandemic with COVID-19 infection, incidence of VAP was found to be higher in COVID-19-infected patients and had a higher

attributable mortality. Attributable mortality for COVID-19 with VAP was 9.17%, whereas attributable mortality for prepandemic and pandemic COVID-19-negative patients was 3.15% and 2.91%, respectively.[124]

The explanation for such a high incidence of VAP in COVID-19 is likely multifactorial. Patients with COVID-19 who are intubated commonly have one or more of the traditional risk factors for VAP such as high lengths of stay, prolonged duration of mechanical ventilation, the presence of ARDS, sedation, neuromuscular blocking agents, and not least the high utilization of prone positioning.[125] Stress on both human and material resources during peak surges has also been argued to have a detrimental impact on the rate of secondary infection.[126]

Diagnosis

HAP/VAP in COVID-19 should be diagnosed in accordance with IDSA/ATS guidelines.[119,120] Although a spot test of procalcitonin on admission to the hospital was not found to be helpful for the diagnosis of bacterial CAP coinfection,[116] a procalcitonin trend for patients in the ICU may be more useful. Richards and colleagues[127] found that a 50% increase in procalcitonin levels from its previous value was independently associated with the presence of a secondary bacterial infection (VAP, ventilator-associated tracheobronchitis, or bacteremia) compared with increases in either white blood cell count or C-reactive peptide.

Treatment

Treatment of suspected bacterial HAP/VAP coinfections should be according to published IDSA/ATS guidelines.[120]

CORONAVIRUS DISEASE 2019 AND OTHER NOSOCOMIAL INFECTIONS
Bloodstream Infections

In a study comparing nosocomial bloodstream infections (BSIs) in non-COVID-19 and COVID-19 patients,[128] *Candida* species accounted for nearly 50% of infections with next commonest being *Enterococcus* (**Table 3**). A comparison between the COVID-19 and non-COVID-19 groups showed that patients with COVID-19 were more than 2 times as likely to have candidemia than non-COVID-19 patients. *Enterococcus* rates were similar; however, the investigators note that the typical risk factors for candidemia and enterococcal BSIs such as gastrointestinal surgeries, malignancies, and chemotherapy were present in the non-COVID-19 patients but tended to be

Table 3
Most common etiologic organisms in coronavirus disease 2019-associated bloodstream infections

Early	Late
S aureus	Enterococcus
Gram-negatives	Candida

absent in the patients with COVID-19, suggesting that these were distinct complications of COVID-19. The investigators also noted that these BSI organisms occurred later in hospitalization, proposing that perhaps antimicrobials, steroids, and the interleukin (IL)-6 inhibitor tocilizumab may have promoted translocations of these organisms over time (see **Table 3**).

In a study of 212 patients with severe COVID-19 in Brazil, Silva and colleagues[129] found bacteremia to carry an odds ratio for mortality of 21. Gago and colleagues[128] went further to specify that although there was not an observed statistically significant difference in mortality among patients with BSI due to Candida or Enterococcus, there was an increase in mortality clustered around cases of BSI that occurred earlier in hospitalization with the less common S aureus and gram-negative organisms.

Bhatt and colleagues[130] published a multicenter case-control study that highlighted some of the risk factors for secondary BSIs in a sample composed of all hospitalized patients: higher need of supplemental oxygen on admission, higher admission serum creatinine levels, and presentation with encephalopathy. Other potential risk factors include the use of antimicrobials, systemic corticosteroids, and IL-6 blockade. The study did, however, have a high proportion of coagulase-negative staphylococci, raising the concern of inappropriately screened contaminants.[130]

CORONAVIRUS DISEASE 2019 AND INVASIVE FUNGAL INFECTIONS

Aspergillosis and mucormycosis are diseases caused by fungal organisms that infect humans as molds. Although they are both recognized entities occurring in patients with COVID-19, considerable debate exists regarding the rate of occurrence, as it concerns COVID-19-associated pulmonary aspergillosis (CAPA).

Coronavirus Disease 2019-Associated Pulmonary Aspergillosis

One autopsy review series reports a CAPA rate of occurrence of approximately 2% in both mechanically ventilated and nonmechanically ventilated COVID-19 decedents.[131] Published incidences of CAPA ranges from 0% to 30% in studies without standardized definitions, and 2% to 11% in studies with standardized definitions.[132]

A definition of "probable CAPA" has been devised to include more than one of the following: new cavitary lung lesions on chest CT without alternative explanation, positive serum galactomannan Enzyme Immunoassay (EIA) index greater than or equal to 0.5, positive BAL galactomannan EIA index greater than or equal to 1.0, or positive aspergillus cultures from BAL specimen.[133–135] In their retrospective analysis of mechanically ventilated patients with COVID-19 in 5 Johns Hopkins Medicine health system hospitals, Permpalung and colleagues[136] added a diagnosis of "possible" CAPA for patients who had more than 1 of the following: positive BAL galactomannan index greater than or equal to 0.5 (lower threshold), positive serum (1, 3)-β-D-glucan (BDG) level greater than or equal to 80 pg/mL without alternate explanation, and/or non-BAL sample culture with growth of Aspergillus. The expanded definition was intended for centers that do not use bronchoscopy for BAL liberally and that use BDG as a fungal marker in addition to galactomannan. **Table 4** shows a comparison of diagnostics in probable versus possible CAPA.

In the study by Permpalung and colleagues,[136] rates of CAPA ranged from 5% to 10% and patients with CAPA had higher severity of illness, need for more ventilatory and hemodynamic support, and longer duration of hospitalization, although mortality was no different from non-CAPA patients. It is worth noting, however, that only 48.7% of patients with CAPA received antifungal therapy, likely representing the challenge of diagnosis.

Treatment of CAPA may be extrapolated from IDSA guidelines for invasive aspergillosis: triazoles (voriconazole, posaconazole, isavuconazole, itraconazole) are recommended as first-line agents, amphotericin B and derivatives can be used for salvage therapy and when voriconazole cannot be used, whereas echinocandins (eg, micafungin, anidulafungin) are not recommended to be used as initial monotherapy but may be effective as salvage therapy either alone or in combination with others.[137]

Coronavirus Disease 2019-Associated Mucormycosis

Mucormycosis is caused by several molds, but species Rhizopus, Lichtheimia, and Mucor account for 75% of infections.[138] Cases of COVID-19-associated mucormycosis are more commonly

Table 4
Diagnostics in "probable" compared with "possible" coronavirus disease 2019-associated pulmonary aspergillosis

	Probable CAPA	Possible CAPA
Imaging	New cavitary lung lesions on chest CT without alternative explanation	Not required
Serum markers	Serum galactomannan EIA index $\geq$ 0.5	Serum (1, 3)-β-ᴅ-glucan $\geq$ 80 pg/mL without alternate explanation
BAL markers	BAL galactomannan EIA index $\geq$ 1.0	BAL galactomannan EIA index $\geq$ 0.5
Lung specimen cultures	Positive *Aspergillus* cultures from BAL	Non-BAL sample culture with growth of *Aspergillus*

sinonasal and rhino-orbito-cerebral than pulmonary or disseminated.[139] Patients in the developing world have accounted for most cases reported thus far.

Mucormycosis is more diagnostically challenging than aspergillosis, in part because there are no approved biomarkers to aid in diagnosis. The etiologic agents of mucormycosis neither produce galactomannan nor do they have BDG in their cell walls. Diagnosis must be undertaken first with clinical suspicion of site of infection (eg, rhino-orbital) followed by surgical sampling and histopathology of the involved site.[140]

Treatment of mucormycosis also differs slightly from aspergillosis, and is likewise more limiting. In contrast to aspergillosis, amphotericin B and derivatives are considered first line for mucormycosis with triazoles being suitable for salvage therapy. Also unlike aspergillosis, echinocandins demonstrate breakthrough infection and may not be appropriate monotherapy for salvage or otherwise. Importantly, voriconazole and itraconazole do not have activity against mucormycosis organisms, therefore a clinician hoping to select coverage for both mucormycosis and aspergillosis without needing to concern themselves with the potential of toxicity from amphotericin B would have only isavuconazole and posaconazole as options.[140] At that point of consideration, consultation with an infectious disease specialist would be recommended.

SUMMARY

The COVID-19 pandemic had a significant impact on the epidemiology of other respiratory infections. The implementation of social distancing and wearing masks and eye protection was associated with a decline in rates of influenza and RSV during 2020 to 2021; now there is a reemergence of these and other community-acquired respiratory viruses. Although coinfections of COVID-19 with other respiratory viruses remain relatively rare, there have been some evidence that coinfection is associated with increased severity of illness. Treatment of coinfections includes a specific antiviral agents if available for the virus and supportive care.

Regarding bacterial pneumonia and COVID-19, CAP and nonintubated HAP are infrequent coinfections; an exception is perhaps merited for CAP caused by *S pneumoniae*. Once patients are endotracheally intubated, however, they become highly susceptible to VAP development in a manner out of proportion to similar patients with non-COVID-19 indications for intubation. About 60% to 70% of COVID-19-related VAPs involve gram-negative organisms[126]; treatment should be according to local antibiograms and resistance patterns in combination with published guidelines.[120] A procalcitonin trend may be a useful adjunct in diagnosis.

Last, nosocomial infections including BSI and opportunistic invasive fungal infections can occur in patients with COVID-19 especially in patients with higher severity of illness.

CLINICS CARE POINTS

- Changes in population behaviour early in the COVID-19 pandemic including; social distancing and masking; were associated with reduced transmission of SARS-CoV-2, influenza, respiratory syncytial virus, along with other seasonal coronavirus and rhinovirus infections.

- Symptoms of many respiratory viral illnesses are similar to SARS-CoV-2 infection. Symptoms that are more unique to SARS-CoV-2 infection than other respiratory viral illness include loss of taste and smell.

- Vaccination and treatment options are available for prevention and management of SARS-CoV-2 and influenza infections.
- Bacterial coinfection and superinfection during SARS-CoV-2 infections have implications for patient outcomes, antibiotic stewardship and health care costs. Bacterial infections include community-acquired pneumonias, hospital-acquired pneumonia, ventilator-associated pneumonias and blood stream infections.
- Fungal infections including COVID-19-associated pulmonary aspergillosis (CAPA) and mucormycosis were identified amongst patients infected with SARS-CoV-2.

DISCLOSURE

Authors involved in this chapter have nothing to disclose.

REFERENCES

1. Li Q, Guan X, Wu P, et al. Early transmission dynamics in Wuhan, China of novel Coronavirus-infected pneumonia. N Engl J Med 2020;382:1199–207.
2. Tyrrell CS AJ, Gkrania-klotsas E. Influenza: epidemiology and hospital management. Medicine (Abingdon) 2021;49:797–804.
3. Shieh W., Blau D., Denison A., et al., 2009 Pandemic influenza A (H1N1): pathology and pathogenesis of 100 fatal cases in the United States, Am J Pathol, 177, 2010, 166–175.
4. Cowling BJ Ali S, Ng T, et al. Impact assessment of non-pharmaceutical interventions against coronavirus disease 2019 and influenza in Hong Kong: an observational study. Lancet Public Health 2020;5(5):e279–88.
5. Tyrrell CS, Allen JLY, Gkrania-Klotsas E. Influenza: epidemiology and hospital management. Medicine (Abingdon) 2021;49(12):797–804.
6. Prevention C. 2020-2021 Flu season summary. 2022. Available from: https://www.cdc.gov/flu/season/faq-flu-season-2020-2021.htm.
7. Prevention, C.f.D.C.a. Archived. Estimated influenza illnesses, medical visits, hospitalizations, and deaths in the United States — 2019–2020 influenza season. 2022. June 10, 2022]; Available from: https://www.cdc.gov/flu/about/burden/2019-2020/archive-09292021.html.
8. Adlhoch C., Mook P., Lamb F., et al., Very little influenza in the WHO European Region during the 2020/21 season, weeks 40 2020 to 8 2021, Euro Surveill, 26 (11), 2021.
9. Olsen S.J., Azziz-Baumgartner E., Budd A., et al., Decreased influenza activity during the COVID-19 pandemic-United States, Australia, Chile, and South Africa, 2020, Am J Transplant, 20 (12), 2020, 3681–3685.
10. Krauland M.G., Galloway D., Raviotta J., et al., Impact of low rates of influenza on next-season influenza infections, Am J Prev Med, 62 (4), 2022, 503–510.
11. Falsey A.R., Hennessey P., Formica M., et al., Respiratory syncytial virus infection in elderly and high-risk adults, N Engl J Med, 352 (17), 2005, 1749–1759.
12. Tin Tin Htar M, Yerramalla M. Moisi J., et al., The burden of respiratory syncytial virus in adults: a systematic review and meta-analysis. Epidemiol Infect 2020;148:e48.
13. Thompson WW, Shay D, Weintraub E, et al. Mortality associated with influenza and respiratory syncytial virus in the United States. JAMA 2003;289(2):179–86.
14. Available at: https://www.cdc.gov/surveillance/nrevss/index.html. Updated January 25, 2023.
15. Alanio C., Verma A., Mathew D., et al., Cytomegalovirus latent infection is associated with an increased risk of COVID-19-related hospitalization, J Infect Dis, 226 (3), 2022, 463–473.
16. Paes BA, Mitchell I, Banerji A, et al. A decade of respiratory syncytial virus epidemiology and prophylaxis: translating evidence into everyday clinical practice. Can Respir J 2011;18(2):e10–e19.
17. Broberg E.K., Waris M., Johansen K., et al., Seasonality and geographical spread of respiratory syncytial virus epidemics in 15 European countries, 2010 to 2016, Euro Surveill, 23 (5), 2018, 00217–00284.
18. Eden JE ea. Off-season RSV epidemics after easing of COVID-19 restrictions. Nat Commun 2022;13(2884):2884.
19. Delestrain C ea. Impact of COVID-19 social distancing on viral infection in France: a delayed outbreak of RSV. Pediatr Pulmonol 2021;56(12):3669–73.
20. Calderaro A, Canto F, Buttrini M, et al. Human respiratory viruses, including SARS-CoV-2, circulating in the winter season 2019-2020 in Parma, Northern Italy. Int J Infect Dis 2021;102:79–84.
21. Sherman A.C., Babiker A., Seiben A., et al., The effect of severe acute respiratory syndrome coronavirus 2 (SARS-CoV-2) mitigation strategies on seasonal respiratory viruses: a tale of 2 large metropolitan centers in the United States, Clin Infect Dis, 72 (5), 2021, e154–e157.
22. Kuitunen I., Artama M., Makela L., et al., Effect of social distancing due to the COVID-19 pandemic on the incidence of viral respiratory tract infections in children in Finland during early 2020, Pediatr Infect Dis J, 39 (12), 2020, e423–e427.
23. Britton P.N., Hu N., Saravanos G., et al., COVID-19 public health measures and respiratory syncytial

virus, *Lancet Child Adolesc Health*, 4 (11), 2020, e42–e43.

24. Yeoh D, Foley D, Minney-Smith C, et al. Impact of coronavirus disease 2019 public health measures on detections of influenza and respiratory syncytial virus in children during the 2020 Australian winter. Clin Infect Dis 2021;72(12):2199–202.

25. Ogilvie M, Vathenen A, Radford M, et al. Maternal antibody and respiratory syncytial virus infection in infancy. J Med Virol 1981;7(4):263–71.

26. Romo V. Children's hospitals grapple with a nationwide surge in RSV infections. 2022. Available from: https://www.npr.org/2022/10/24/1130764314/childrens-hospitals-rsv-sur.

27. Nichols GL. Coronavirus seasonality, respiratory infections and weather. BMC Infect Dis 2021; 21(1011):1101.

28. Ljubin-Sternak S ea. Seasonal coronaviruses and other neglected respiratory viruses: a global perspective and a local snapshot. Front Public Health 2021;9:691163.

29. Wan W, Thoon K, Loo L, et al. Trends in respiratory virus infection during the COVID-19 pandemic in Singapore, 2020. JAMA Netw Open 2021;4: e2115873.

30. Teo KW ea. Rhinovirus persistence during the COVID-19 pandemic on pediatric acute wheezing presentations. J Med virology 2022;94(11):5547–52.

31. Groves HE, Piche-Renaud P, Peci A, et al. The impact of the COVID-19 pandemic on influenza, respiratory syncytial virus, and other seasonal respiratory virus circulation in Canada: a population-based study, Lancet Reg Health Am 2021;1: 100015.

32. Poole S, Brendish NJ, Clark TW. SARS-CoV-2 has displaced other seasonal respiratory viruses: results from a prospective cohort study. J Infect 2020;81(6):966–72.

33. Fong M.W., Gao H., Wong J., et al., Nonpharmaceutical measures for pandemic influenza in non-healthcare settings-social distancing measures, Emerg Infect Dis, 26 (5), 2020, 976–984.

34. Cowling BJ, Ng D, Ip D, et al. Community psychological and behavioral responses through the first wave of the 2009 influenza A(H1N1) pandemic in Hong Kong. J Infect Dis 2010;202(6):867–76.

35. Ali S., Cowling B., Lao E., et al., Mitigation of influenza B epidemic with school closures, Hong Kong, 2018, Emerg Infect Dis, 24 (11), 2018, 2071–2073.

36. Honein M., Christie A.M, Rose D., et al., Summary of guidance for public health strategies to address high levels of community transmission of SARS-CoV-2 and related deaths, december 2020, *MMWR Morb Mortal Wkly Rep*, 69 (49), 2020, 1860–1867.

37. Chu D, Akl E, Duda S, et al. Physical distancing, face masks, and eye protection to prevent person-to-person transmission of SARS-CoV-2 and COVID-19: a systematic review and meta-analysis. Lancet 2020;395:1973–87.

38. Jefferson T, Del Mar C, Dooley L, et al. Physical interventions to interrupt or reduce the spread of respiratory viruses. Cochrane Database Syst Rev 2020;11:CD006207.

39. Chan KF MT, Ip MS, Ho PL. Invasive pneumococcal disease, pneumococcal pneumonia and all-cause pneumonia in Hong Kong during the COVID-19 pandemic compared with the preceding 5 years: a retrospective observational study. BMJ Open 2021;11(10):e055575.

40. Crichton ML SA, Chalmers JD. The impact of the COVID-19 pandemic on exacerbations and symptoms in bronchiectasis: a prospective study. Am J Respir Crit Care Med 2021;204:857–9.

41. Hawkins E., Fertal B., Muir S., et al., Adding eye protection to universal masking reduces COVID-19 among frontline emergency clinicians to the level of community spread, Am J Emerg Med, 46, 2020, 792–793.

42. Mermel L., Eye protection for preventing transmission of respiratory viral infections to healthcare workers, *Infect Control Hosp Epidemiol*, 39, 2018, 1387.

43. Javanian M., Barary M., Ghebrehewat S., et al., A brief review of influenza virus infection, J Med Virol, 93 (8), 2021, 4638–4646.

44. Khorramdelazad H, Kozemi M, Najafi A, et al. Immunopathological similarities between COVID-19 and influenza: investigating the consequences of Co-infection. Microb Pathog 2021;152:104554.

45. Liu Y., Gayle A., Wilder-Smith A., et al., The reproductive number of COVID-19 is higher compared to SARS coronavirus, *J Trav Med*, 27 (2), 2020, taaa021.

46. Rahman A, Sathi NJ. Risk factors of the severity of COVID-19: a meta-analysis. Int J Clin Pract 2021; 75(7):e13916.

47. Hobbs A., Turner N., Omer I.,et al., Risk factors for mortality and progression to severe COVID-19 disease in the Southeast region in the United States: a report from the SEUS Study Group, *Infect Control Hosp Epidemiol*, 42 (12), 2021, 1464–1472.

48. Celewicz A., Celewicz M., Michalczyk M., et al., Pregnancy as a risk factor of severe COVID-19, J Clin Med, 10 (22), 2021, 5458.

49. Guan W., Ni Z., Hu Y., et al., Clinical characteristics of coronavirus disease 2019 in China, N Engl J Med, 382 (18), 2020, 1708–1720.

50. Gao Z., Xu Y., Sun C., et al., A systematic review of asymptomatic infections with COVID-19, *J Microbiol Immunol Infect*, 54 (1), 2021, 12–16.

51. Esakandari H, Nabi-Afjadi M, Fakkari-Afjadi J, et al. A comprehensive review of COVID-19 characteristics. Biol Proced Online 2020;22:19.

52. Mehta P., McAuley D., Brown M., et al., COVID-19: consider cytokine storm syndromes and immunosuppression, *Lancet*, 395 (10229), 2020, 1033–1034.

53. Mehandru S, Merad M. Pathological sequelae of long-haul COVID. Nat Immunol 2022;23(2): 194–202.

54. Biggerstaff M, Cauchemaz S, Reed C, et al. Estimates of the reproduction number for seasonal, pandemic, and zoonotic influenza: a systematic review of the literature. BMC Infect Dis 2014;14:480.

55. Van Kerkhove MD, Vandemaele K, Shinde V, et al. Risk factors for severe outcomes following 2009 influenza A (H1N1) infection: a global pooled analysis. Plos Med 2011;8(7):e1001053.

56. Mertz D, Kim T, Johnstone J, et al. Populations at risk for severe or complicated influenza illness: systematic review and meta-analysis. BMJ 2013;347: f5061.

57. Clark NM, Lynch JP 3rd. Influenza: epidemiology, clinical features, therapy, and prevention. Semin Respir Crit Care Med 2011;32(4):373–92.

58. Julkunen I., Melen K., Nyqvist M., et al., Inflammatory responses in influenza A virus infection, Vaccine, 19 (Suppl 1), 2000, S32–S37.

59. Altamirano-Lagos MJ, Diaz F, Manseilla MA, et al. Current animal models for understanding the pathology caused by respiratory syncytial virus. Front Microbiol 2019;10:873.

60. Otomaru H, Kamigaki T, Tamaki R, et al. Transmission of respiratory syncytial virus among children under 5 Years in households of rural communities, the Philippines. Open Forum Infect Dis 2016;6: ofz045.

61. Weber A, Milligan P. Modeling epidemic caused by respiratory syncytial virus. Math Biosci 2001;172: 95–113.

62. Piroth L., Cottenet J., Marriet A-S., et al., Comparison of the characteristics, morbidity, and mortality of COVID-19 and seasonal influenza: a nationwide, population-based retrospective cohort study, Lancet Respir Med, 9 (3), 2021, 251–259.

63. Pormohammad A., Ghorbani S., Khatami A., et al., Comparison of influenza type A and B with COVID-19: a global systematic review and meta-analysis on clinical, laboratory and radiographic findings, *Rev Med Virol*, 31 (3), 2021, e2179.

64. Crotta S, Davidson S, Mahlakoiv T, et al. Type I and type III interferons drive redundant amplification loops to induce a transcriptional signature in influenza-infected airway epithelia. Plos Pathog 2013; 9(11):e1003773.

65. Okoli GN, Otete H, Beck C, et al. Use of neuraminidase inhibitors for rapid containment of influenza: a systematic review and meta-analysis of individual and household transmission studies. PLoS One 2014;9(12):e113633.

66. Grijalva C.G., Feldstein L., Talbot H., et al., Influenza vaccine effectiveness for prevention of severe influenza-associated illness among adults in the United States, 2019-2020: a test-negative study, *Clin Infect Dis*, 73 (8), 2021, 1459–1468.

67. Tenforde M.W., Talbot H., Trabue C., et al., Influenza vaccine effectiveness against hospitalization in the United States, 2019-2020, *J Infect Dis*, 224 (5), 2021, 813–820.

68. Candelli M., Pignataro G., Torelli E., et al., Effect of influenza vaccine on COVID-19 mortality: a retrospective study, *Intern Emerg Med*, 16 (7), 2021, 1849–1855.

69. Fiore AE, Bridges CB, Cox NJ. Seasonal influenza vaccines. Curr Top Microbiol Immunol 2009;333:43–82.

70. Mascellino MT, Timoteo F, Angelis M, et al. Overview of the main anti-SARS-CoV-2 vaccines: mechanism of action, efficacy and safety. Infect Drug Resist 2021;14:3459–76.

71. MD J. Mechanism of action of the janssen COVID-19 vaccine. 2022. June 29, 2022]; Available from: https://www.janssenmd.com/janssen-covid19-vaccine/pharmacology/mechanism-of-action/mechanism-of-action-of-the-janssen-covid19-vaccine.

72. Chong WH, Saha BK, Medarov BI. A systematic review and meta-analysis comparing the clinical characteristics and outcomes of COVID-19 and influenza patients on ECMO. Respir Investig 2021;59(6):748–56.

73. Taquet M., Dercon Q., Luciano S., et al., Incidence, co-occurrence, and evolution of long-COVID features: a 6-month retrospective cohort study of 273,618 survivors of COVID-19, *Plos Med*, 18 (9), 2021, e1003773.

74. Dadashi M, Khaleghnejad S, Elkhichi P, et al. COVID-19 and influenza Co-infection: a systematic review and meta-analysis. Front Med (Lausanne) 2021;8:681469.

75. Dao T.L., Hoang V., Colson P., et al., Co-infection of SARS-CoV-2 and influenza viruses: a systematic review and meta-analysis, *J Clin Virol Plus*, 1 (3), 2021, 100036.

76. Wu Q., Xing Y., Shi L., et al., Coinfection and other clinical characteristics of COVID-19 in children, *Pediatrics*, 146 (1), 2020, e20200961.

77. Schweitzer KS, Crue T, Nall J, et al. Influenza virus infection increases ACE2 expression and shedding in human small airway epithelial cells. Eur Respir J 2021;58(1):2003988.

78. Lai Y, Han T, Lao Z, et al. Phillyrin for COVID-19 and influenza Co-infection: a potential therapeutic strategy targeting host based on bioinformatics analysis. Front Pharmacol 2021;12:754241.

79. Rynda-Apple A, Robinson KM, Alcorn JF. Influenza and bacterial superinfection: illuminating the immunologic mechanisms of disease. Infect Immun 2015;83(10):3764–70.

80. Brady M, Byington C, Davies D, et al. Updated guidance for palivizumab prophylaxis among infants and young children at increased risk of hospitalization for respiratory syncytial virus infection. Pediatrics 2014;134:e620–38.

81. Brand S, Munywoki P, Walumbe D, et al. Reducing respiratory syncytial virus hospitalization in a lower-income country by vaccinating mothers-to-be and their households. eLife 2020;9:e47003.

82. Tang M., Li Y., Chen X., et al., Co-Infection with common respiratory pathogens and SARS-CoV-2 in patients with COVID-19 pneumonia and laboratory biochemistry findings: a retrospective cross-sectional study of 78 patients from a single center in China, Med Sci Monit, 27, 2021, e929783-1-e929783-8.

83. Zandi M, Soltani S, Fani M, et al. Severe acute respiratory syndrome coronavirus 2 and respiratory syncytial virus coinfection in children. Osong Public Health Res Perspect 2021;12:286–92.

84. Tang ML, Li Y, Chen X, et al. Co-infection with common respiratory pathogens and SARS-CoV-2 in patients with COVID-19 pneumonia and laboratory biochemistry findings: a retrospective cross-sectional study of 78 patients from a single center in China. Med Sci Monit 2021;27:e929783.

85. Alvares PA. SARS-CoV-2 and respiratory syncytial virus coinfection in hospitalized pediatric patients. Pediatr Infect Dis J 2021;40(4):e164–6.

86. Chekuri S., Szymczak W., Goldstein D., et al., SARS-CoV-2 coinfection with additional respiratory virus does not predict severe disease: a retrospective cohort study, J Antimicrob Chemother, 76 (Supplement_3), 2021, iii12-iii19.

87. Ma L, Wang W, Le Grange J, et al. Coinfection of SARS-CoV-2 and other respiratory pathogens. Infect Drug Resist 2020;13:3045–53.

88. Goldberg E.M., Hasegawa K., Lawrence A., et al., Viral coinfection is associated with improved outcomes in emergency department patients with SARS-CoV-2, West J Emerg Med, 22 (6), 2021, 1262–1269.

89. Chen T., Song J., Liu H., et al., Positive Epstein-Barr virus detection in coronavirus disease 2019 (COVID-19) patients, Sci Rep, 11 (1), 2021, 10902.

90. Nadeem A, Suresh K, Awais H, et al. Epstein-barr virus coinfection in COVID-19. J Investig Med High Impact Case Rep 2021;9. 23247096211040626.

91. Meng M., Zhang S., Dong X., et al., COVID-19 associated EBV reactivation and effects of ganciclovir treatment, Immun Inflamm Dis, 10 (4), 2022, e597.

92. Gold J.E., Okyay R., Licht W., et al., Investigation of long COVID prevalence and its relationship to epstein-barr virus reactivation, Pathogens, 10 (6), 2021, 763.

93. Nunn A., Guy G., Botchway S., et al., SARS-CoV-2 and EBV; the cost of a second mitochondrial "whammy"?, Immun Ageing, 18 (1), 2021, 40.

94. Amaral P, Ferraira B, Roll S, et al. COVID-19 and cytomegalovirus Co-infection: a challenging case of a critically ill patient with gastrointestinal symptoms. Eur J Case Rep Intern Med 2020;7(10):001911.

95. Gatto I., Biagioni E., Coloretti I., et al., Cytomegalovirus blood reactivation in COVID-19 critically ill patients: risk factors and impact on mortality, Intensive Care Med, 48 (6), 2022, 706–713.

96. Naendrup J, Borrega J, Eichenauer D, et al. Reactivation of EBV and CMV in severe COVID-19 epiphenomena or trigger of hyperinflammation in need of treatment? A large case series of critically ill patients. J Intensive Care Med 2021;37(9):1152–8.

97. Paolucci S., Cassaniti I., Novazzi F., et al., EBV DNA increase in COVID-19 patients with impaired lymphocyte subpopulation count, Int J Infect Dis, 104, 2021, 315–319.

98. Pluss M, Mese K, Kowallick J, et al. Case report: cytomegalovirus reactivation and pericarditis following ChAdOx1 nCoV-19 vaccination against SARS-CoV-2. Front Immunol 2021;12:784145.

99. Katsikas Triantafyllidis K., Giannos P., Mian I., et al., Varicella zoster virus reactivation following COVID-19 vaccination: a systematic review of case reports, Vaccines (Basel), 9 (9), 2021, 1013.

100. Munasinghe B, Fernando U, Mathurageethan M, et al. Reactivation of varicella-zoster virus following mRNA COVID-19 vaccination in a patient with moderately differentiated adenocarcinoma of rectum: a case report. SAGE Open Med Case Rep 2022;10. 2050313X221077737.

101. Abu-Rumeileh S., Mayer B., Still V., et al., Varicella zoster virus-induced neurological disease after COVID-19 vaccination: a retrospective monocentric study, J Neurol, 269 (4), 2022, 1751–1757.

102. Buranasakda M, Kotruchin P, Phanthachai K, et al. Varicella zoster meningitis following COVID-19 vaccination: a report of two cases. Int J Infect Dis 2022;119:214–6.

103. Touzard-Romo F,TC, Lonks JR. Co-infection with SARS-CoV-2 and human metapneumovirus. R Med J 2020;103(6):23–4.

104. He H, Liao C, Wang R, et al. Co-infection with SARS-CoV-2 and parainfluenza virus in a hemodialysis patient: a Case report. Clin Nephrol 2020;94:207–11.

105. Swets M, Russell C, Harrison E, et al. SARS-CoV-2 co-infection with influenza viruses, respiratory syncytial virus, or adenoviruses. Lancet 2022;399(10334):1463–4.

106. Motta JC GC. Adenovirus and novel coronavirus (SARS-Cov2) coinfection: a case report. ID Cases 2020;22:e00936.

107. Morens DM TJ, Fauci AS. Predominant role of bacterial pneumonia as a cause of death in pandemic influenza: implications for pandemic influenza preparedness. J Infect Dis 2008;198(7):962–70.

108. Roquilly A., Torres A., Villadangos J.A., et al., Pathophysiological role of respiratory dysbiosis in hospital-acquired pneumonia, *Lancet Respir Med*, 7 (8), 2019, 710–720.

109. Howard L. Is there an association between severe acute respiratory syndrome coronavirus 2 (SARS-CoV-2) and Streptococcus pneumoniae? Clin Infect Dis 2021;72(5):e76–8.

110. Sweere J.,Van Bellenghem H.J., Ishak H., et al.,-Bacteriophage trigger antiviral immunity and prevent clearance of bacterial infection, Science, 363, (6434), 2019,eaat9691.

111. Boumaza A., Gay L., Mezouar S., et al., Monocytes and macrophages, targets of severe acute respiratory syndrome coronavirus 2: the clue for coronavirus disease 2019 immunoparalysis, *J Infect Dis*, 224 (3), 2019, 395–406.

112. Metlay J, Waterer G, Long A, et al. Diagnosis and treatment of adults with community-acquired pneumonia. An official clinical practice guideline of the American Thoracic Society and Infectious Diseases Society of America. Am J Respir Crit Care Med 2019;200(7):e45–67.

113. Jain S, Self W, Wunderink R, et al, CDC EPIC Study Team. Community-acquired pneumonia requiring hospitalization among U.S. adults. N Engl J Med 2015;373:415–27.

114. Lehmann C, Pho M, Lehmann C, Pitrak D, et al. Community-acquired coinfection in coronavirus disease 2019: a retrospective observational experience. Clin Infect Dis 2021;72(8):1450–2.

115. Amin-Chowdhury Z., Aiano F., Mensah A., et al., Impact of the coronavirus disease 2019 (COVID-19) pandemic on invasive pneumococcal disease and risk of pneumococcal coinfection with severe acute respiratory syndrome coronavirus 2 (SARS-CoV-2): prospective national cohort study, England, Clin Infect Dis, 72 (5), 2021, e65–e75.

116. Relph K, Russel C, Fairfield C, et al. International severe acute respiratory and emerging infections consortium coronavirus clinical characterization consortium (ISARIC4C) investigators. Procalcitonin is not a reliable biomarker of bacterial coinfection in people with coronavirus disease 2019 undergoing microbiological investigation at the time of hospital admission. Open Forum Infect Dis 2022;9(5):ofac179.

117. Hani C., Trieu N., Saab I., et al., COVID-19 pneumonia: a review of typical CT findings and differential diagnosis, *Diagn Interv Imaging*, 101 (5), 2020, 263–268.

118. Bhimraj A. Infectious diseases society of America guidelines on the treatment and management of patients with COVID-19. Infect Dis Soc America 2022;ciaa478. Version 9.0.1.

119. Ryder J, Kalil A. The puzzles of ventilator-associated pneumonia and COVID-19: absolute knowns and relative unknowns. Crit Care Med 2022;50(5):894–6.

120. Kalil A, Metersky M, Klompas M, et al. Management of adults with hospital-acquired and ventilator-associated pneumonia: 2016 clinical practice guidelines by the infectious diseases society of America and the american thoracic society. Clin Infect Dis 2017;63(5):e61–111.

121. Clancy C., Schwartz I., Kula B., et al., Bacterial superinfections among persons with coronavirus disease 2019: a comprehensive review of data from postmortem studies, *Open Forum Infect Dis*, 8 (Suppl 1), 2021, 296.

122. Castañeda-Méndez P, Cabrera-Ruiz M, Barragán-Reyes A, et al. Epidemiologic and microbiologic characteristics of hospital-acquired infections in patients with COVID-19 at intensive care unit, Mexico City. Open Forum Infect Dis 2021;8:296.

123. Pickens C.O., Gao C., Cuttica M.J., et al., Bacterial superinfection pneumonia in patients mechanically ventilated for COVID-19 pneumonia, *Am J Respir Crit Care Med*, 204 (8), 2021, 921–932.

124. Vacheron C, Lepape A, Savey A, et al. Attributable mortality of ventilator-associated pneumonia among COVID-19 patients. Am J Respir Crit Care Med 2022;206(2):161–9.

125. Povoa P M-LI, Nseir S. Secondary pneumonias in critically ill patients with COVID-19: risk factors and outcomes. Curr Opin Crit Care 2021;27:468–73.

126. Kalil AC Cawcutt K. Is ventilator-associated pneumonia more frequent in patients with coronavirus disease 2019? Crit Care Med 2022;50(3):522–4.

127. Richards O, Pallman P, King C, et al. Procalcitonin increase is associated with the development of critical care-acquired infections in COVID-19 ARDS. Antibiotics (Basel) 2021;10(11):1425.

128. Gago J, Filardo T, Conderino S, et al. Pathogen species is associated with mortality in nosocomial bloodstream infection in patients with COVID-19. Crit Care Med 2022;9:ofac083.

129. Silva D.L., Lima C.,Magalhães V.,et al., Fungal and bacterial coinfections increase mortality of severely ill COVID-19 patients, *J Hosp Infect*, 113, 2021, 145–154.

130. Bhatt PJ, Shiau S, Brunetti L, et al. Risk factors and outcomes of hospitalized patients with severe coronavirus disease 2019 (COVID-19) and secondary bloodstream infections: a multicenter case-control study. Clin Infect Dis 2021;72:e995–1003.

131. Kula BE, Clancy C, Hong Nguyen M, et al. Invasive mould disease in fatal COVID-19: a systematic review of autopsies. Lancet Microbe 2021;2:e405–14.

132. Clancy CJ, Hong Nguyen M. Coronavirus disease 2019-associated pulmonary aspergillosis: reframing the debate. Open Forum Infect Dis 2022;9: ofac081.

133. Bartoletti M, Pascale R, Cricca M, et al, PREDICO Study Group. (2021), Epidemiology of invasive pulmonary aspergillosis among intubated patients with COVID-19: a prospective study. Clin Infect Dis 2021;73:e3606–14.

134. Koehler P, Cornerly O, Böttiger BW, et al. COVID-19 associated pulmonary aspergillosis. Mycoses. Mycoses 2020;63:528–34.

135. White P Dhillon R, Cordey A, et al. A national strategy to diagnose coronavirus disease 2019-associated invasive fungal disease in the intensive care unit. Clin Infect Dis 2021;73:e1634–44.

136. Permpalung N., Po-Yu Chiang T., Massie A., et al., Coronavirus disease 2019-associated pulmonary aspergillosis in mechanically ventilated patients, *Clin Infect Dis*, 74, 2022, 83–91.

137. Patterson T, Thompson G, Denning DW, et al. Practice guidelines for the diagnosis and management of aspergillosis: 2016 update by the infectious diseases society of America. Clin Infect Dis 2016;63: e1–60.

138. Patel A, Agarwal R, Rudramurthy SM, et al. Muco-Covi Network3, Multicenter epidemiologic study of coronavirus disease-associated mucormycosis. Emerg Infect Dis 2021;27:2349–59.

139. Narayanan S, Chua J, Baddley JW. Coronavirus disease 2019-associated mucormycosis: risk factors and mechanisms of disease. Clin Infect Dis 2022;74:1279–83.

140. Farmakiotis D. Mucormycoses. Infect Dis Clin North Am 2016;30:143–63.

Lessons Learned from Health Disparities in Coronavirus Disease-2019 in the United States

Alejandro A. Diaz, MD, MPH[a],*, Neeta Thakur, MD, MPH[b],
Juan C. Celedón, MD, DrPH[c]

KEYWORDS

- Health disparities • Race/ethnicity • Covid-19 • Black • Latinx • Latino • Hispanic

KEY POINTS

- The coronavirus disease-2019 (COVID-19) pandemic has disproportionally affected historically marginalized populations, including minorities, immigrants, and economically disadvantaged individuals.
- COVID-19 cases, hospitalizations, and deaths are higher in Black, Latinx, and Indigenous populations than in non-Latinx white individuals, yet vaccination rates in minority groups are lower than the national average.
- COVID-19 disparities are rooted in longstanding health inequities due to structural determinants of health (eg, racism, low socioeconomic status) that affect education, housing, employment, and access to high-quality health care.
- Short-term (eg, subsidies for heavily affected communities) and long-term (eg, universal health care) policies to mitigate the negative impact of structural and socioeconomic barriers have the potential to reduce health disparities in general, and for COVID-19 outcomes in particular.

INTRODUCTION

As of June 2022, 2 years into the coronavirus disease-2019 (COVID-19) pandemic, 84.2 million people in the United States have been infected, and over 1 million have died.[1] The impact of this calamity has been felt across our society, but the burden of hospitalizations and deaths has disproportionally affected historically marginalized populations, including minorities, immigrants, and economically disadvantaged individuals. Black, Latinx, and Indigenous populations have the infection and death rates higher than non-Latinx White groups (heretofore referred to as "White").[2,3]

As we have passed the grim 1-million death mark for the ongoing pandemic, the age-adjusted death rates from COVID-19 in younger people are approximately twice as high in Black and Latinx populations than in White groups.[4] In the first year of the pandemic, vaccines were quickly developed and became an effective tool to reduce transmission, hospitalization, and deaths from COVID-19. Since the initial rollout, however, vaccination rates have been lower in Black and Latinx communities. As of June 2022, only 48% and 63% of eligible Black and Latinx people have received at least one vaccine

[a] Division of Pulmonary and Critical Care Medicine, Brigham and Women's Hospital, Harvard Medical School, 75 Francis Street, Boston, MA 02115, USA; [b] Department of Medicine, University of California at San Francisco, 505 Parnassus Avenue, Box 0841, San Francisco, CA 94143, USA; [c] Division of Pediatric Pulmonary Medicine, UPMC Children's Hospital of Pittsburgh, Suite 9130, Rangos Building, 4401 Penn Avenue, Pittsburgh, PA 15224, USA
* Corresponding author.
E-mail address: ADiaz6@bwh.harvard.edu

Clin Chest Med 44 (2023) 425–434
https://doi.org/10.1016/j.ccm.2022.11.021
0272-5231/23/© 2022 Elsevier Inc. All rights reserved.

dose, well below the national average of 78%.[5] Among Black and Latinx populations, a long-standing mistrust in the health care system and the research enterprise, language barriers, immigration issues, and lack of health insurance in low-paying jobs magnified non-access to vaccines.[6]

Health disparities during the COVID-19 pandemic are not random but rather due to long-standing racial/ethnic and socioeconomic inequities caused by structural racism and discriminatory policies regarding access to high-quality education, employment, housing, and health care.[7] Although access to health care improved following the passage of the Affordable Care Act, millions of people remain uninsured, which compromises the capacity of the US health care system to deliver equitable care, particularly in a health crisis. Moreover, the pandemic overwhelmed hospitals that predominantly care for Black, Latinx, and Indigenous communities, exacerbating already strained, low-resourced health systems and limiting access to advanced treatments and critical care services. This article discusses the challenges faced by marginalized and underserved populations, and the lessons learned from the COVID-19 pandemic.

Structural and Social Determinants of Health

Structural and social determinants of health (SDOH) are "the circumstances in which people live and the systems and structures that model their experience and access to health care."[7] In prior work, we have used the World Health Organization (WHO) Conceptual framework for Action on Social Determinants of Health (WHO CSDH)[8] to simultaneously examine root causes of existing disparities while also identifying opportunities for action (**Fig. 1**).[7] This framework proposes that structural bases (eg, social class) impact the socioeconomic and political context (eg, government, policies, and cultures), influencing structural determinants (eg, policies, socioeconomic status, and racism), which shape exposure to intermediary social determinants. The intermediary determinants include health care access, occupational and housing conditions, and psychosocial stress that, in the end, determine an individual's unique social circumstances that shape behavior and risk for disease.[7] This framework helps us evaluate the immediate circumstances of living while also considering the broader context that impacted COVID-19 outcomes. This article focuses on structural determinants that were essential drivers of health disparities during the COVID-19 pandemic.

Disparities in Coronavirus Disease-2019 Infection

Since the early phases of the pandemic, COVID-19 has disproportionally affected minorities living in hotspot counties. The mean difference between the proportion of cases and the proportion of the population was 30.2% and 14.5% for Blacks and Latinx, respectively.[9] In California, Latinx residing in less-advantaged neighborhoods (ie, low median household income, low median educational attainment, and high household density) experienced exponential growth in COVID-19 cases during a 6-week period of observation at the beginning of the pandemic, with the highest increase in low-income areas.[10] This observation was also seen in cities across the United States (eg, Chicago, New York City, Philadelphia, and Newark), where the number of reported COVID-19 was higher in less-advantaged neighborhoods than in more-advantaged ones.[11] Compared with the rates of COVID-19 in White populations, those in Black and Latinx populations were 1.5 to 3.5 times and 1.3 to 28 times higher, respectively.[2,12] Community transmission was up to 28 times higher for Latinx than White populations, whereas in the hospital or health care settings Latinx had 1.3 to 7.7 times higher risk for COVID-19 than White populations.[2] **Fig. 2** shows that, regardless of the timepoint in the pandemic, Latinx (green line) and American Indians/Alaska Natives (yellow line) generally had the highest incident cases from early 2020 to June of 2022.[13]

Several structural and socioeconomic factors (neighborhood and household characteristics, income, education, and work conditions) have fueled disease transmission. Black and Latinx populations are disproportionately represented among the poor and are more likely to be frontline workers with low-paying jobs, leading to high levels of COVID-19 exposure but limited job-sponsored benefits.[6,7] Nearly half of Black and Latinx female health care workers earn <$15 per hour, and more than 10% are uninsured.[14] Black individuals are less likely to telecommute and more likely to work in the service sector and to use public transportation than members of other racial/ethnic groups (Black, 23%; Latinx, 15%; and White, 7%).[15] Moreover, Black individuals were more likely to report leaving the home in the prior 3 days of infection than White individuals,[16] increasing opportunities for transmission. Fueled by economic hardship, Latinx immigrants continued to work in high-transmission jobs while expressing gratitude that lockdown orders did not extend to their construction, cleaning, and cooking jobs, as they were often ineligible for unemployment benefits or income relief because of

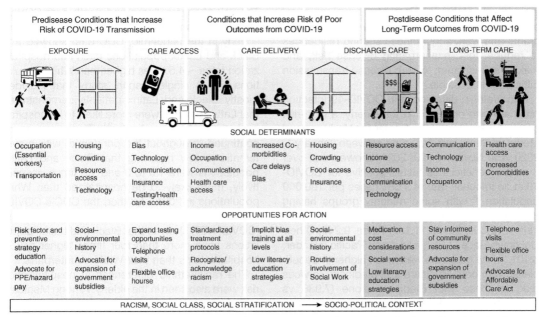

Fig. 1. Structural and social determinants of health contributing to the racial and ethnic disparities in the coronavirus disease (COVID-19) pandemic in the United States and proposed areas for action, as informed by the World Health Organization Conceptual Framework for Action. PPE, personal protective equipment. (*From* Thakur N, Lovinsky-Desir S, Bime C, Wisnivesky JP, Celedón JC. The Structural and Social Determinants of the Racial/Ethnic Disparities in the U.S. COVID-19 Pandemic. What's Our Role?. Am J Respir Crit Care Med. 2020;202(7):943-949.)

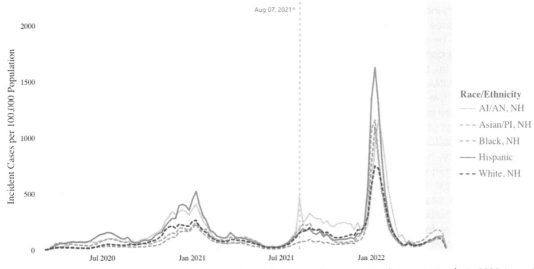

Fig. 2. COVID-19 weekly cases per 100,000 population by race/ethnicity, United States, March 1, 2020-June 4, 2022. Percentage of cases reporting race, 63.1%. Demographic data for COVID-19 cases is based on a subset of individuals where state and territorial jurisdictions have reported case-level data to the CDC since January 21, 2020. Demographic data have varying degrees of missing data and are not generalizable to the entire population of individuals with COVID-19. All displayed counts include confirmed COVID-19 cases as reported by US states, US territories, New York City (NYC), and the District of Columbia from the previous day. Counts for certain jurisdictions also include probable COVID-19 cases. Case rates displayed for the week ending 08/07/2021 reflect a large data influx. The clinical dates for these data were not available. These data are provisional and will be updated as CDC receives additional information. AI/AN, American Indian/Alaska Native; NH, non-hispanic; PI, Pacific Islander. (*From* Center for Disease Control and Prevention. COVID-19 Weekly Cases and Deaths per 100,000 Population by Age, Race/Ethnicity, and Sex. Available at: https://covid.cdc.gov/covid-data-tracker/#demographicsovertime. Accessed Jun 3 2022.)

their legal status.[17] Unstable housing compounded the situation, with low-income immigrants and work acquittances sharing residences to reduce cost, exacerbating disease risk, and making self-isolation to curb disease transmission difficult or impossible.[17]

Racial/ethnic differences in COVID-19 infection rates are also observed in the elderly, a high-risk group. An analysis of the Center for Medicare and Medicaid Services (CMS) data between January 1, 2020, and November 20, 2021, showed that over 6 million beneficiaries tested positive for COVID-19 at an infection rate of 9,587 cases per 100,000 population,[18] with some minority groups having the highest rates: Indigenous Populations, 14,413; Latinx, 12,300; Black, 11,182; White, 9,242; Other/Unknown Race, 7,017; and Asian/Pacific Islander, 6,101.[18] The case rate was much higher in beneficiaries with both Medicare and Medicaid Services than in those with Medicare alone (7,936 vs 16,583 per 100,000).[18] People having both services were generally impoverished and experienced higher rates of chronic illness and need for long-term care than those with only Medicare.[18]

Black, Indigenous, Latinx, and economically disadvantaged individuals are 1.1 to 2.8 times more likely to be at high risk for complications from COVID-19 infection by virtue of comorbidities than White or high-income individuals.[19] This high-risk group includes approximately 18.2 million people who may be uninsured or underinsured,[19] a condition more common in Black and Latinx individuals than in their White counterparts.[19] Despite the positive impact of the Affordable Care Act, one in five Latinx or Indigenous people under 65 years still lacks health insurance.[20]

The intersection of different structural factors— socioeconomic status, race/ethnicity, English language proficiency, housing type and transportation, and household composition and disability— are included in the Social Vulnerability Index of CDC, a validated measure of community resilience during disease outbreaks.[21] The conjunction of adverse structural factors impact exposure and disease risk. People living in the most vulnerable counties, which were driven by minority status and non-English language use, had a greater risk of COVID-19 diagnosis than those in the least vulnerable counties (**Fig. 3**).[21]

Disparities in Coronavirus Disease-2019 Outcomes

Most people affected with COVID-19 present with mild disease or are asymptomatic, whereas some became severely ill and require hospitalization.

The risk of severe illness and death from COVID-19 is higher in the unvaccinated and older adults.

Early in the pandemic, CDC data showed that Black and Latinx populations each had hospitalization rates ~4.5 times higher than White populations.[22,23] A single-hospital study that included mostly Black and Latinx patients demonstrated that Latinx patients were more likely to be hospitalized than White patients.[24] This early trend continued throughout the pandemic, with a systematic review reporting that Black and Latinx populations were 1.5 to 3 and 1.5 times, respectively, more likely to be hospitalized than White populations in 2021.[2] Further, the CDC's COVID-Associated Hospitalization Surveillance Network (COVID-NET) showed that Black and Latinx populations have more than four times higher risk of hospitalizations than their White counterparts.[2]

The racial/ethnic differences in hospitalization risk were also seen in the elderly. Among Medicare and Medicaid beneficiaries, an analysis of over 1.6 million COVID-19 hospitalizations showed that Indigenous, Black, and Latinx populations had 1.5 to 2.3 times higher hospitalization rates than White populations.[18]

Minority communities also have higher mortality rates from COVID-19 than White communities. Although there is substantial variability across states, aggregate data demonstrate that the risk of death from COVID-19 was significantly higher in Black (standardized mortality ratio [SMR] = 3.57) and Latinx (SMR = 1.88) populations than in White populations.[25] A systematic review including American Public Media data corroborated the increased mortality in minorities, reporting the following rate ratios for minority groups compared with Whites: Asian, 1.2; Pacific Islanders, 2.4; Indigenous, 3.1; Black, 3.2; and Latinx, 3.2.[2] Such mortality risk was particularly striking in non-elderly individuals. Among individuals younger than 65 years, the percentage of Latinx (35%) and non-White (30%) individuals who died from COVID-19 was much higher than that in Whites (13%).[4] Consistent with these differences, the risk of death from COVID-19 was ~7 to 9 times higher in Black individuals aged 25 to 54 years than that in Whites in the same age group.[26] Increased mortality risk estimates (ranging from 5.5 to 7.9) were also reported for Latinx individuals aged 25 to 54 years.[26] Thus, Black and Latinx individuals lost more years of potential life than their White counterparts. The estimated years of potential life lost using a cutoff point of 65 years were 33,446, 45,777, and 48,204 years for White, Black, and Latinx people.[26]

Structural factors, including neighborhood type, contributed to health disparities in COVID-19 outcomes. Among the boroughs of New York City, the

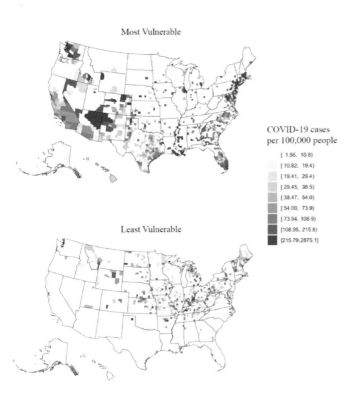

Most Vulnerable

Least Vulnerable

COVID-19 cases
per 100,000 people

[1.56, 10.8)
[10.82, 19.4)
[19.41, 29.4)
[29.45, 38.5)
[38.47, 54.0)
[54.00, 73.9)
[73.94, 108.9)
[108.95, 215.8)
[215.79, 2875.1]

Fig. 3. COVID-19 cases per capita between most and least socially disadvantaged counties. This data represents cases from the onset of the pandemic through April 19, 2020. The most vulnerable quartile of counties (n = 706, top) and the least vulnerable quartile of counties (n = 625, bottom), as indicated by the minority status and language domain of the US Centers for Disease Control's Social Vulnerability Index. Counties without linked Federal Information Processing Standard code or reported COVID-19 cases were excluded. Darker shades represent counties with more cases per capita. (*From* Khazanchi R, Beiter ER, Gondi S, Beckman AL, Bilinski A, Ganguli I. County-Level Association of Social Vulnerability with COVID-19 Cases and Deaths in the USA. J Gen Intern Med. 2020;35(9):2784-2787.)

Bronx (which has the highest proportion of Black and Latinx residents) and Manhattan have the lowest and highest average income, respectively. Illustrating the impact of economic disadvantage on health outcomes, the Bronx and Manhattan also had the highest (224 per 100,000) and lowest (122 per 100,000) mortality rates from COVID-19.[27] Further, patients cared for in New York's less-resourced, community hospitals were three times more likely to die that those cared for at well-resourced hospitals.[28] A multicenter study of 65 medical centers across the US demonstrated that patients admitted to hospitals with fewer (<50 beds) intensive care units (ICU) beds had a higher risk of death than those admitted to hospitals with higher number (≥100 beds) of ICU beds (odds ratio [OR] = 3.28, 95% confidence interval [CI] = 2.16 to 4.99),[29] exposing health care system failures that may continue to contribute to mortality during times of capacity strain (eg, influenza season) well after the COVID-19 pandemic.

Structural discrimination limits employment and education opportunities for minority communities in the United States, ultimately limiting their socioeconomic growth.[30] In the first year of the pandemic, US counties with a higher proportion of residents who were Black, who had less than a high school diploma education, or who had lower household income reported more deaths from COVID-19 than other counties.[31,32] In addition,

language barriers impacted COVID-19 outcomes, as ecological studies showed that counties with a greater proportion of minorities and non-English-speaking people had increased COVID-19 mortality.[21] Although further data on these "invisible" non-English-speaking communities are needed, language barriers might be considered a key social determinant of health in the United States.

Disparities in Coronavirus Disease-2019 Care

At the beginning of the pandemic, a study in Louisiana showed that Black patients were more likely to be on Medicaid, to be hospitalized, and to be tested for COVID-19 in the emergency department than White patients, who were more often diagnosed by a primary care provider.[33] In Los Angeles, the case fatality rate for COVID-19 patients requiring intubation was higher for a low-resourced safety-net hospital than that for a well-resourced academic hospital. This facility regularly serves mostly Black and economically disadvantaged populations and during the winter 2020 to 2021 COVID-19 surge, most patients who died at this safety-net hospital were Latinx.[28] Similarly, during the November 2020 surge in Chicago, small community hospitals that predominantly care for Medicaid beneficiaries or uninsured populations were overwhelmed by the number and complexity of patients, whereas large academic hospitals had open intensive care unit beds. Such disparities in health care can be attributed to longstanding un-addressed issues such as structural racism,[28] the totality of ways in which societies foster racial discrimination through mutually reinforcing systems of housing, education, employment, earnings, benefits, credit, media, health care, and criminal justice. Such patterns and practices in turn reinforce discriminatory beliefs, values, and distribution of resources.[30]

Racial health disparities are rooted in the Jim Crow Laws (eg, a collection of state and local statutes that legalized racial discrimination, starting after the Civil War, and continuing until 1965), when health care institutions were segregated by law. Following the Civil Rights Act of 1964[34,35] Medicare mandated that US hospitals receiving federal funding were racially integrated, yet today many hospitals in predominantly Black communities still operate with lower revenues because of charity care, limiting resources for staffing, training, and quality improvement initiatives, and reducing their capacity to respond to increased care needs. All this likely led to worse COVID-19 outcomes among Black communities in the US Southeast.[34,35]

Language barriers can impede optimal health care. In the United States, over 25 million people report "limited English poficiency" (LEP) and may thus require interpreter services during medical encounters.[36] LEP affects access and use of health care and communication with health care providers, which can worsen health outcomes such as hospitalization length.[37] Title VI of the Civil Rights Act of 1964 requires health care institutions to provide language services for people with LEP, a task facilitated by recording the patients' preferred language in the medical record and using technology to increase the availability of interpreters (eg, video and telephone).[38] However, many health care systems still struggle to ensure appropriate interpreter services,[39,40] a fact magnified during the COVID-19 pandemic.

During the initial COVID-19 surge, interpreter services at an academic hospital in Boston could not meet the in-person language needs of the overwhelming number of patients with LEP, predominantly Spanish-speaking patients. Although the challenge prompted physicians to create a Spanish Language Care Group in response to the crisis, improving health care for people with LEP requires a multipronged approach. Such an approach includes expanding access to language services by increasing their reimbursement and maximizing their availability.[36] Speaking the patients' language (**Fig. 4**) and having a culturally

humble approach to their concerns is a powerful component of care for non-English-speaking populations.

Disparities in Coronavirus Disease-2019 Vaccination

The development of vaccines was a breakthrough in the fight against the COVID-19 pandemic, as they proved effective in reducing the risk of severe disease, hospitalization, and death. As of May 2022, 257.8 million (~78%) of 330 million people in the United States had received at least one dose of a COVID-19 vaccine, and slightly less than a third of those vaccinated had received at least one additional dose (booster).[5] Despite the disproportionate burden of COVID-19 on minority populations, only 48% of Black individuals and 63% of Latinx individuals had received at least one vaccine dose. Surveys have shown that vaccine uptake was lower among Black participants than White participants, even in those who self-reported willingness to get the vaccine.[41] Vaccination hesitancy has decreased in Black populations[42] but poverty and younger age (18 to 49 years) remain as risk factors for vaccine hesitancy in this group.[43]

Vaccination is an act of trust in science and the health care system. Minority survey participants reported that they did not trust the COVID-19 vaccine development process and wanted more transparent information, an attitude justified by prior abuses of trust by researchers and physicians.[44] The year 2022 marked the fiftieth anniversary of the uncovering of the Tuskegee syphilis study, in which Black participants were not given treatment of this life-threatening disease for

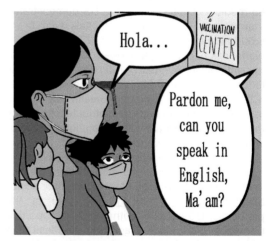

Fig. 4. Spanish-speaking mother at an English-speaking-only vaccination site. (*Courtesy of* A. Payá Mora, BS, Santiago, Chile.)

decades despite substantial evidence of the therapy's efficacy.[45] Researchers working for the same agency (the Public Health Service, a precursor of the CDC) that conducted the Tuskegee study purposely infected Guatemalan study participants with syphilis and gonorrhea to develop preventive methods for these infections.[45] Contemporary vaccine hesitancy is not only explained by historical facts but also by ongoing instances of racism in health care. Black patients are more likely to have their pain negated, their illnesses misdiagnosed, and even treatment denied by health care providers.[46] Trust is earned through long-term patient-provider relationships and may be more easily built with racial concordance with health care providers. Black participants had increased information-seeking behavior after listening to videos about COVID-19 from Black physicians.[47]

Language barriers are an important obstacle to vaccination efforts, even in people with LEP who have health insurance. A study of Medicare Advantage beneficiaries demonstrated that Latinx individuals with LEP were less likely to anticipate getting the vaccines than those with English proficiency, despite having a higher rate of a positive COVID-19 test.[48] This disparity was mainly attributed to differences in income but LEP was likely a contributory factor.[48] LEP, inadequate health literacy, and limited Internet access are potential barriers to online initiatives to increase vaccination rates in vulnerable populations, as one study showed that only 10.6% of patients with LEP scheduled an appointment through patient portals.[49]

In the United States in 2018, 43.5 million people, 13.5% of the total population, are non-US born residents,[50] of whom over 10 million were undocumented in 2021.[51] Immigrants are more likely to have high-risk, essential jobs and less likely to seek medical care. Additional barriers to vaccination include lack of time off work, financial resources, and health insurance.[51] Because vaccination sites often require documenting personal information, undocumented immigrants fear that their personal information might be shared with immigration authorities and that deportation may follow.[6] Thus, being an immigrant is both a risk factor for COVID-19 and non-vaccination status in the United States.

Lesson Learned and Opportunities for Action

Improving access to health care
In the United States, the COVID-19 pandemic further exposed profound health disparities caused by structural and social determinants, such as racism and misguided policies on

education, health, and housing.[7] As a society, we must commit to providing medical care for all. Curbing disease outbreaks requires treating all people based on their health needs, regardless of insurance status, race or ethnicity, immigration status, and other attributes. Although implementing medical care will require a considerable investment of money, time, and resources, health equity leads to enormous cost savings and improved overall health in the long term.[52–54]

In the absence of universal health care, short-term policies are needed to mitigate the impact of the pandemic in underserved groups. First, economically disadvantaged communities should continue to receive cash benefits for COVID-related expenses from state and federal sources, and such benefits should be clearly outlined by health care providers serving historically marginalized, underserved communities.[17] This reassurance is relevant, as fear of medical bills can lead to avoidance or delays in seeking preventive and therapeutic care. Second, the Affordable Care Act should be expanded to cover COVID-19 care, including emergency department visits, hospitalizations, and access to virtual services, would improve outcomes in historically disadvantaged communities.[7] Third, safety-net hospitals that care for the urban poor—a group predominantly composed of Black, Latinx, and immigrant populations—should receive adequate resources (eg, protective equipment, equipment for intensive care units, medical and nonmedical staff) to face the health crisis posed by the current pandemic and foreseeable potential catastrophes.[7] Fourth, hospitals and academic institutions should clearly state and improve upon their charity policies. COVID-19 mortality seemed to be higher in counties with predominantly non-English communities, a group mainly composed of low-income immigrants.[21] Fifth, migrants and refugees should receive culturally and language-appropriate care, including for vaccinations. Although data on this vulnerable population are not routinely collected, making them an invisible group, leaders of vaccination campaigns must clarify that personal information is kept confidential to avoid vaccination hesitancy due to fear of deportation.

Tackling Racism and Implicit Biases

In the United States, the racial injustices and subsequent protests that occurred during the pandemic highlighted the continued negative impact of structural racism on our society.[7] Scientific evidence has linked structural racism, such as historical redlining of neighborhoods, to unequal environmental exposures leading to a heavy burden of asthma in Black communities.[55] During the pandemic, movements to address ethnoracial inequities through implicit bias training and implementation of equity, diversity, and inclusion efforts were invigorated at the community level and at academic hospitals and in medical societies.[7] As researchers, educators, and health care providers, we can explicitly tackle disparities at the individual level. For instance, we can apply processes to select trainees and faculty to better represent the rich diversity of our society and provide financial compensation to support these individuals.[7] To better serve migrants and refugees, medical institutions should consider sponsoring highly qualified immigrant trainees.

Job Protections

Essential workers, who take the risk of keeping our society functioning, need job protections, such as paid medical leave and child and elder care support. State and local officials should implement policies and work with employers to protect frontline workers and give appropriate paid medical leave.

Improving Communication and Facilitating Access to Vaccines

Messaging about COVID-19 preventive measures, testing resources, vaccines, and general guidance should consider strategies for populations with low health literacy and in multiple languages to reach people with LEP. The use of trusted messengers is one strategy to provide accurate information and has proven to encourage behavior changes, such as seeking information about COVID-19.[6,47]

Vaccination rates should continue to rise for all, as vaccine boosters are needed to keep protection against COVID-19. Using non-English-speaking personnel at vaccination sites, giving transportation vouchers and incentives, employing navigators to help with online appointments, and installing vaccination sites in disadvantaged neighborhoods are some strategies that could increase vaccination rates.

SUMMARY

The COVID-19 pandemic has disproportionately affected historically marginalized communities, such as minority populations, immigrants, and economically disadvantaged individuals. Black, Latinx, and Indigenous people have higher rates of COVID-19 infections, hospitalizations, and deaths than White populations. The pandemic has exacerbated health disparities rooted in historical structural inequalities that our society has chosen

to neglect. Thus, policies that tackle structural inequities (racism, housing, education), ensure access to health care and health information, and protect vulnerable populations should be prioritized. Preventive and therapeutic care for COVID-19 should be provided through an equity lens to ensure that everybody is treated and protected based on their unique needs. Reducing the devastating effects of the ongoing COVID-19 pandemic on underserved and historically disadvantaged communities should be a high priority in our journey to achieve health equity and social justice.

FUNDING/SUPPORT

Dr A.A. Diaz is supported by funding from the US National Heart, Lung, and Blood Institute (R01-HL133137, R01-HL14986, R01-HL164824) and the Brigham and Women's Hospital Minority Faculty Career Development Award. Dr N. Thakur is supported by funding from the US National Institutes of Health (R01-HL161049), Robert Wood Johnson Foundation, United States, and the Nina Ireland Program for Lung Health. Dr J.C. Celedón is supported by grants HL117191 and HL152475 from the US National Institutes of Health.

DISCLOSURE

Dr A.A. Diaz declares speaker fees from Boehringer Ingelheim outside of submitted work; Dr N. Thakur has no disclosures to declare. Dr J.C. Celedón reports research materials from Pharmavite (vitamin D and placebo capsules), and GSK and Merck (inhaled steroids) to provide medications free of charge to participants in his NIH-funded studies, outside of this submitted work.

ACKNOWLEDGMENTS

The authors thank Ms Anastasia Payá Mora for creating **Fig. 4**. Note: To test oneself and learn about implicit bias, visit https://implicit.harvard.edu.

REFERENCES

1. Center for Disease Control and Prevention. United States COVID-19 cases, deaths, and laboratory testing (NAATs) by state, territory, and jurisdiction. Available at: https://covid.cdc.gov/covid-data-tracker/#cases_casesper100klast7days. Accessed on 2 June 2022.
2. Mackey K, Ayers CK, Kondo KK, et al. Racial and ethnic disparities in COVID-19-related infections, hospitalizations, and deaths : a systematic review. Ann Intern Med 2021;174(3):362–73.

3. Hatcher SM, Agnew-Brune C, Anderson M, et al. COVID-19 among American Indian and Alaska native persons - 23 states, january 31-july 3, 2020. MMWR Morb Mortal Wkly Rep 2020;69(34):1166–9.

4. Wortham JM, Lee JT, Althomsons S, et al. Characteristics of persons who died with COVID-19 - United States, february 12-may 18, 2020. MMWR Morb Mortal Wkly Rep 2020;69(28):923–9.

5. USA Facts. US Coronavirus vaccine tracker. Available at: https://usafacts.org/visualizations/covid-vaccine-tracker-states. Accessed June 3, 2022.

6. Diaz AA, Celedon JC. COVID-19 vaccination: helping the latinx community to come forward. EClinicalMedicine 2021;35:100860.

7. Thakur N, Lovinsky-Desir S, Bime C, et al. The structural and social determinants of the racial/ethnic disparities in the U.S. COVID-19 pandemic. What's our role? Am J Respir Crit Care Med 2020;202(7):943–9.

8. Solar O, Inwin A. A conceptual framework for action on the social determinants of health: social determinants of health discussion paper 2. Geneva, Switzerland: World Health Organization; 2010.

9. Moore JT, Ricaldi JN, Rose CE, et al. Disparities in incidence of COVID-19 among underrepresented racial/ethnic groups in counties identified as hotspots during June 5–18, 2020 — 22 states february–june 2020. MMWR Morb Mortal Wkly Rep 2020;69(33):1122–6.

10. Chow DS, Soun J, Gavis-Bloom J, et al. The disproportionate rise in COVID-19 cases among Hispanic/Latinx in disadvantaged communities of Orange County, California: A socioeconomic case-series. Pre-print. Posted online on 7 May 2020. medRxiv. doi: 10.1101/2020.05.04.20090878.

11. Okoh AK, Sossou C, Dangayach NS, et al. Coronavirus disease 19 in minority populations of Newark, New Jersey. Int J Equity Health 2020;19(1):93.

12. Adegunsoye A, Ventura IB, Liarski VM. Association of black race with outcomes in COVID-19 disease: a retrospective cohort study. Ann Am Thorac Soc 2020;17(10):1336–9.

13. Center for Disease Control and Prevention. COVID-19 weekly cases and deaths per 100,000 population by age, race/ethnicity, and sex. Available at: https://covid.cdc.gov/covid-data-tracker/#demographicsovertime. Accessed June 3, 2022.

14. Himmelstein KEW, Venkataramani AS. Economic vulnerability among us female health care workers: potential impact of a $15-per-hour minimum wage. Am J Public Health 2019;109(2):198–205.

15. Anderson M. Who relies on public transit in the U.S. Pew Research Center. 2016. Available at: https://www.pewresearch.org/fact-tank/2016/04/07/who-relies-on-public-transit-in-the-u-s/. Accessed June 27, 2022.

16. Alsan M, Stantcheva S, Yang D, et al. Disparities in coronavirus 2019 reported incidence, knowledge, and behavior among US adults. JAMA Netw Open 2020;3(6):e2012403.

17. Page KR, Flores-Miller A. Lessons we've learned - covid-19 and the undocumented latinx community. N Engl J Med 2021;384(1):5–7.

18. Centers for Medicare and Medicaid Services. Preliminary Medicare COVID-19 data snapshot. Available at: https://www.cms.gov/files/document/medicare-covid-19-data-snapshot-fact-sheet.pdf. Accessed June 2, 2022.

19. Gaffney AW, Hawks L, Bor DH, et al. 18.2 million individuals at increased risk of severe COVID-19 illness are un- or underinsured. J Gen Intern Med 2020;35(8):2487–9.

20. Artiga S, Hill L, Orgera K, et al. Health coverage by race and ethnicity, 2010-2019. Available at: https://www.kff.org/racial-equity-and-health-policy/issue-brief/health-coverage-by-race-and-ethnicity/. Accessed June 3, 2022.

21. Khazanchi R, Beiter ER, Gondi S, et al. County-level association of social vulnerability with COVID-19 cases and deaths in the USA. J Gen Intern Med 2020;35(9):2784–7.

22. Centers for Disease Control and Prevention. COVID view summary ending on June 20, 2020. Available at: https://www.cdc.gov/coronavirus/2019-ncov/covid-data/covidview/past-reports/06262020.html. Accessed July 20, 2020.

23. Gold JAW, Wong KK, Szablewski CM, et al. Characteristics and clinical outcomes of adult patients hospitalized with COVID-19 - Georgia, March 2020. MMWR Morb Mortal Wkly Rep 2020;69(18):545–50.

24. Hsu HE, Ashe EM, Silverstein M, et al. Race/ethnicity, underlying medical conditions, homelessness, and hospitalization status of adult patients with COVID-19 at an urban safety-net medical center - Boston, Massachusetts, 2020. MMWR Morb Mortal Wkly Rep 2020;69(27):864–9.

25. Gross CP, Essien UR, Pasha S, et al. Racial and ethnic disparities in population-level covid-19 mortality. J Gen Intern Med 2020;35(10):3097–9.

26. Bassett MT, Krieger N, Chen JT. The unequal toll of COVID-19 mortality by age in the United States: quantifying racial/ethnic disparities. Available at: https://www.hsph.harvard.edu/social-and-behavioral-sciences/2020/06/23/the-unequal-toll-of-covid-19-mortality-by-age-in-the-united-states-quantifying-racial-ethnic-disparities/. Accessed on 20 July 20. Accessed.

27. Wadhera RK, Wadhera P, Gaba P, et al. Variation in COVID-19 hospitalizations and deaths across New York city boroughs. JAMA 2020;323(21):2192–5.

28. Kelly C, Parker WF, Pollack HA. Low-income COVID-19 patients die needlessly because they are stuck in the wrong hospitals—while the right hospitals too often shut them out. Available at: https://www.

healthaffairs.org/do/10.1377/forefront.20210401.95800/full/. Accessed Jun 13, 2022.

29. Gupta S, Hayek SS, Wang W, et al. Factors associated with death in critically ill patients with coronavirus disease 2019 in the US. JAMA Intern Med 2020; 180(11):1436–47.

30. Bailey ZD, Krieger N, Agenor M, et al. Structural racism and health inequities in the USA: evidence and interventions. Lancet 2017;389(10077):1453–63.

31. Khanijahani A. Racial, ethnic, and socioeconomic disparities in confirmed COVID-19 cases and deaths in the United States: a county-level analysis as of November 2020. Ethn Health 2021;26(1):22–35.

32. Tan AX, Hinman JA, Abdel Magid HS, et al. Association between income inequality and county-level COVID-19 cases and deaths in the US. JAMA Netw Open 2021;4(5):e218799.

33. Price-Haywood EG, Burton J, Fort D, et al. Hospitalization and mortality among black patients and white patients with covid-19. N Engl J Med 2020;382(26):2534–43.

34. Krishnan L, Ogunwole SM, Cooper LA. Historical insights on coronavirus disease 2019 (COVID-19), the 1918 influenza pandemic, and racial disparities: illuminating a path forward. Ann Intern Med 2020;173(6):474–81.

35. Hua CL, Bardo AR, Brown JS. Mistrust in physicians does not explain black-white disparities in primary care and emergency department utilization: the importance of socialization during the Jim Crow era. J Natl Med Assoc 2018;110(6):540–6.

36. Herzberg EM, Barrero-Castillero A, Matute JD. The healing power of language: caring for patients with limited English proficiency and COVID-19. Pediatr Res 2022;91(3):526–8.

37. Flores G. The impact of medical interpreter services on the quality of health care: a systematic review. Med Care Res Rev 2005;62(3):255–99.

38. Office of Civil Rights. Guidance to federal financial assistance recipients regarding title vi and the prohibition against national origin discrimination affecting limited English proficient persons - summary. Available at: https://www.hhs.gov/civil-rights/for-providers/laws-regulations-guidance/guidance-federal-financial-assistance-title-vi/index.html. Accessed June 2, 2022.

39. Flores G, Torres S, Holmes LJ, et al. Access to hospital interpreter services for limited English proficient patients in New Jersey: a statewide evaluation. J Health Care Poor Underserved 2008;19(2):391–415.

40. Ryan J, Abbato S, Greer R, et al. Rates and predictors of professional interpreting provision for patients with limited English proficiency in the emergency department and inpatient ward. Inquiry 2017;54. 46958017739981.

41. Nguyen LH, Joshi AD, Drew DA, et al. Self-reported COVID-19 vaccine hesitancy and uptake among participants from different racial and ethnic groups in the United States and United Kingdom. Nat Commun 2022;13(1):636.

42. Funk C, Tyson A, Pew Research Center. Growing share of Americans say they plan to get a COVID-19 vaccine – or already have. Available at: https://www.pewresearch.org/science/2021/03/05/growing-share-of-americans-say-they-plan-to-get-a-covid-19-vaccine-or-already-have/. Accessed June 3, 2022.

43. Nguyen KH, Anneser E, Toppo A, et al. Disparities in national and state estimates of COVID-19 vaccination receipt and intent to vaccinate by race/ethnicity, income, and age group among adults >/= 18 years, United States. Vaccine 2022;40(1):107–13.

44. Jimenez ME, Rivera-Nunez Z, Crabtree BF, et al. Black and latinx community perspectives on COVID-19 mitigation behaviors, testing, and vaccines. JAMA Netw Open 2021;4(7):e2117074.

45. Tobin MJ. Fiftieth anniversary of uncovering the tuskegee syphilis study: the story and timeless lessons. Am J Respir Crit Care Med 2022;205(10):1145–58.

46. Bajaj SS, Stanford FC. Beyond tuskegee - vaccine distrust and everyday racism. N Engl J Med 2021; 384(5):e12.

47. Alsan M, Stanford FC, Banerjee A, et al. Comparison of knowledge and information-seeking behavior after general COVID-19 public health messages and messages tailored for black and latinx communities : a randomized controlled trial. Ann Intern Med 2021;174(4):484–92.

48. Himmelstein J, Himmelstein DU, Woolhandler S, et al. COVID-19-Related care for hispanic elderly adults with limited English proficiency. Ann Intern Med 2022;175(1):143–5.

49. Fuchs JR, Fuchs JW, Tietz SE, et al. Older adults with limited English proficiency need equitable COVID-19 vaccine access. J Am Geriatr Soc 2021;69(4):888–91.

50. United States Census Bureau. Narrative profiles: 2014-2018 American community surevy. https://www.census.gov/acs/www/data/data-tables-and-tools/narrative-profiles/2018/report.php?geotype=nation&usVal=us. Accessed Aug 3, 2022.

51. Mulasi I. E Pluribus Unum. N Engl J Med. 386 (21), 2022, 1969-1971.

52. LaVeist TA, Gaskin D, Richard P. Estimating the economic burden of racial health inequalities in the United States. Int J Health Serv 2011;41(2):231–8.

53. Celedon JC, Roman J, Schraufnagel DE, et al. Respiratory health equality in the United States. The American thoracic society perspective. Ann Am Thorac Soc 2014;11(4):473–9.

54. Bhatt J, Batra N, Davis A, et al. US health care can't afford health inequities. Available at: https://www2.deloitte.com/us/en/insights/industry/health-care/economic-cost-of-health-disparities.html. Accessed June 24, 2022.

55. Schuyler AJ, Wenzel SE. Historical redlining impacts contemporary environmental and asthma-related outcomes in black adults. Am J Respir Crit Care Med 2022;206(7):824–37.

Lessons Learned from a Global Perspective of Coronavirus Disease-2019

Viren Kaul, MD[a], Japjot Chahal, MD[b], Isaac N. Schrarstzhaupt, PhD[c],
Heike Geduld, MBChB[d], Yinzhong Shen, MD[e], Maurizio H. Cecconi, MD[f],
Andre M. Siqueira, MD, PhD[g], Melissa M. Markoski, PhD[h],
Leticia Kawano-Dourado, MD, PhD[i,j],*

KEYWORDS

- COVID-19 • SARS-CoV-2 • Lessons learned • Socioeconomic status • Global spread
- Resource allocation

KEY POINTS

- Non-pharmacological measures (NPMs) are effective in containing the spread of the severe acute respiratory syndrome coronavirus 2 virus.
- Robust peer-reviewed research played an integral role in responding to the coronavirus disease-2019 (COVID-19) pandemic, from studying the role of NPM to treatments and vaccines.
- Collaboration of regional, national, and international public health organizations and social media or mass communication platforms is vital to decrease the spread of misinformation.
- COVID-19 vaccines were the central element in reducing the morbidity and mortality of the COVID-19 pandemic. Vaccine equity is a top priority to ensure the most vulnerable are also protected.
- Access to appropriate health care and preventative measures reduced morbidity and mortality from COVID-19.

INTRODUCTION

On March 11, 2020, the World Health Organization (WHO) declared the spread of severe acute respiratory syndrome coronavirus 2 (SARS-CoV-2) infection (coronavirus disease-2019 [COVID-19]), a pandemic (**Table 1**).[1] A few months before this declaration, a cluster of severe pneumonia cases was reported in Wuhan, China. As of September 30, 2022, the WHO recorded 614,385,693 cases worldwide of COVID-19 with 6,522,600 cumulative deaths.[2]

The Wuhan seafood wholesale market was shut down with the hopes of local mitigation. China's

[a] Department of Pulmonary and Critical Care Medicine, Crouse Health/Upstate Medical University, 736 Irving Avenue, Syracuse, NY, 13210, USA; [b] Department of Pulmonary and Critical Care Medicine, SUNY Upstate Medical University, 750 East Adams Street, Syracuse, NY, 13210, USA; [c] Capixaba Institute of Health Education, Research and Innovation (ICEPi), Rua Duque de Caxias, 267 - Centro, Vitória/ES, 29010-120, Brazil; [d] Division of Emergency Medicine, Faculty of Medicine and Health Sciences, Room 5006 Clinical Building, Stellenbosch University Tygerberg Campus, Cape Town 7505, South Africa; [e] Department of Infection and Immunity, Shanghai Public Health Clinical Center, Fudan University, 2901 Caolang Road, Jinshan District, Shanghai, 201508, China; [f] Department of Anesthesia and Intensive Care, IRCCS Instituto Clinico Humanitas, Via Manzoni 56, Rozzano (Milano), Italy; [g] Instituto Nacional de Infectologia Evandro Chagas, Fundação Oswaldo Cruz, Avenida Brasil 4365, CEP 21040-900, Rio de Janeiro RJ Brazil; [h] UFCSPA - Federal University of Health Sciences of Porto Alegre. Sarmento Leite, 245 - Centro Histórico, Porto Alegre - RS, 90050-170, Brazil; [i] Hcor Research Institute, Hospital do Coracao, R. Des Eliseu Guilherme, 200, 8o andar, Sao Paulo, SP 04004-030, Brazil; [j] Pulmonary Division, InCor, University of Sao Paulo
* Corresponding author. Hcor Research Institute, Hospital do Coracao, R. Des Eliseu Guilherme, 200, 8o andar, Sao Paulo, SP 04004-030, Brazil.
E-mail address: ldourado@hcor.com.br

Clin Chest Med 44 (2023) 435–449
https://doi.org/10.1016/j.ccm.2022.11.020
0272-5231/23/© 2022 Elsevier Inc. All rights reserved.

Table 1
Lessons learned from coronavirus disease-2019: summary of considerations for future respiratory virus pandemics

Global spread	• Non-pharmacological measures are effective in containing the spread of the virus • Contact tracing can help limit the spread • Face masks, in conjunction with other public health measures can tangibly reduce transmission
Impact on health care	• Rapid and generous sharing of information between researchers, clinicians, agencies, and countries is instrumental in planning, preparation, treatment, and prevention • Resource allocation strategies should be considered at all levels to prepare for equitable distribution of resources between areas suffering varying degrees of impact • Supply chain challenges can be effectively addressed by robust deployment of public-private collaborations • Telehealth can be effectively used to provide care • Attention needs to be paid to the mental and physical well-being of health care workers • Evaluation of health care worker needs, provision of meaningful incentives, and infusing effort into training future generation of health care workers should be prioritized to ensure long-term retention
Dissemination of knowledge	• Preprint articles provide rapid dissemination of information but the need for rapidity must be balanced with robust peer-review to avoid inaccurate publications • Peer-reviewed research plays an integral role to ensure accurate science is shared between stakeholders • Living guidelines promote unity and availability of timely evidence-based guidance • Collaboration of regional, national, international public health organizations along with mass media channels is vital to decrease the spread of misinformation
Vaccination	• Equitable sharing of vaccines and other resources among countries is a top priority • Misinformation hinders vaccination efforts globally • Low- and middle-income areas can have lower vaccinations rates than the high-income areas, further exacerbating the socioeconomic disparity
Socioeconomic impact	• Disparity in access to robust health care in areas of low socioeconomic status can lead to worse outcomes • Despite increases in hospital beds, good quality care is limited by availability of trained personnel and appropriate resources • Pandemics can have a significant impact on the financial well-being of society and balancing mitigation strategies with socio-economic feasibility remains an ongoing learning curve

Viral Pneumonia of Unknown Etiology system, which was created after the SARS epidemic, was activated by January 3, 2020, followed by a limitation of travel in and out of the region by January 23, 2020.[3–5] Around the same time, patients with symptoms of the virus were asked to quarantine. These measures required the individual to stay isolated for up to 14 days to curb the spread of the virus.

On January 13, 2020, a case of SARS-CoV-2 infection was reported in Thailand. This was the first report of a case outside of China.[6] Without a known vaccine or cure available, stricter measures were implemented including holiday extensions, city-wide lockdowns, and quarantine of suspected patients.[7]

On February 20, 2020, a young patient in Codogno hospital (Lombardy, Italy) with no known risk factors for SARS-CoV-2 infection tested positive for the virus. By February 21, 2020, there was a rapid rise in the number of cases of COVID-19 in the Northern part of Italy. Intensive care units (ICUs) had to double their pre-pandemic capacity in less than 6 weeks to accommodate the large number of patients arriving at the hospital with severe COVID-19.[8,9] By March 17, 2020, there were 31,506 positive cases despite the whole country of Italy having been placed under lockdown by

March 9, 2020.[10] Lockdowns were similarly instituted by numerous countries. By March 25, 2020, a third of countries in the world were in lockdown.[11]

The virus was spreading unabated by now. Thailand declared a State of Emergency Decree on March 26, 2020. Additional measures included a stay-at-home policy, canceled national holidays, imposed school closures, and suspended international flights.[12] Nevertheless, COVID-19 continued to spread.

NON-PHARMACOLOGICAL MEASURES

Containment of SARS-CoV-2 spread was necessary to reduce morbidity and mortality from COVID-19 and to reduce the pressure on the health care system. Non-pharmacological measures (NPMs) aimed at transmission mitigation were implemented including quarantines, mobility restrictions, socioeconomic restrictions, physical distancing measures, face masking, and hygiene measures. Many countries used travel restrictions to varying degrees throughout the pandemic, ranging from complete isolation as implemented by the Australian and New Zealand Governments to temporary border closures implemented by countries like France, the United Kingdom, and the United States. A study model showed that sustained 90% travel restrictions to and from mainland China, for example, were only modestly effective unless they were also associated with behavioral changes, likely due to the ability of the virus to be transmitted by asymptomatic and oligosymptomatic individuals in an airborne route.[13,14] Travel restrictions applied reactively to countries that were reporting variants and ignoring countries with little or no reported surveillance data worsened the inequity of the global response.[15]

On the basis of the now accumulated data on the transmissibility of the SARS-CoV-2, it is now known that travel restriction measures in isolation failed to halt the spread of the pandemic. Rather, demanding mask use during traveling, a proof of a negative COVID-19 test shortly before airline boarding, and more recently—demanding a complete vaccination status—seem to be more reasonable measures to help reduce transmissibility without unreasonably compromising travel mobility.

Contact Tracing

Contact tracing was another measure adopted by some countries with varying levels of strictness to identify probable or confirmed cases. Individuals in contact with those diagnosed with or exposed to COVID-19 were instructed to quarantine. Accessibility to testing and rapid turnaround times were crucial to the success of contact tracing and proved to be a challenge. It took many months for countries committed to contact tracing to be able to effectively implement it. The disparity in the availability of testing highlighted the known biases in global health.[16–18]

Mobility Restrictions

Mobility is a variable associated with the spread of the virus spread. Mobility restrictions included limitations on public transportation use, air traffic travel, and indoor as well as outdoor activities.[19] Although these measures appeared to be effective initially at limiting the spread outside of the Wuhan region, there has been evidence of SARS-CoV-2 present in the United States since at least January 20, 2020. The impact of the pandemic on mobility was either determined by governments or by the population themselves perceiving the risk, which varied significantly throughout the world.

Brazil, for example, saw a natural decline in mobility in March 2020, when the first official death was reported in the country. This had a direct impact on slowing the increase in the number of cases during the first wave of the pandemic in the country, when vaccines didn't exist.

The United Kingdom also saw a significant impact on its mobility; however, the population changed its behavior at each lockdown. The first lockdown came into effect on March 26, 2020; gradual reopening started on June 1 of the same year. The second and third national lockdowns were enforced on May 5, 2021 and August 3, 2021. Mobility during those lockdowns was 47% higher than in the first lockdown, where the mobility dropped to 73% lower than in the pre-pandemic period (**Fig. 1**).

The Delta variant surge in India offered another example where cases started to rise exponentially in the second week of March 2021. As a result, deaths began to rise at the beginning of April 2021, whereas the mobility dropped only in the second week of April 2021 – after deaths increased exponentially by more than a week (**Fig. 2**).

Mobility reductions have had a clear impact in reducing the transmission of COVID-19. When informed by changes in trends in COVID-19 case monitoring, mobility restrictions were useful in controlling the effective reproduction number (Rt) and preventing deaths, especially before widespread use of vaccination.

United Kingdom - Transit stations - Google Mobility

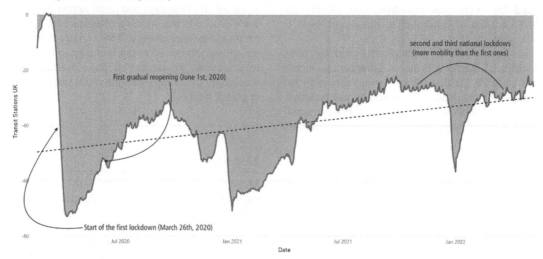

Fig. 1. Mobility in the United Kingdom over time. The zero mark in the *y*-axis refers to pre-pandemic mobility levels. Note an attenuated reduction in mobility from the first, second, and third lockdowns. (*From* Rede Análise Available at: http://bit.ly/Rede_MobilitySymptoms. Accessed Jun 22 2022.)

Socioeconomic Restrictions

Socioeconomic restrictions refer to the placement of limitations on or closure of community gatherings such as schools, workplaces, daycares, elderly housing, swimming pools, bars/restaurants, banks, grocery stores, etc. Complete lockdowns had large effects in controlling COVID-19 community transmission; however, these measures come with significant impacts in the economy and in the mental health of the population, disproportionately affecting resource-poor areas[20,21] Restrictions lighter than a complete lockdown proved effective for control of community transmission in 2020 (to drive the reproduction number – Rt – below 1).[22] On the basis of the data from Reuters, Italy, and Spain had a 94% decrease in retail and recreational trips during the pandemic. A reduction of over 60% was noted in physical presence in workplaces. It is evident that these measures contributed to decreased transmission but at high socioeconomic costs that led countries to implement these changes in different degrees.[13]

Physical Distancing

Physical distancing, also known as social distancing, is a regulation of the distance and number of people per square meter in a location. On the basis of the studies published during the SARS outbreak, six feet was determined to be potentially effective in the reduction of transmission.[23] A significant focus was placed on reducing mass gatherings, closing of workplaces, and isolating households, towns, and cities. A

combination of these measures has been reported to have an approximately 60% reduction in transmission.[24] Similarly, personal hygiene measures were implemented and aimed to reduce other routes of SARS-CoV-2 transmission, such as fomites. These measures included hand washing, avoidance of contact with contaminated surfaces, appropriate utilization of personal protective equipment (PPE) such as eye and hand protection with the use of face shields/goggles with gloves, protective glass, and temperature checks upon entrance.

Facemasks

Facemasks played a notable role in shaping the course of the pandemic. The utility of universal face masks was gradually learned leading to various mask mandates across the globe.[25] At the beginning of the pandemic, with a lack of indepth knowledge about how transmission occurred (whether by aerosols or direct/indirect contact, or both) and with concern about the scarcity of masks for health professionals, the WHO delayed recommending the use of masks to the general population. On April 3, 2020, the Centers for Disease Control (CDC) recommended wearing a face covering to reduce the spread in the community.[26] This recommendation was followed by similar advice from the WHO on April 6, 2020.[27] However, these initial recommendations encouraged the use of masks that could be manufactured by hand, even with the folding of cotton cloths, and used with elastics, albeit without clarification on the issue of adjustment and filtration efficiency.

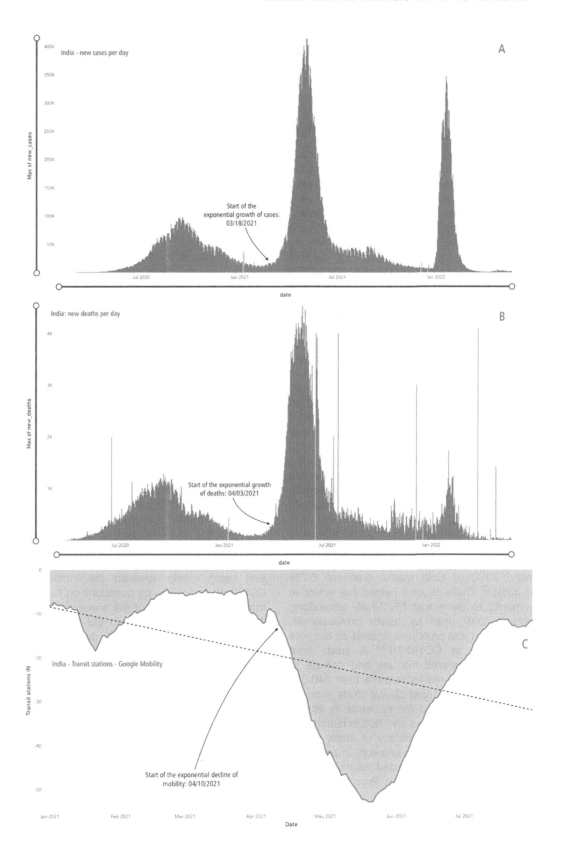

On June 5, WHO published an updated guide, including placing a table with the filtration efficiencies of masks made with different fabrics (ranging from 0.7% to 26%).[27] In 2020, the number of fabric masks made by the textile industry increased, mainly in developing countries.[28] A systematic review and meta-analysis published by Sharma and colleagues[29] in 2020 noted that the effectiveness of cloth masks was very low for the prevention of COVID-19, but that they could be used in outdoor public spaces to reduce transmission. However, a portion of the population with greater purchasing power chose to use professional masks (surgical or FFP2/N95). The most penetrating particle size (MPPS) for N95s ranges from 30 to 100 nm, whereas that for surgical masks ranges from 200 to 500 nm. The MPPS for cloth masks is similar as surgical masks. The particle filtration efficiency (PFE) for various masks however depends on several factors including type of the mask, condition of the mask, and mask fit.[30] A study in patients with seasonal coronaviruses showed that the surgical face masks significantly reduced the detection of viral RNA in both respiratory droplets and aerosols in the air. Those who did not use masks were found to have a 40% rate of aerosol detection, compared with a zero detection rate in those who used face masks.[31]

Since the pandemic, many studies evaluated the efficiency of masks. Experiments performed using particle counters and probes coupled to different models of masks to simulate coughing, speech, sneezing, or breathing[32] showed that the filtration efficiencies of masks/respirators FFP2/N95 were much higher (92% to 98%) than those obtained with the use of surgical masks (around 70%) or cloth masks (between 0.7% and 30%).[33] These studies helped the scientific community to claim that FFP2/N95 respirators, previously only used by health professionals, would be the most protective against an airborne disease such as COVID-19.[34] A study from Bangladesh compared the use and nonuse of cloth and surgical masks in more than 340,000 people, and a randomized clinical study in health professionals published for influenza in 2019[35] comparing surgical masks and N95 in health professionals, showed the efficacy of mask use in reducing SARS-CoV-2 transmission. Importantly, masks should not be regarded as single measures or with 100% efficiency. Proof-of-concept

studies, experimental laboratory projections, and mathematical and physical models, have shown that the effectiveness of masks is related not only to their filtration efficacy, but to proper fitting, the viral load of infectious sources, environment aeration, and the reproduction rate of the predominant viral variant.[36] For this reason, it is challenging to make projections regarding the "percentage" of generalized protection, as different combinations of the aforementioned factors yield different risks. Nevertheless, well-aerated outdoor environments, even with many infected sources, provide less transmission risk, which allows the use of masks of lower efficacy but with relative safety. On the contrary, indoor environments, such as public transport and medical centers that treat patients with COVID-19, require more efficient masks. Finally, as SARS-CoV-2 is highly dispersed through aerosol droplets, in general terms, the more efficient the mask is (in terms of filtration), the better the protection.[37]

Surveillance

Surveillance was pivotal for understanding the pandemic and giving early warnings to the population, so that risk management could be more effective. Several initiatives were launched, like the Covid Trends and Impacts Survey (CTIS), developed by the University of Maryland and Facebook Health.[38] This survey inquired Facebook users on the presence of COVID-like symptoms. COVID-like symptoms were a sum of fever, cough, and shortness of breath. A rise in COVID-like symptoms anticipated official data by approximately 15 days The CTIS survey showed that using masks lowered the incidence of COVID-19 symptoms as questions on the use of masks were also part of the survey.[39] The data from Brazil's Rio Grande do Sul state showed the impact of mask mandates on the incidence of symptoms (**Fig. 3**).

During the COVID-19 pandemic, we have learned about the colossal impact of contact tracing, mobility and socioeconomic restrictions, physical distancing, face masking, and surveillance. These NPMs to control disease transmission came with their own difficulties, such as real and perceived limitations in personal freedom. Public dissatisfaction also stemmed from the impacts of social isolation on the economy,

Fig. 2. Relationship between new daily cases of COVID-19 in India (A), daily deaths (B), and mobility (C). Note the mobility reduction following an exponential rise in deaths after one week. The zero mark in the mobility graph refers to pre-pandemic mobility levels.

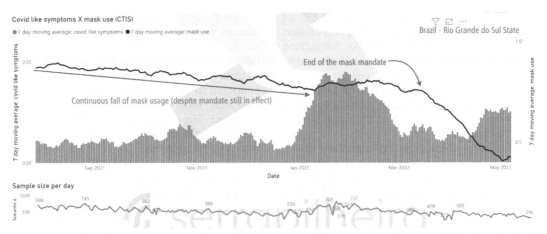

Fig. 3. Impact of mask mandates on mask-wearing reports on CTIS survey. On the state of Rio Grande do Sul, Brazil. The graph shows patients with COVID-like symptoms and the dark blue line depicts persons reporting mask usage outside of their homes. On the wave depicted in May 2022, a rise in symptoms is noted when the mask usage reporting is the lowest. (*From* Rede Análise Available at: http://bit.ly/Rede_MobilitySymptoms. Accessed June 22, 2022.)

behavioral and mental health.[40] Wide-ranging debates on ideal long-term strategies to limit transmission while maintaining sustainable social, financial, and mental health are ongoing.

IMPACT ON HEALTH CARE AND RESOURCE ALLOCATION

Temporal heterogeneity marked the pandemic worldwide, which meant that there were regions experiencing a spike in cases, weeks or months before others (as was the case for China followed by Europe and then the Americas). Rising cases led to a rise in emergency room visits followed by hospitalizations, including utilization of the ICUs. During the "surges" the wise use of rapid and generously shared information by countries helped some regions to prepare for these acute burdens on health care. Allocation of scarce resources such as the supply of oxygen and ventilators were great challenges and in some highly burdened areas led to catastrophic system collapse such as in Brazil, India, or in Iran.[41,42] As the pandemic progressed, and the medical systems were overwhelmed on a wider scale, countries going through periods of increased transmission and case burden struggled to keep up with the needs of the patients.

During the initial wave, the lack of PPE and medical devices such as ventilators was an important limiting factor. The lack of resources was less stark during subsequent waves compared with the deficit of trained personnel.[43] Regional and wide-scale redeployment of personnel from noncritical care areas was necessary. These redeployments led to physical, mental, emotional, and financial strain on health care personnel, with an increased rate of burnout. These challenges highlighted the importance of proactive personnel management during future pandemics.

The lack of evidence-based strategies for resource allocation and the most appropriate models for local, regional, national, and international resource sharing was starkly evident.[44,45] The sparse existing guidelines for resource allocation were revisited.[46] What stood out was the variation in guidelines across various states even within one country.[47] Evidence abounds on the overburdening of health system posed by COVID-19. Lack of appropriate public health measures to control disease transmission and the ICU bed occupancy in Sao Paulo state in Brazil illustrates that after the ICU bed occupancy reached approximately 100%, there was a rapid increase in new deaths despite the added ICU beds. These newly available ICU beds could not provide high-standard ICU care as critical care health professionals were not available to staff them. This shortage of health care workers resulted from a significant burden of stress and negative socioeconomic, psychological, and physical impacts across the spectrum of health care workers with successive waves during the pandemic.[48] Studies reported a significant increase in the turnover intention in nurses, which was also noted among the rest of the health care workers.[49] By the spring of 2020, Canadian health care workers reported more than 30% prevalence of severe burnout.[50] Half of the health care workers reported decreased likelihood of maintaining their current occupation due to the pandemic in the United

States while a study found that only 4.8% of nurses at a hospital in Egypt reported no intention to leave their current job.[51,52] As institutions recover in the aftermath of the pandemic, workforce retention, and well-being will prove to be an uphill battle while providing quality care to the community making workforce satisfaction and well-being a top priority at all levels of policy making in health care.

In the out-of-hospital setting, outpatient clinics pivoted to providing telehealth services to allow social distancing measures that in turn limited in-person health care. A retrospective study noted an 80% reduction of utilization in outpatient resources compared with pre-pandemic years with a four-fold increase in telehealth resources.[53] A large review of countries implementing telehealth during the pandemic had a positive sentiment about its use going forward – an enormous 84.9%. This was based on data from high-income countries: 43.6% of the articles reviewed originated in the United States. On the contrary, the feasibility of telehealth in countries that are low- and middle-income or resource-scarce may continue to be an issue.[54]

Governments took unprecedented measures to address resource shortages. In the United States, the Defense Production Act was invoked to allow robust public-private partnerships to accelerate the development and testing of therapeutics, ventilators, vaccines, and time-sensitive release of funds for the same.[55] In the United Kingdom, companies produced 14,000 ventilators in 3 months as part of the "Ventilator Challenge", one part of the government's three-pronged approach to increase ventilator production in a short period of time.[56]

The international health care supply chain is a dynamic multi-tiered process. It involves manufacturers, vendors, purchasers, storage, distribution, and providers. As the chain requires constant flow without disruption, the consequences of the pandemic were felt worldwide due to the multifactorial impact on every single step of the supply chain across various countries. A shortage of PPE due to a drastic uptick in use and limited global supplies was the hallmark of resource limitation at the beginning of the pandemic. With China as the primary producer, as well as the pandemic epicenter, international efforts shifted toward reclaiming, reusing, and repurposing the existing supply. Manufacturing infrastructure was repurposed to bolster supply and fulfill the deficits.[57] As an example, India stopped the export of 26 active pharmaceutical ingredients due to the fear of shortages for use within the country.[58]

With the unsettling rise in cases globally, many lessons were learned from the direct and indirect impact on health care delivery. Information sharing between countries is vital and constant evaluation of local and national resource allocation plans is important to stay prepared for future pandemics. Telehealth visits rose as resource shortages were observed. The importance of public-private partnership to address shortages will serve as benchmarks for future crises.

LITERATURE IN CORONAVIRUS DISEASE AND RESEARCH EFFORTS

The COVID-19 pandemic, with its unprecedented needs, led to an acceleration in research on COVID-19 and concomitant rise in the number of scientific articles. The rapid spread of COVID-19 was paralleled by the speed of literature being published. The first publication on COVID-19 was on January 2, 2020 and the rate of published articles related to COVID-19 hit an all-time high of 2276 in a week by the 22nd week of 2020. Between January 2, 2020 and July 21, 2020 the mean number of publications per week was 990.[59] Both researchers and journals were over-stretched by COVID-19. The use of preprint online platforms to speed up the release of information was another consequence of the pandemic that had its own pros and cons. Publishing on preprint platforms allowed for rapid dissemination of data by overcoming that limitation of traditional publishing processes including slow timelines of peer-review, time to publication, and challenges with formatting per different journals' guidelines. However, the importance of robust peer-review became evident as incomplete, fabricated, or improperly analyzed data led to spread of information that eventually was proven to be incorrect.[60] Although open to public comment which serves as form of peer-review, about 5% of pre-print articles were commented on, usually with only one comment per article.[61] Traditional publications also suffered from the challenges of need of rapid publication such as the retracted article regarding use of hydroxycholoroquine in COVID-19.[62]

Impressive robust scientific initiatives were also launched. A highlight was the implementation of adaptive platforms to run multiple research questions in COVID-19 simultaneously, such as RECOVERY,[63,64] REMAP-CAP[65] and the ACTT.[66] Adaptive trials such as these allowed rapid reaction to changing knowledge and therapeutics while evaluating different target candidates for the treatments. These trials subsequently provided guidance and clarity on the role of multiple therapeutics such as the role of antivirals, systemic steroids, and other immunomodulators, among others.

Another critical achievement of the global medical research community was the creation and maintenance of the "living" guidelines on therapeutics for COVID-19 published by the WHO.[67] The first version of these guidelines was published in September 2020 and most recently the twelfth iteration of the guidelines was released on September 26, 2022. Curated by a review committee with global representation, these guidelines provided front-line clinicians with the ability to deliver evidence-based care that was in keeping with the most recent high-quality literature.

Misinformation

COVID-19 is the first pandemic in history during which technology and social media were used on a large scale to keep people safe, informed, productive, and connected. At the same time, the technology we rely on to keep us connected and informed enabled and amplified a deluge of inaccurate information that undermined the global response and jeopardized the measures to control the pandemic due to conflicting messaging.

With the deluge of data and information came a similarly impressive amount of confusion and misinformation.[59] Although the discordance in statements from official sources was based on available literature, the interpretation and implementation of the information were often askew by the populace leading to confusion in the community. From vital information on the origin and therapies of a pandemic to ongoing published literature, we saw the emergence of an "infodemic".[68] In a rapidly changing situation, with millions of individuals in isolation, social media became a frontrunner source for major updates. Research conducted in Italy showed that in March of 2020, an average of daily 46,000 Twitter posts were linked to misinformation.[69] A survey published in the UK indicated that 46% of adults had seen misleading information about the pandemic; 40% reported finding it hard to know what is true or false.[70] Over a quarter of the most-viewed 75 videos regarding COVID-19 in March 2020 on YouTube contained misinformation.[71]

Misinformation also stemmed from poor conduct of research; examples include studies published by researchers in both pre-print and traditional publications who claimed passionately that hydroxychloroquine or proxalutamide were effective.[72,73] Medical journals faced a herculean task of processing submitted manuscripts while ensuring standards.[74,75]

This pandemic highlighted the importance of rapid development and sharing of research findings while ensuring consistent messaging. The role of social media was significant and provided impetus for health care personnel to actively participate in ensuring accurate information dissemination.[76] Health care agencies recognized the importance of cohesive messaging as noted by increased connectivity of messaging between different stakeholder agencies on Twitter as the pandemic progressed.[77]

VACCINATION

The development of vaccines required unprecedented efforts to bring resources, manpower, and intellectual strengths together. As discussed earlier, the public-private partnerships fostered across the globe were critical for this endeavor. In December 2020, two mRNA vaccines were approved for administration in the United States.[78] Since then several types of vaccines against COVID-19 have been developed and deployed across the globe including nucleic acid vaccines, viral vector vaccines, inactivated vaccines, and protein-based vaccines.[79] The WHO COVAX initiative declared that "no one is safe, unless everyone is safe", in a bid to ensure equitable distribution of vaccines globally.[80] The goal was to fundraise capital to ensure vaccine access for 100 low- to middle-income countries.[81] By mid-December 2020, approximately half of the expected production of 5.3 billion doses of vaccines for 2021 had been preordered by the 27 countries of the European Union, the United States, the United Kingdom, Canada, Australia, and Japan. Cumulatively these high-income countries represented only 13% of the global population.[82] In contrast, the COVAX facility had only reserved a few hundred million doses.[81] Several countries developed vaccines indigenously and provided a robust vaccine program for their population, demonstrating the importance of engaging all shareholders internationally. India launched its vaccine program in January of 2021 and as of April 2, 2022 reported 91% of the whole population was at least partially vaccinated.[81] By the end of 2021, Latin America was one of the leaders in vaccination numbers globally, where existing resources for vaccine deployment were crucial for the success of vaccination campaigns.[83]

The global vaccination efforts have been hindered by hesitancy, among other reasons, with misinformation playing a significant role.[84] As of April 2022, vaccination efforts across the globe have reached a plateau, with many countries such as the United States reporting only 67% of the population as being completely immunized. Countries such as Nigeria and Ethiopia at the same time reported 10% to 20% vaccination rates, starkly bringing into focus the impact of resource limitation, imbalance of sharing these resources, and factors such as hesitancy causing a dent in acceptance.[85]

The vaccine coverage in some countries revealed these inequities. In May of 2022, the African continent had 17% of its population vaccinated with two doses and 1.65% of its population vaccinated with three doses. In Brazil, a low-middle income country (LMIC), with significant socioeconomic disparities, vaccine inequity has been clearly shown. The southeast and south regions had the most robust coverage: Sao Paulo State was the most vaccinated state, with 84% of its total population vaccinated with two doses. The north region had the lowest coverage, with less than 50% of the population in states like Amapá and Roraima vaccinated with two doses. When the third dose coverage was analyzed, the northern states in Brazil had less than 15% of their total population covered, which was directly associated with worse socioeconomic status in the north and northeast of Brazil. Lower-income regions, like the north, reported an average of 55% of two doses of vaccinal coverage, and the higher-income regions, like south and southeast, reported an average of 75% of two doses (**Fig. 4**).

As we have learned from the pandemic, age-based vaccine distribution strategies were crucial for mortality reduction.[86,87] Countries globally adopted this recommendation prioritizing older-age individuals and health care workers.[86,87] As the vaccine supply is currently plentiful, nations with low vaccine supplies have become the focal point for vaccination efforts. Models have shown that dose sharing between countries with high and low vaccine availability is beneficial from a global perspective as vaccine sharing lessens the costs of surveillance such as from border testing and genomic surveillance as well as decreases the risk of evolution of the virus.[88] In certain populations, specific targeting such as social media campaigns, slogans, and trusted messengers proved beneficial. Vaccine uncertainty was eased by involving communities hit the hardest by the pandemic.[89] Africa, a continent that has experience vaccinating large numbers of its population, had systems in place to effectively implement vaccinations. Such efforts include storing vaccines at cold temperatures, a requirement for the Ebola vaccine, and establishing vaccine sites such as churches, mosques, banks, and markets.[90]

Vaccination efforts continue to heighten. Access to vaccines plagued the initial rollout, but governments quickly combated the issue. During future pandemics, ensuring equitable access to

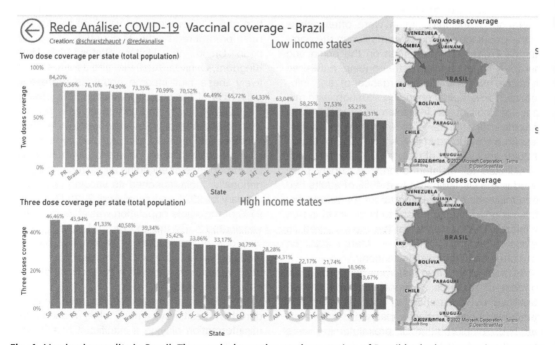

Fig. 4. Vaccine inequality in Brazil. The graph shows the northern region of Brazil had a lower vaccine coverage than the southeast (mainly São Paulo, the richest state of the country). (*From* Rede Análise Available at: https://redeanalise.com.br/. Accessed June 22, 2022.)

vaccines will be key to address the global spread of agents.

SOCIOECONOMIC IMPACT

The socioeconomic impact of this pandemic was evident early in the pandemic. In Brazil, for example, regional health disparities played a massive role in disease burden and mortality. In low-income areas, the mortality rates in the young were similar to the rates seen in the elderly, in contrast to regions with a high-income status and greater availability of higher quality of care. The need for high-quality care in these disadvantaged regions of critically ill patients was highlighted. These findings can be extrapolated to other low-income and middle-income countries with similar socioeconomic status.[91] Brazil had remarkable differences between the first (March-October 2020) and second (January-May 2021) waves. During the second wave, Brazil faced the Gamma variant of SARS-CoV-2 and an increase in mobility likely due to pandemic fatigue, whereas the vaccine coverage was still very low. This led to an increase in admissions for invasive and noninvasive ventilation by 192%. However, the admissions to the ICU were similar, suggesting a limitation in access to critical care. Also noted was a decrease in admissions in the state capitals, which again pointed toward socioeconomic challenges in specific regions.[92] The second wave proved to be more devastating with an increased burden of severe cases resulting in a higher mortality. Similar situations were seen in both the UK and Africa.[93] In Africa, despite the first wave, many countries had not instituted similar degrees of public health measures, and those that had instituted them, experienced fatigue in adherence to the measures which contributed in part to the subsequent waves.[94]

In South Africa, women experienced increased vulnerability to domestic trauma.[95] Police reported 87,000 cases of violence during the first week of lockdown. This further suggested an increased need for mental health professionals during these stressful times,[96] whereas a significant decrease in motor vehicle accidents, pedestrian-vehicle accidents, and assaults was seen. In particular, assaults involving a knife decreased dramatically.[97] The unemployment rate was a striking 30.1% during the lockdown. Measures such as social distancing, mask-wearing, and avoiding close contact were more consistently implemented by individuals of educated and higher socioeconomic status, as opposed to those of lower socioeconomic status.[98]

The profound socioeconomic impact of the pandemic is a major lesson learned. High-income regions have access to high-quality care which in turn decreases mortality rates as highlighted. To reiterate: addressing inequities is as important to delivery of health care as innovation in therapies and preventative strategies.

THE PATH FORWARD

Progress in technology, diagnostics, networks, and preparedness for pandemics must continue. Following the 2009 influenza pandemic, the Member States of the WHO adopted the Pandemic Influenza Preparedness (PIP) Framework, which supports fair access to measures to alleviate threats and financing. Each country has a different risk profile. Going forward, attention needs to be placed on an immediate response plan to implement national strategies similar to the WHO-adopted method, keeping existing inequities in mind so as not to exacerbate them during a pandemic situation.[99]

Continued research on public health and mitigation measures will accelerate the positive impact we have noted and minimize harm going forward. The mistrust in science and health care will likely be restored as vaccines and effective COVID-19 treatments become established. Reliance on interorganizational consistency, trusted leaders, and accessible, evidence-based guidelines will pave the way toward rebuilding public trust. Lastly, ongoing efforts are needed to protect the health and safety of health care workers who experienced the burdens of burn-out, discrimination, risk of occupational exposure, and illness from COVID-19.[99]

The use of facemasks, indoor aeration, and distancing can mitigate the airborne transmission of virus. Early implementation of quarantine and contact tracing in conjunction with common-sense public health measures are effective in controlling transmission. A global effort to keep resources, knowledge, and implementation equitably distributed and available at all levels is critical for success.

Many possible scenarios exist going forward. Endemicity similar to influenza and other human coronaviruses is entirely possible.[100] Vaccinations and previous infections may achieve herd immunity. However, a broad application of vaccines worldwide and accurate and available diagnostic testing is needed for accurate monitoring and local mitigation.[101] As for now, COVID-19 will continue to circulate for the foreseeable future.

CONFLICTS OF INTEREST AND DISCLOSURE STATEMENT

None of the authors have conflicts of interest to declare.

REFERENCES

1. WHO Director-General's opening remarks at the media briefing on COVID-19. 2020. Available at: https://www.who.int/director-general/speeches/detail/who-director-general-s-opening-remarks-at-the-media-briefing-on-covid-19—11-march-2020. Accessed April 5, 2022.
2. WHO coronavirus (COVID-19) dashboard. Available at: https://covid19.who.int. Accessed October 3, 2022.
3. Singh S, McNab C, Olson RM, et al. How an outbreak became a pandemic: a chronological analysis of crucial junctures and international obligations in the early months of the COVID-19 pandemic. Lancet 2021;398(10316):2109–24.
4. Worobey M. Dissecting the early COVID-19 cases in Wuhan. Science 2021;374(6572):1202–4.
5. A national fight against COVID-19: lessons and experiences from China, 2020, Aust N Z J Public Health. Available at: https://onlinelibrary.wiley.com/doi/full/10.1111/1753-6405.13042. Accessed April 29, 2022.
6. Thailand-c19-case-study-20-september.pdf. Available at: https://www.who.int/docs/default-source/coronaviruse/country-case-studies/thailand-c19-case-study-20-september.pdf. Accessed April 29, 2022.
7. Lin Q, Zhao S, Gao D, et al. A conceptual model for the coronavirus disease 2019 (COVID-19) outbreak in Wuhan, China with individual reaction and governmental action. Int J Infect Dis 2020;93:211–6.
8. Grasselli G, Pesenti A, Cecconi M. Critical care utilization for the COVID-19 outbreak in Lombardy, Italy: early experience and forecast during an emergency response. JAMA 2020;323(16):1545–6.
9. Baseline characteristics and outcomes of 1591 patients infected with SARS-CoV-2 admitted to ICUs of the Lombardy region, Italy | critical care medicine, JAMA. Available at: https://jamanetwork.com/journals/jama/fullarticle/2764365. Accessed July 20, 2022.
10. Marca AL, Niederberger C, Pellicer A, et al. COVID-19: lessons from the Italian reproductive medical experience. Fertil Steril 2020;113(5):920–2.
11. UPDATED: timeline of the coronavirus | think global health. Council on foreign relations. Available at: https://www.thinkglobalhealth.org/article/updated-timeline-coronavirus. Accessed June 22, 2022.
12. Rajatanavin N, Tuangratananon T, Suphanchaimat R, et al. Responding to the COVID-19 second wave in Thailand by diversifying and adapting lessons from the first wave. BMJ Glob Health 2021;6(7):e006178.
13. Bruinen de Bruin Y, Lequarre AS, McCourt J, et al. Initial impacts of global risk mitigation measures taken during the combatting of the COVID-19 pandemic. Saf Sci 2020;128:104773.
14. The effect of travel restrictions on the spread of the 2019 novel coronavirus (COVID-19) outbreak. Available at: https://www.science.org/doi/full/10.1126/science.aba9757. Accessed May 13, 2022.
15. Preiser W, Engelbrecht S, Maponga T. No point in travel bans if countries with poor surveillance are ignored. Lancet 2022;399(10331):1224.
16. Thornton J. Covid-19: lack of testing in Brazil is a "major failure," says MSF. BMJ 2020;370:m2659.
17. Donors bet on a US firm to fix testing in Africa. Then COVID-19 hit. Reuters. Available at: https://www.reuters.com/investigates/special-report/health-coronavirus-africa-cepheid/. Accessed May 13, 2022.
18. Praharaj I, Jain A, Singh M, et al. Pooled testing for COVID-19 diagnosis by real-time RT-PCR: a multi-site comparative evaluation of 5- & 10-sample pooling. Indian J Med Res 2020;152(1–2):88–94.
19. Caruso PF, Angelotti G, Greco M, et al. Early prediction of SARS-CoV-2 reproductive number from environmental, atmospheric and mobility data: a supervised machine learning approach. Int J Med Inf 2022;162:104755.
20. Atalan A. Is the lockdown important to prevent the COVID-19 pandemic? effects on psychology, environment and economy-perspective. Ann Med Surg 2020;56:38–42.
21. Butterworth P, Schurer S, Trinh TA, et al. Effect of lockdown on mental health in Australia: evidence from a natural experiment analysing a longitudinal probability sample survey. Lancet Public Health 2022;7(5):e427–36.
22. Denis F, Septans AL, Le Goff F, et al. Analysis of COVID-19 transmission sources in France by self-assessment before and after the partial lockdown: observational study. J Med Internet Res 2021;23(5):e26932.
23. CDC. COVID-19 and Your Health. Centers for Disease Control and Prevention. 2021. Available at: https://www.cdc.gov/coronavirus/2019-ncov/prevent-getting-sick/how-covid-spreads.html. Accessed June 28, 2022.
24. Anderson RM, Heesterbeek H, Klinkenberg D, et al. How will country-based mitigation measures influence the course of the COVID-19 epidemic? Lancet 2020;395(10228):931–4.
25. Mitze T, Kosfeld R, Rode J, et al. Face masks considerably reduce COVID-19 cases in Germany. Proc Natl Acad Sci 2020;117(51):32293–301.
26. Recommendation regarding the use of cloth face coverings, especially in areas of significant community-based transmission. Available at: https://stacks.cdc.gov/view/cdc/86440. Accessed May 13, 2022.
27. World Health Organization, Advice on the use of masks in the context of COVID-19: interim

guidance, 6 April 2020, 2020, World Health Organization: Geneva, Switzerland. Available at: https://apps.who.int/iris/handle/10665/331693, Accessed May 13, 2022.

28. Produção de máscaras cria alternativa para negócios. Agência Brasil. 2020. Available at: https://agenciabrasil.ebc.com.br/economia/noticia/2020-05/producao-de-mascaras-cria-alternativa-para-negocios. Accessed June 22, 2022.

29. Sharma SK, Mishra M, Mudgal SK. Efficacy of cloth face mask in prevention of novel coronavirus infection transmission: a systematic review and meta-analysis. J Educ Health Promot 2020;9:192.

30. Ju JTJ, Boisvert LN, Zuo YY. Face masks against COVID-19: standards, efficacy, testing and decontamination methods. Adv Colloid Interface Sci 2021;292:102435.

31. Leung NH, Chu DK, Shiu EY, et al. Respiratory virus shedding in exhaled breath and efficacy of face masks. Nat Med 2020;26(5):676–80.

32. Clapp PW, Sickbert-Bennett EE, Samet JM, et al. Evaluation of cloth masks and modified procedure masks as personal protective equipment for the public during the COVID-19 pandemic. JAMA Intern Med 2021;181(4):463–9.

33. Konda A, Prakash A, Moss GA, et al. Aerosol filtration efficiency of common fabrics used in respiratory cloth masks. ACS Nano 2020;14(5):6339–47.

34. Asadi S, Cappa CD, Barreda S, et al. Efficacy of masks and face coverings in controlling outward aerosol particle emission from expiratory activities. Sci Rep 2020;10(1):15665.

35. N95 respirators vs medical masks for preventing influenza among health care personnel: a randomized clinical trial JAMA. Available at: https://jamanetwork.com/journals/jama/fullarticle/2749214. Accessed June 22, 2022.

36. Face masks effectively limit the probability of SARS-CoV-2 transmission. Available at: https://www.science.org/doi/10.1126/science.abg6296. Accessed June 22, 2022.

37. Two metres or one: what is the evidence for physical distancing in covid-19? | The BMJ. Available at: https://www.bmj.com/content/370/bmj.m3223. Accessed June 22, 2022.

38. UMD Global CTIS. Available at: https://covidmap.umd.edu/. Accessed June 22, 2022.

39. Nguyen M. Mask mandates and COVID-19 related symptoms in the US. Clinicoecon Outcomes Res 2021;13:757–66.

40. Hanna K, Giebel C, Tetlow H, et al. Emotional and mental wellbeing following COVID-19 public health measures on people living with dementia and carers. J Geriatr Psychiatry Neurol 2022;35(3):344–52.

41. Coronavirus COVID-19 collapses health system in manaus, Brazil | MSF. Médecins sans frontières (MSF) international. Available at: https://www.msf.org/coronavirus-covid-19-collapses-health-system-manaus-brazil. Accessed June 28, 2022.

42. Fassihi F. Iran's health system 'beyond disastrous' from Covid surge. The New York times. 2021. Available at: https://www.nytimes.com/2021/08/13/world/middleeast/iran-virus-delta-variant.html. Accessed June 28, 2022.

43. Schaller SJ, Mellinghoff J, Cecconi M. Education to save lives: C19SPACE, the COVID19 skills PrepAration CoursE. Intensive Care Med 2022;48(2):227–30.

44. Hempel S, Burke R, Hochman M, et al. Allocation of scarce resources in a pandemic: rapid systematic review update of strategies for policymakers. J Clin Epidemiol 2021;139:255–63.

45. Ramachandran P, Swamy L, Kaul V, et al. A national strategy for ventilator and ICU resource allocation during the coronavirus disease 2019 pandemic. Chest 2020;158(3):887–9.

46. Zucker HA, Adler KP, Berens DP. Current members of the New York state task force on life and the law. 272. Available at: chrome-extension://efaidnbmnnnibpcajpcglclefindmkaj/https://www.health.ny.gov/regulations/task_force/reports_publications/docs/ventilator_guidelines.pdf. Accessed June 28, 2022.

47. Variation in ventilator allocation guidelines by US state during the coronavirus disease 2019 pandemic: a systematic review | critical care medicine, JAMA. Available at: https://jamanetwork.com/journals/jamanetworkopen/fullarticle/2767360. Accessed May 13, 2022.

48. Kolié D, Semaan A, Day LT, et al. Maternal and newborn health care providers' work-related experiences during the COVID-19 pandemic, and their physical, psychological, and economic impacts: findings from a global online survey. PLOS Glob Public Health 2022;2(8):e0000602.

49. Falatah R. The impact of the coronavirus disease (COVID-19) pandemic on nurses' turnover intention: an integrative review. Nurs Rep 2021;11(4):787–810.

50. Burnout in hospital-based health care workers during COVID-19. Ontario COVID-19 Sci Advisory Table. Available at: https://covid19-sciencetable.ca/sciencebrief/burnout-in-hospital-based-healthcare-workers-during-covid-19/ . Accessed June 28, 2022.

51. Hendrickson RC, Slevin RA, Hoerster KD, et al. The impact of the COVID-19 pandemic on mental health, occupational functioning, and professional retention among health care workers and first responders. J Gen Intern Med 2022;37(2):397–408.

52. Said RM, El-Shafei DA. Occupational stress, job satisfaction, and intent to leave: nurses working on front lines during COVID-19 pandemic in

Zagazig City, Egypt. Environ Sci Pollut Res 2021; 28(7):8791–801.

53. Journal of medical internet research—impact of the COVID-19 pandemic on health care utilization in a large integrated health care system: retrospective cohort study. Available at: https://www.jmir.org/2021/4/e26558/. Accessed May 13, 2022.

54. Doraiswamy S, Abraham A, Mamtani R, et al. Use of telehealth during the COVID-19 pandemic: scoping review. J Med Internet Res 2020;22(12): e24087.

55. Defense production Act | FEMA.gov. Available at: https://www.fema.gov/disaster/defense-production-act. Accessed May 13, 2022.

56. Ventilator Challenge hailed a success as UK production finishes. GOV.UK. Available at: https://www.gov.uk/government/news/ventilator-challenge-hailed-a-success-as-uk-production-finishes. Accessed May 13, 2022.

57. Livingston E, Desai A, Berkwits M. Sourcing personal protective equipment during the COVID-19 pandemic. JAMA 2020;323(19):1912–4.

58. Impact of the coronavirus pandemic on the supply chain in health care | British Journal of Health care Management. Available at: https://www.magonlinelibrary.com/doi/full/10.12968/bjhc.2020.0047. Accessed May 13, 2022.

59. Abd-Alrazaq A, Schneider J, Mifsud B, et al. A comprehensive overview of the COVID-19 literature: machine learning–based bibliometric analysis. J Med Internet Res 2021;23(3):e23703.

60. Kaul V, Gallo de Moraes A, Khateeb D, et al. Medical education during the COVID-19 pandemic. Chest 2021;159(5):1949–60.

61. Kodvanj I, Homolak J, Virag D, et al. Publishing of COVID-19 preprints in peer-reviewed journals, pre-printing trends, public discussion and quality issues. Scientometrics 2022;127(3):1339–52.

62. Mehra MR, Ruschitzka F, Patel AN. Retraction—hydroxychloroquine or chloroquine with or without a macrolide for treatment of COVID-19: a multinational registry analysis. Lancet 2020;395(10240): 1820.

63. RECOVERY Trial—using adaptive designs to help identify treatments for COVID-19. MRC Biostatistics Unit. 2020. Available at: https://www.mrc-bsu.cam.ac.uk/blog/recovery-trial-using-adaptive-designs-to-help-identify-treatments-for-covid-19/. Accessed May 13, 2022.

64. RECOVERY Collaborative Group, Horby P, Lim WS, et al. Dexamethasone in hospitalized patients with covid-19. N Engl J Med 2021;384(8):693–704.

65. Response to COVID-19 pandemic. REMAP-CAP trial. Available at: https://www.remapcap.org/coronavirus. Accessed May 13, 2022.

66. National Institute of Allergy and Infectious Diseases (NIAID). A multicenter, adaptive, randomized blinded controlled trial of the safety and efficacy of investigational therapeutics for the treatment of COVID-19 in hospitalized adults. clinicaltrials.gov. 2022. Available at: https://clinicaltrials.gov/ct2/show/NCT04280705. Accessed May 12, 2022.

67. Therapeutics and COVID-19: living guideline. Available at: https://www.who.int/publications-detail-redirect/WHO-2019-nCoV-therapeutics-2022.3. Accessed May 13, 2022.

68. Naeem SB, Bhatti R. The Covid-19 'infodemic': a new front for information professionals. Health Info Libr J 2020;37(3):233–9.

69. Mostrous A, Cummings B, Hollowood E. The infodemic fake news coronavirus. Tortoise. 2020. Available at: https://www.tortoisemedia.com/2020/03/23/the-infodemic-fake-news-coronavirus/. Accessed May 13, 2022.

70. Covid-19 news and information: consumption and attitudes. 5. Available at: https://www.ofcom.org.uk/research-and-data/tv-radio-and-on-demand/news-media/coronavirus-news-consumption-attitudes-behaviour. Accessed May 13, 2022.

71. Li HOY, Bailey A, Huynh D, et al. YouTube as a source of information on COVID-19: a pandemic of misinformation? BMJ Glob Health 2020;5(5): e002604.

72. Gautret P, Lagier JC, Parola P, et al. Hydroxychloroquine and azithromycin as a treatment of COVID-19: results of an open-label non-randomized clinical trial. Int J Antimicrob Agents 2020;56(1): 105949.

73. Taylor L. Covid-19: trial of experimental "covid cure" is among worst medical ethics violations in Brazil's history, says regulator. BMJ 2021;375: n2819.

74. Eisen MB, Akhmanova A, Behrens TE, et al. Publishing in the time of COVID-19. eLife 2020;9: e57162.

75. COVID-19 research: pandemic versus "paper-demic", integrity, values and risks of the "speed science". Available at: https://www.tandfonline.com/doi/epub/10.1080/20961790.2020.1767754?needAccess=true. Accessed May 13, 2022.

76. Topf JM, Williams PN. COVID-19, social media, and the role of the public physician. Blood Purif 2021; 50(4–5):595–601.

77. Wang Y, Hao H, Platt LS. Examining risk and crisis communications of government agencies and stakeholders during early-stages of COVID-19 on Twitter. Comput Human Behav 2021;114:106568.

78. CDC Museum COVID-19 timeline. Centers for disease control and prevention. 2022. Available at: https://www.cdc.gov/museum/timeline/covid19.html. Accessed May 13, 2022.

79. COVID-19 clinical resources | COVID-19 resource center. American college of chest physicians. Available at: https://www.chestnet.org/topic-

collections/covid-19/clinical-resources. Accessed May 13, 2022.

80. Covax. Available at: https://www.who.int/initiatives/act-accelerator/covax. Accessed May 13, 2022.

81. Deployment of COVID-19 vaccines. In: Wikipedia. 2022. Available at: https://en.wikipedia.org/w/index.php?title=Deployment_of_COVID-19_vaccines&oldid=1084870211. Accessed May 13, 2022.

82. Mullard A. How COVID vaccines are being divvied up around the world. Nature 2020. https://doi.org/10.1038/d41586-020-03370-6.

83. Lotta G, Fernandez M, Kuhlmann E, et al. COVID-19 vaccination challenge: what have we learned from the Brazilian process? Lancet Glob Health 2022;10(5):e613–4.

84. Sharma K, Zhang Y. and Liu Y. COVID-19 vaccine misinformation campaigns and social media narratives, 2022. arXiv:2106.08423.

85. Ritchie H, Mathieu E, Rodés-Guirao L, et al. Coronavirus pandemic (COVID-19). Our World Data. 2020. Available at: https://ourworldindata.org/covid-vaccinations. Accessed May 13, 2022.

86. Bubar KM, Reinholt K, Kissler SM, et al. Model-informed COVID-19 vaccine prioritization strategies by age and serostatus. Science 2021;371(6532):916–21.

87. Fitzpatrick MC, Galvani AP. Optimizing age-specific vaccination. Science 2021;371(6532):890–1.

88. Vaccine nationalism and the dynamics and control of SARS-CoV-2. Available at: https://www.science.org/doi/10.1126/science.abj7364. Accessed May 13, 2022.

89. AuYoung M, Rodriguez Espinosa P, ting Chen W, et al. Addressing racial/ethnic inequities in vaccine hesitancy and uptake: lessons learned from the California alliance against COVID-19. J Behav Med 2022. https://doi.org/10.1007/s10865-022-00284-8.

90. Key lessons from africa's COVID-19 vaccine rollout. WHO | regional office for Africa. Available at: https://www.afro.who.int/news/key-lessons-africas-covid-19-vaccine-rollout. Accessed May 13, 2022.

91. Ranzani OT, Bastos LSL, Gelli JGM, et al. Characterisation of the first 250,000 hospital admissions for COVID-19 in Brazil: a retrospective analysis of nationwide data. Lancet Respir Med 2021;9(4):407–18.

92. Bastos LS, Ranzani OT, Souza TML, et al. COVID-19 hospital admissions: Brazil's first and second waves compared. Lancet Respir Med 2021;9(8):e82–3.

93. Challen R, Brooks-Pollock E, Read JM, et al. Risk of mortality in patients infected with SARS-CoV-2 variant of concern 202012/1: matched cohort study. BMJ 2021;372:n579.

94. Salyer SJ, Maeda J, Sembuche S, et al. The first and second waves of the COVID-19 pandemic in Africa: a cross-sectional study. Lancet 2021;397(10281):1265–75.

95. Piquero AR, Jennings WG, Jemison E, et al. Domestic violence during the COVID-19 pandemic—evidence from a systematic review and meta-analysis. J Crim Justice 2021;74:101806.

96. Nguse S, Wassenaar D. Mental health and COVID-19 in South Africa. South Afr J Psychol 2021;51(2):304–13.

97. Zsilavecz A, Wain H, Bruce JL, et al. Trauma patterns during the COVID-19 lockdown in South Africa expose vulnerability of women. South Afr Med J 2020;110(11):1110–2.

98. Kollamparambil U, Oyenubi A. Behavioural response to the Covid-19 pandemic in South Africa. PLoS One 2021;16(4):e0250269.

99. Strategic preparedness, readiness and response plan to end the global COVID-19 emergency in 2022. Available at: https://www.who.int/publications-detail-redirect/WHO-WHE-SPP-2022.1. Accessed May 13, 2022.

100. After the pandemic: perspectives on the future trajectory of COVID-19, nature. Available at: https://www.nature.com/articles/s41586-021-03792-w. Accessed May 13, 2022.

101. Aschwanden C. Five reasons why COVID herd immunity is probably impossible. Nature 2021;591(7851):520–2.

Moving?

Make sure your subscription moves with you!

To notify us of your new address, find your **Clinics Account Number** (located on your mailing label above your name), and contact customer service at:

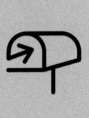

Email: journalscustomerservice-usa@elsevier.com

800-654-2452 (subscribers in the U.S. & Canada)
314-447-8871 (subscribers outside of the U.S. & Canada)

Fax number: 314-447-8029

Elsevier Health Sciences Division
Subscription Customer Service
3251 Riverport Lane
Maryland Heights, MO 63043

ELSEVIER